Ultrastructure of Male Urogenital Glands

ELECTRON MICROSCOPY IN BIOLOGY AND MEDICINE

Current Topics in Ultrastructural Research

SERIES EDITOR: P.M. MOTTA

Already published in this series

Vol. 1 Motta, P.M. (ed.): Ultrastructure of Endocrine Cells and Tissues. ISBN: 0-89838-568-7.
Vol. 2 Van Blerkom, J. and Motta, P.M. (eds.): Ultrastructure of Reproduction: Gametogenesis, Fertilization, and Embryogenesis. ISBN: 0-89838-572-5.
Vol. 3 Ruggeri, A. and Motta, P.M. (eds.): Ultrastructure of the Connective Tissue Matrix. ISBN: 0-89838-600-4.
Vol. 4 Motta, P.M. and Fujita, H. (eds.): Ultrastructure of the Digestive Tract. ISBN: 0-89838-893-7.
Vol. 5 Van Blerkom, J. and Motta, P.M. (eds.): Ultrastructure of Human Gametogenesis and Early Embryogenesis. ISBN: 0-89838-383-8.
Vol. 6 Riva, A. and Motta, P.M. (eds.): Ultrastructure of the Expatraparietal Glands of the Digestive Tract. ISBN: 0-7923-0303-2.
Vol. 7 Bonucci, E. and Motta, P.M. (eds.): Ultrastructure of Skeletal Tissue. ISBN: 0-7923-0373-3.
Vol. 8 Motta, P.M. (ed.): Ultrastructure of Smooth Muscle. ISBN: 0-7923-0480-2.
Vol. 9 Familiari, G., Makabe, S., and Motta, P.M. (eds.): Ultrastructure of the Ovary. ISBN: 0-7923-1003-9.
Vol. 10 Motta, P.M., Murakami, T., and Fujita, H. (eds.): Scanning Electron Microscopy of Vascular Casts: Methods and Applications. ISBN: 0-7923-1297-X.

Ultrastructure of the Male Urogenital Glands: Prostate, Seminal Vesicles, Urethral, and Bulbourethral Glands

edited by

Alessandro Riva, M.D.
Department of Cytomorphology, University of Cagliari,
Cagliari, Italy

and

Francesca Testa Riva, Ph.D.
Department of Cytomorphology, University of Cagliary
Cagliari, Italy

and

Pietro Motta, M.D., Ph.D.
Department of Human Anatomy, Faculty of Medicine, University of Rome "La Sapienza"
Rome, Italy

Springer-Science+Business Media, LLC

Library of Congress Cataloging-in-Publication Data

Ultrastructure of the male urogenital glands prostate, seminal vesicles, urethral, and bulbourethral glands / edited by Alessandro Riva, Francesca Testa Riva, Pietro Motta
p cm — (Electron microscopy in biology and medicine, EMBM 11)
Includes bibliographical references and index
ISBN 978-1-4613-6125-1 **ISBN 978-1-4615-2624-7 (eBook)**
DOI 10.1007/978-1-4615-2624-7
1 Generative organs, Male—Ultrastructure 2 Andrology
I Riva, Alessandro II Testa Riva, Francesca III Motta, Pietro M IV Series
[DNLM 1 Genitalia, Male—ultrastructure WJ 701 U47 1994]
QP257 U58 1994
611' 63—dc20
DNLM/DLC
for Library of Congress 94-11636
CIP

Originally published by Kluwer Academic Publishers, New York in 1994
Softcover reprint of the hardcover 1st edition 1994

Printed on acid-free paper

Preface

Male urogenital glands (also termed *male accessory sex glands*) have received relatively little attention from electron microscopists, with perhaps the exception of the prostate gland. Moreover, even though comparative studies have clearly shown that these glands exhibit species dependent features, very few studies, scattered among various publications, are available on the urogenital glands of man.

This volume, the 11th of the series *Electron Microscopy in Biology and Medicine*, presents an unprecedented collection of information on the functional microanatomy and cytoarchitecture of these organs in humans.

Through the integration of transmission and scanning electron microscopy with a variety of modern techniques, it documents the most important aspects of the histophysiology of these glands from their development to some pathological alterations. In order to cover some key mechanisms of their cell biology, such as the action of sex hormones, the epithelio-mesenchymal interactions, and the dynamic of the secretory process, reports on human organs have been supplemented by some studies on experimental animals.

On the basis of the outstanding level of the contributions and the quality of the illustrations, we believe that this book, which has been compiled by some of the world authorities on the topic, will serve not only as a reference work for students, scientists, and professionals interested in biomedical foundations of andrology, but also as a stimulus for future research in this exciting and relatively neglected chapter of human reproduction.

Finally, we wish to thank Mr. J.K. Smith and his staff, who once again have fully demonstrated their professional skill in the production of the book.

A. Riva, P.M. Motta, and F. Testa-Riva

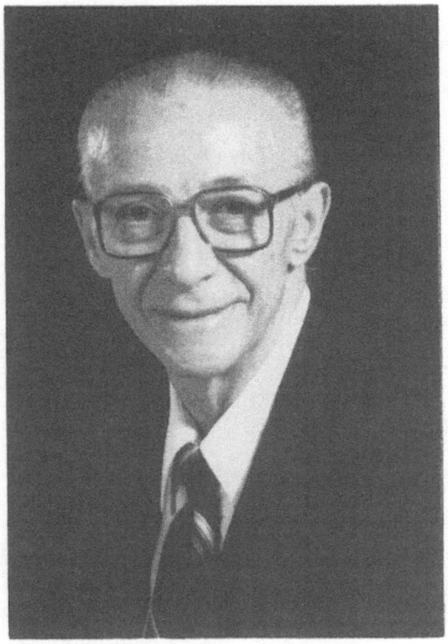

Prof Liberato J A DiDio

This book is dedicated to our friend Prof. Dr. Liberato J.A. DiDio as a tribute to the first Honorary President of the International Federation of Associations of Anatomists (1989), Emeritus Professor and Emeritus Dean of the Medical College of Ohio

A. Riva, F. Testa-Riva, and P.M. Motta, editors

Contents

Contents

Contributing Authors

Amselgruber, Werner, 2nd Chair of Veterinary Anatomy, Universität München, Veterinärstrasse 13, D 8000 München 22, Germany

Aumüller, Gerhard, Department of Anatomy and Cell Biology, Klinikum der Philipps Universität, Robert Koch Strasse 6, D 35033 Marburg, Germany

Bono, Aldo, Division of Urology, Multizonal Hospital of Varese, Viale L. Borri 57, I 21100 Varese, Italy

Capella, Carlo, Department of Human Pathology, 2nd Faculty of Medicine, University of Pavia at Varese, Viale L. Borri 57, I 21100 Varese, Italy

Congiu, Terenzio, Department of Cytomorphology, University of Cagliari, Via Porcell 2, I 09124, Cagliari, Italy

Correr, Silvia, Department of Anatomy, Faculty of Medicine, University "La Sapienza", Via A. Borelli 50, I 00161 Rome, Italy

Cossu, Margherita, Department of Cytomorphology, University of Cagliari, Via Porcell 2, I 09124, Cagliari, Italy

Cunha, Gerald R., Anatomy Department, University of California, San Francisco, California, 94143 USA

De Lisa, Antonello, Clinic of Urology, University of Cagliari, Ospedale SS Trinità, I 09100 Cagliari, Italy

De Mesy Jensen, Karen L., University of Rochester School of Medicine and Dentistry, Department of Pathology and Laboratory Medicine, 575 Elmwood Ave., Rochester, New York 14642, USA

DiDio, Liberato J.A., Department of Morphology, Escola Paulista de Medicina, Rua Botucatu 740, Sãu Paulo, SP 04023-900 Brasil

Di Sant'Agnese, P. Antony, University of Rochester School of Medicine and Dentistry, Department of Pathology and Laboratory Medicine, 575 Elmwood Ave., Rochester, New York 14642, USA

Finzi, Giovanna, Department of Pathology, Multizonal Hospital of Varese, Viale L. Borri 57, I 21100 Varese, Italy

Frigerio, Bruno, Department of Pathology, General Hospital of Saronno, Piazzale Borella 3, I 21047 Saronno (Varese), Italy

Kellokumpu-Lehtinen, Pirkko, Department of Clinical Medicine/Oncology, University of Tampere, SF 33101 Tampere, Finland

Lantini, Maria Serenella, Department of Cytomorphology, University of Cagliari, Via Porcell 2, I 09124, Cagliari, Italy

Mata, Lucinda, Cell Biology Department, Gulbenkian Institute of Science, Apartado 14, 2781 Oeiras of Codex, Portugal

Motta, Pietro M., Department of Anatomy, Faculty of Medicine, University "La Sapienza", Via A. Borelli 50, I 00161 Rome, Italy

Migliari, Roberto, Clinic of Urology, University of Cagliari, Ospedale SS Trinità, I 09100 Cagliari, Italy

Riva, Alessandro, Department of Cytomorphology, University of Cagliari, Via Porcell 2, I 09124, Cagliari, Italy

Salvadore, Maurizio, Department of Pathology, Multizonal Hospital of Varese, Viale L. Borri 57, I 21100 Varese, Italy

Seitz, Jürgen, Department of Anatomy and Cell Biology, Klinikum der Philipps Universität, Robert Koch Strasse 6, D 35033 Marburg, Germany

Sinowatz, Fred, 2nd Chair of Veterinary Anatomy, Universität München, Veterinärstrasse 13, D 8000 München 22, Germany

Testa-Riva, Francesca, Department of Cytomorphology, University of Cagliari, Via Porcell 2, I 09124, Cagliari, Italy

Vaalasti, Annikki, Department of Biomedical Sciences, University of Tampere, Box 2000, SF 33521 Tampere, Finland

Ultrastructure of Male Urogenital Glands

CHAPTER 1

Normal and Abnormal Development of Human Male Accessory Sex Glands

FRED SINOWATZ, PIRKKO KELLOKUMPU-LEHTINEN, & WERNER AMSELGRUBER

1. Introduction

Development of the male accessory sex glands in humans follows the same pattern as observed in most mammals (Fig. 1). Prostate and bulbourethral glands develop as derivatives of the urogenital sinus. Seminal vesicles and ampullary glands originate from the lower end of the Wolffian (mesonephric) duct. Although the fine structure of the adult male accessory sex glands has been studied in various species, including man, relatively few studies on the development of these organs have used electron microscopy. This is a short review of the ultrastructural changes occurring in the prostate, seminal vesicles, ampulla ductus deferentis, and bulbourethral glands of man during prenatal and postnatal differentiation under physiological and selected pathological conditions.

2. Prenatal and Postnatal Development of the Prostate

2.1. Morphology of the Prostatic Primordium

The prostate gland is formed from the upper part of the definitive urogenital sinus in the region into which the mesonephric and paramesonephric ducts open [10,13]. At 7 weeks, male embryos have a colliculus seminalis in the cranial part of the urethra [11]. Mesonephric and paramesonephric ducts open into a narrow urethral lumen. The epithelium of the urethra is composed of two to three cell layers. On the apical surface of the epithelial cells a few microvilli and occasional cilia can be seen. In their apical parts, adjacent epithelial cells are connected by well-developed junctional complexes consisting of the zonula occludens, zonula adhaerens, and desmosomes. Lateral plasma membranes of the epithelial cells are straight and mostly closely apposed. Only in the basal area are the intercellular spaces slightly extended. The centrally or basally located nuclei are oval and show a smooth outline. They occupy one half to two thirds of the cell volume, are rich in euchromatin, and have a distinct nucleolus. Within the cytoplasm, small, round mitochondria are mainly located in the apical part of the cells. Short profiles of rough endoplasmic reticulum, many ribosomes, and some stacks of Golgi cisternae can be also observed.

The urethral mesenchyme is loosely packed and composed of rounded primitive cells [13]. The large round nuclei possess one or two distinct nucleoli. Small mitochondria, polysomes, and some elements of granular endoplasmic reticulum occur within the cytoplasm. A Golgi apparatus is not regularly seen. Myoblasts have not yet developed. Occasionally, nerve cells are observed in the periphery of the urethral mesenchyme.

At the age of 9 weeks, the colliculus seminalis is well developed at the level of the openings of the mesonephric and paramesonephric ducts into the urethral lumen. The urethral epithelium usually consists of two to five layers of cuboidal cells. Only a monolayer of columnar epithelial cells is seen on the colliculus seminalis. Urethral

Riva, A., Testa Riva, F., and Motta, P.M., (eds.), Ultrastructure of the Male Urogenital Glands: Prostate, Seminal Vesicles, Urethral, and Bulbourethral Glands. *ISBN 0-7923-2800-0.*

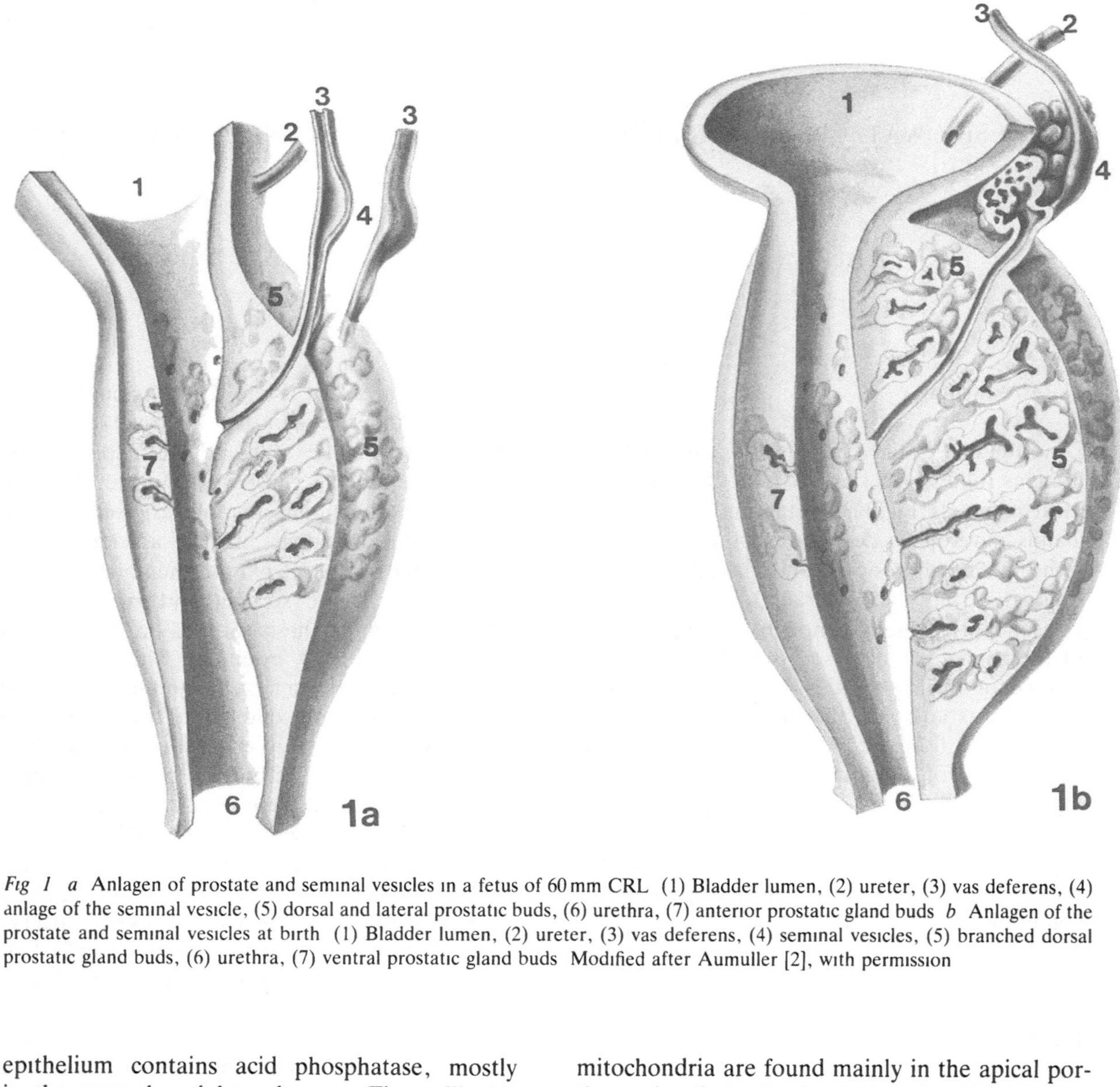

Fig 1 *a* Anlagen of prostate and seminal vesicles in a fetus of 60 mm CRL (1) Bladder lumen, (2) ureter, (3) vas deferens, (4) anlage of the seminal vesicle, (5) dorsal and lateral prostatic buds, (6) urethra, (7) anterior prostatic gland buds *b* Anlagen of the prostate and seminal vesicles at birth (1) Bladder lumen, (2) ureter, (3) vas deferens, (4) seminal vesicles, (5) branched dorsal prostatic gland buds, (6) urethra, (7) ventral prostatic gland buds Modified after Aumuller [2], with permission

epithelium contains acid phosphatase, mostly in the ventral and lateral parts. The colliculus seminalis differs in that aspect [10]. At the beginning of the 10th week, the epithelium still contains several cell layers [13]. The number of microvilli on the surface of the apical cells has increased. Slender cytoplasmic processes project into the widened intercellular spaces between neighboring luminal epithelial cells. Cells of the middle and basal cell layers possess large round nuclei that are centrally located. The cytoplasm of the epithelial cells contains many ribosomes and short strands of endoplasmic reticulum. Oval or round mitochondria are found mainly in the apical portions of cells in the luminal and middle layers. Mitochondria are generally close to the basement membrane in the basal cells.

In the urethral mesenchyme, cellular density has increased considerably and differentiation into three concentric zones is observed. The inner zone consists of elongated fibroblastic cells (Fig. 2a) with a well-developed rough endoplasmic reticulum. The increased synthetic capacity of these cells is confirmed by the accumulation of collagen fibers in the intercellular space. The interface between the urethral epithelium and

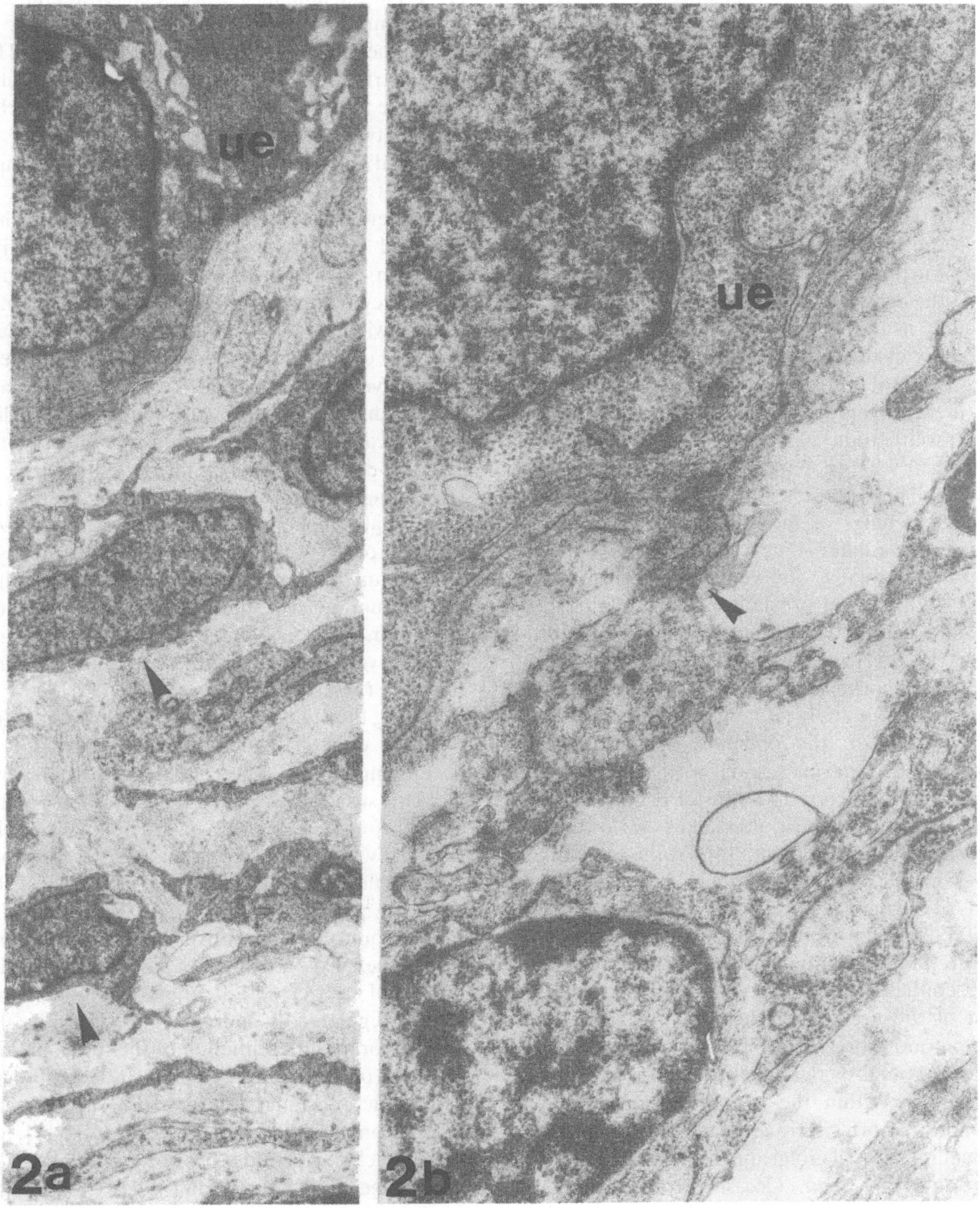

Fig 2 *a* Well-differentiated mesenchymal fibroblastic cells (arrows) of a 9-week old male fetus near the urethral epithelium (ue) at the level of the openings of paramesonephric and mesonephric ducts (×5000) *b* Direct epithelio mesenchymal contact (arrow) in a 10 week old male fetus (×15,000)

mesenchyme now shows distinct morphological signs of interaction. The basal lamina is folded. Quite frequently, cytoplasmic processes of the fibroblasts come into close contact with the basal lamina (Fig. 2b). The intermediate zone is composed of primitive mesenchymal cells. In the outer zone, myoblasts can be seen and the amount of intercellular collagen has increased. Differentiation of the mesenchyme adjacent to the epithelium of the urethra is taken to be the first ultrastructural sign of incipient prostatic development.

At the age of 10 weeks prostatic glands start to develop near the openings of the mesonephric ducts, as evidenced by the formation of several outgrowths of urethral epithelium in the surrounding mesenchyme [12,14]. The location, number, and proliferation of prostatic gland buds vary significantly between individuals. Usually, one or two gland buds per side grow laterally and caudally to the openings of the Wolffian and Müllerian ducts. At a later time, similar buds develop laterally, cranially, and ventrally. The epithelial outgrowths of the prostatic portion of the fetal urethrae can be divided into five groups, according to the area in which they develop [16]: anterior (from the ventral urethral wall), lateral (from the lateral walls), middle (from the posterior urethral wall, cranial to the openings of mesonephric ducts), and posterior (caudal to the openings of mesonephric ducts). The ventral gland buds are only transitory in most individuals and recede or vanish by the fourth month [2]. At the same time, the seminal vesicles start their development as buds of the mesonephric ducts, while the bulbourethral glands begin to appear as outgrowths from the urethral epithelium distal to the prostatic buds. The epithelium of the prostatic buds resembles that of the urethral epithelium, but appears to contain more organelles. The prostatic cells have a large, round or oval nucleus with a prominent nucleolus. Within the cytoplasm, round mitochondria, short cisternae of rough endoplasmic reticulum, a small Golgi apparatus, and numerous ribosomes are seen. Occasional electron-dense granules are observed in the basal parts of the cells.

By the end of the 11th week, a lumen appears in the terminal portions of some prostatic buds, completing the acinar structure for the first time [14]. At that time secretory vesicles (Fig. 3) containing acid phosphatase can be observed [10,14] at the luminal surface. Cells with granular cytoplasmic vesicles located in the basal part of the epithelium can be observed at this stage. The size, distribution, and morphology of the granules resemble those of catecholamine-storing particles [14]. Between weeks 11 and 14, the number of epithelial outgrowths from the urethral epithelium increases. Most of these acquire a lumen (Fig. 3) and differentiate into tubulo-acinar glands with a stratified epithelium made up of three to five cell layers. The majority of epithelial cells have slender cytoplasmic processes that project into slightly widened intercellular spaces. Some apical cells are columnar and appear clearly polarized. They have a large oval nucleus and a Golgi apparatus in a supranuclear location. In some cells, the apical cytoplasm contains granules with electron-dense flocculent material, indicative of impending secretory activity. Microvilli and an occasional cilium occur on their apical surface. At the age of 13 weeks, a few cells with a basal nucleus and many opaque secretory granules that fill the supranuclear and apical portions of their cytoplasm are seen within the luminal epithelium. Mesenchymal cells form fibroblast layers around the acini (Fig. 4).

During the 15th and 16th weeks, the number of prostatic epithelial buds increases, further [14] developing lumina. The histological organization and ultrastructure of the epithelium is not greatly altered compared to prior stages. Triangular cells (Fig. 5), which could represent an early developmental stage of future columnar epithelial cells, are seen in the basal portion of the epithelium. The amount of connective tissue surrounding the epithelial outgrowths increases steadily. The process of early cytodifferentiation of human prostate is regulated by androgens, as shown by the contemporary differentiation of the testis, and its secretion of androgens [2], and the acceleration of embryonic prostatic differentiation in vitro by testosterone and dihydrotestosterone [15,17].

Three characteristic processes can be observed in specimens of 120–190 mm CRL (i.e., 16–22 weeks of gestation): (a) a reduction in anterior glands; (b) development of the utriculus prostaticus into a large cystic structure, often lined by a stratified squamous epithelium (observed in some of the prostatic ducts near their junction with the urethra as well); and (c) commencement

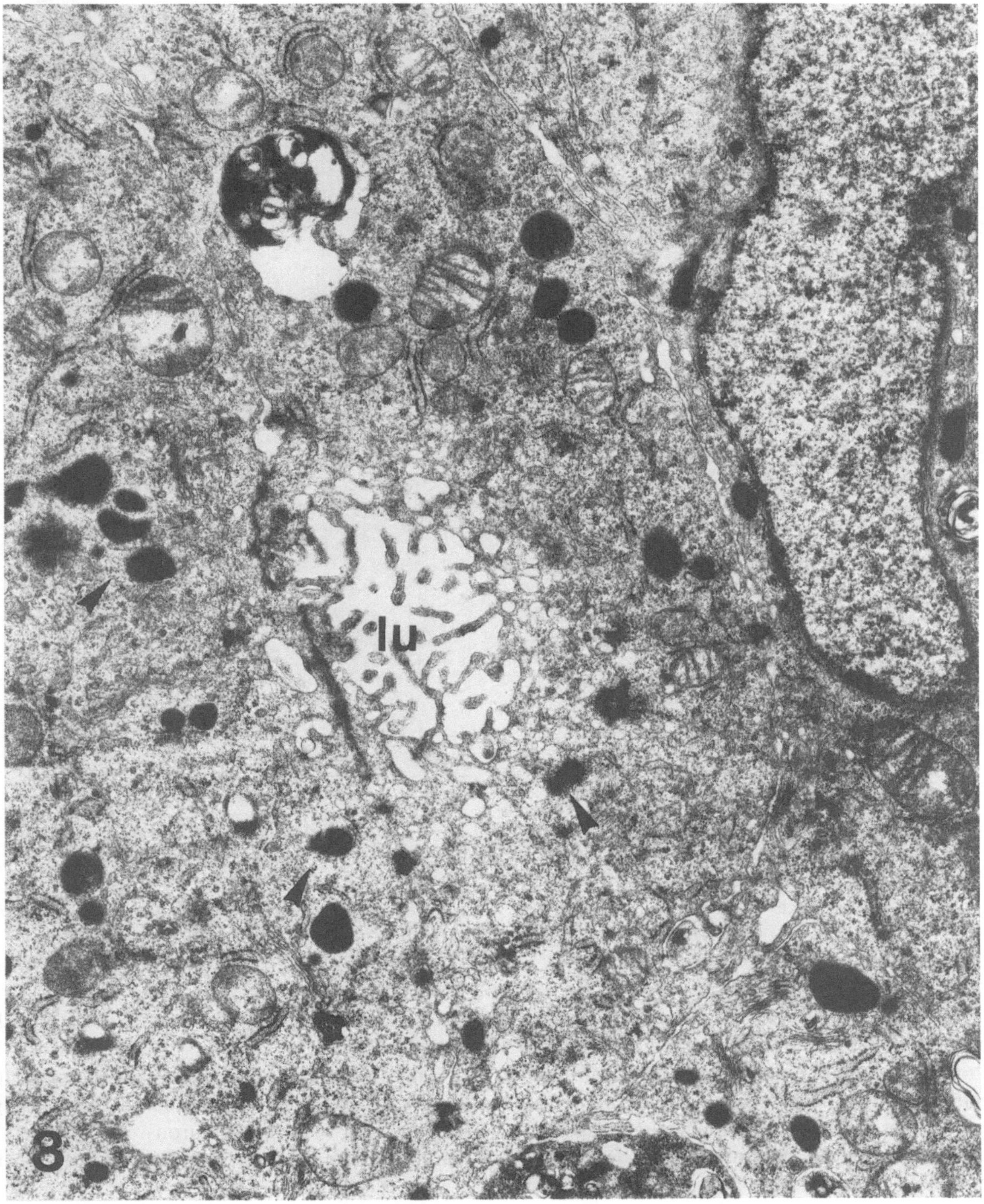

Fig. 3. At the age of 10 weeks secretory granules (arrows) can be observed at the luminal part of developing prostatic cells (lu = lumen) (×15,000).

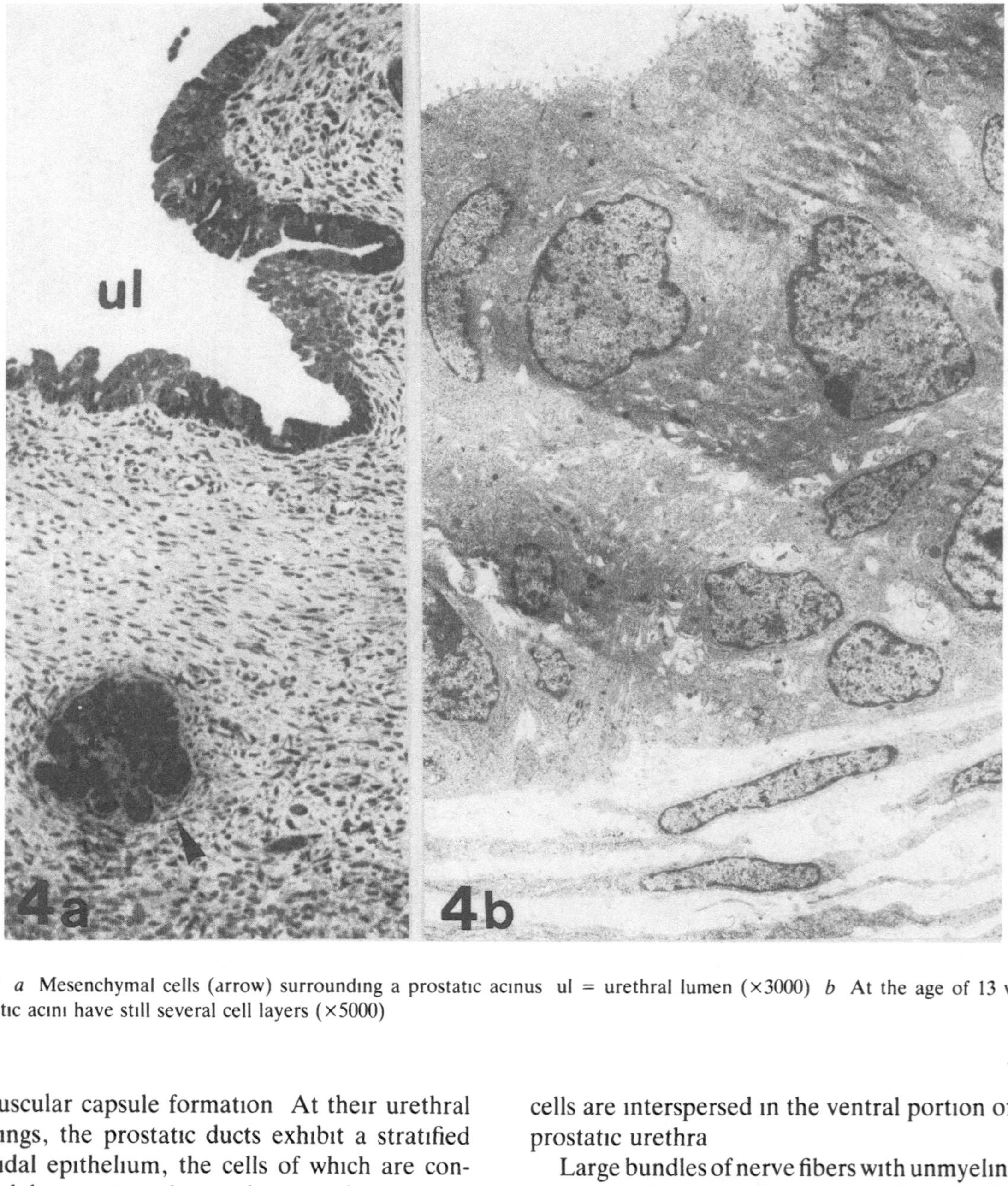

Fig 4 a Mesenchymal cells (arrow) surrounding a prostatic acinus ul = urethral lumen (×3000) *b* At the age of 13 weeks prostatic acini have still several cell layers (×5000)

of muscular capsule formation At their urethral openings, the prostatic ducts exhibit a stratified cuboidal epithelium, the cells of which are connected by junctional complexes and numerous desmosomes Their nuclei are large and irregularly shaped The cytoplasm contains mitochondria, a small Golgi apparatus, short profiles of rough endoplasmic reticulum, and glycogen deposits The prostatic stroma now consists of loosely arranged bundles of collagen fibers, numerous fibroblasts and myoblasts which form parallel layers around the epithelium Striated muscle cells are interspersed in the ventral portion of the prostatic urethra

Large bundles of nerve fibers with unmyelinated axons are found in the interstitial tissue Large ganglia with binucleate neurons, as described in earlier light microscopical studies, are also seen

2 2 *Postnatal Development*

Postnatal development can be characterized as follows [1,2]

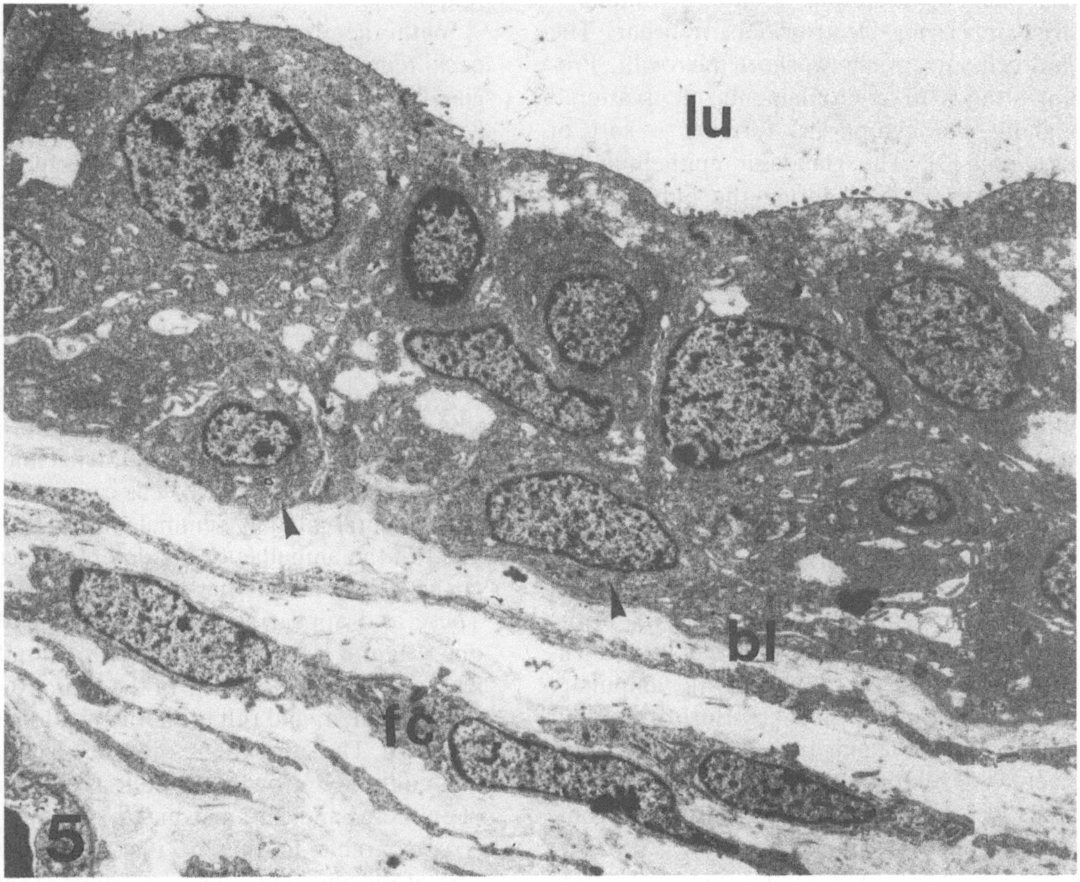

Fig 5 Prostatic epithelium, flattened at the age of 16 weeks A few triangular cells (arrow) at the basal part of the epithelium can be observed bl = basal lamina, fc = fibroblasts, lu = lumen (×5000)

1. Perinatal phase (8th month of pregnancy to 1st postnatal month)
2. Postnatal involution phase (1st to 2nd postnatal month)
3. Infantile resting phase (2nd postnatal month to 10–12 years)
4. Pubertal differentiation phase (12–18 years)
5. Maturation phase (18–21 years)

Several precise light microscopical studies on postnatal prostatic development have been performed [17,23,28]. During postnatal development a differentiation gradient within the epithelial ducts can be observed. Morphogenesis and differentiation starts in the intermediate portion of the epithelial anlage and proceeds to the urethral and subcapsular portions. The latter is reached by about 17–18 years [2]. Epithelial anlagen initially consist of a multilayered squamous or cuboidal epithelium. During the pubertal differentiation phase, it is transformed into a pseudostratified epithelium with secretory cells, basal cells, and neuroendocrine cells [2]. Electron microscopical data are only available for a few of the above-mentioned phases [25], as it is generally quite difficult to obtain normal human prostatic tissue from juveniles. During the infantile resting phase, the prostatic epithelium consists of low columnar cells with large oval nuclei that make up two thirds of the cellular volume. Round to elongate mitochondria are dispersed within the cytoplasm. Short strands of rough endoplasmic reticulum and numerous free ribosomes surround the nuclei. A small, supranuclear Golgi appparatus consisting of four to five flattened cisternae and associated vesicles is evident. Within the apical cytoplasm, a fair number of secretory granules containing material of varying electron density occur. The luminal cell surface shows short microvilli. Prominent strands of microfilaments are scattered throughout the cytoplasm, forming a sort of cytoskeleton [2]. The glandular epithelium becomes pseudostratified during the pubertal differentiation phase, being composed of columnar secretory and small basal cells. The latter are usually triangular.

3. Prenatal and Postnatal Development of the Seminal Vesicles and the Ampulla Ductus Deferentis

3.1. Prenatal Development

An initially diffuse, and later spindle-shaped, widening of the Wolffian ducts in the area of the incipient seminal vesicles (Fig. 1a) can be taken as the first indication of these and the ampullary glands. This finding was made by Burkl [5] in four different embryos ranging from 40 to 50 mm CRL. The actual development of the seminal vesicles becomes clearly evident by the third embryonic month (60 mm CRL, 17; 65 mm CRL, 5; 65 mm CRL) [4,19], when longitudinal folds arise from the Wolffian ducts at the level of the cervix vesicae. Initially, these laterally oriented folds are only set off from the Wolffian duct by two shallow furrows. Their further development is characterized by a widening and deepening of the diverticula. The continuous transition from the impending vesicular glands to the Wolffian ducts is replaced by increasingly well-demarcated structures. The previously small diverticula appear sacculelike [5].

Continued elongation and growth in the cranial and dorsolateral directions can be seen during development of the glands in the following weeks and lead to the irregular shape of the impending organs, where narrow regions alternate with sacculelike and plicated diverticula. The openings of the glands become increasingly narrow until finally, in the fourth month, the lateral portion has largely been pinched off as a caudally oriented, raised furrow, which forms the seminal vesicle. Only the caudal connection to the deferent duct remains.

With the exception of the medially located neck region, the entire length of the vesicular gland shows numerous evaginations and plicae at $5\frac{1}{2}$ months (175 mm CRL) [4]. A primitive lamina propria has formed beneath the surface epithelium, and the surrounding mesenchyme has taken on a primarily circular orientation to the longitudinal axis of the organ. Finally, at the age of 7 months (204 mm CRL) [4], there is a distinct increase in the volume of the central lumen in a proximo-distal direction.

Further development through birth is characterized by continued growth in length and circumference, whereby cells of the epithelial lining show columnar character. Basal cells cannot be seen in the prenatal human seminal vesicle. Development of the ampullae of the deferent duct occurs at the same time as that of the vesicular glands. These also appear as widenings of the Wolffian ducts at the beginning of the third month. The first mucosal folds appear in the initially spindle-shaped lumen, and run primarily in a longitudinal direction. The subsequent formation of diverticula and continued growth, as well as differentiation of epithelial and mesenchymal tissue components, is comparable to that of the seminal vesicles. Therefore, this developmental stage is called the *ampullo-vesiculo-ductal complex* [3].

The epithelial linings of the fetal glandula vesicularis, ampulla ductus deferentis, and ductus ejaculatorius are similar to one another. The central lumen, folds, and alveoli are covered with a simple columnar epithelium. Individual epithelial cells are roughly 30 μm high and 7 μm wide. The nuclei of the glandular cells are round to elongated, with a karyoplasm rich in euchromatin and a distinct nucleolus. Free ribosomes mitochondria with numerous cristae, profiles of rough endoplasmic reticulum, and glycogen particles are randomly distributed throughout the cytoplasm. A weakly developed Golgi apparatus, with a maximum of 3–4 lamellae, is found in a supranuclear location [2]. In the apical third of the cell, zonulae occludentes and desmosomes with irradiating filaments provide intercellular contact. At the level of these junctional complexes, the cells contain a pair of centrioles, dense bodies of varying size, and a thick network of microfilaments, microtubules, and smooth vesicles. No secretory granules are seen. Striking features of the prenatal gland include the absence of basal cells and the appearance of large numbers of degenerative cells.

3.2. Postnatal Maturation

The vesicular gland of the neonate is characterized by numerous [3,9,10,13,14] mucosal folds and invaginations (Fig. 1b). Within the lamina propria, the mesenchyme forms fine strands of connective tissue, while a simultaneous differentiation of intramural mesenchymal cells into smooth muscle is taking place. The first clear proof of this came from Aumüller and Riva [3], who were able to demonstrate actin using immunohistochemical methods. In both neonates and prepubescents, the vesicular and ampullary glands possess a secretory epithelium made up of columnar main cells; and isolated basal cells can be seen for the first time [2,4]. This latter type of cell remains a constant feature of the vesicular gland in adults. These cells are wedge shaped in cross section, with their broader surface abutting the basement membrane. They do not extend to the free epithelial surface. The nucleus is large in relation to the cytoplasm. Its chromatin is densely packed, thereby causing the nuclei of the basal cells to take on a darker appearance than those of the columnar main cells. In the narrow, light-colored cytoplasm there are only rudimentary complements of organelles, made up primarily of various-sized mitochondria and free ribosomes. Only a few cisternae of rough endoplasmic reticulum, occasional small vesicles, and osmiophilic granules can be seen. The Golgi apparatus is either missing or poorly developed. No signs of secretory processes can be discerned.

The slender main cells are columnar in character, resting on the basement membrane and contacting the basal cells. The ovoid nuclei exhibit a variable number of nucleoli. The cytoplasm contains mitochondria with many cristae, often surrounded by cisternae of rough endoplasmic reticulum. Lysosomes and small lipid droplets represent an additional feature. In a supranuclear location, a moderately developed Golgi apparatus can be found. The lumen of the seminal vesicles contains small amounts of PAS-positive material in the newborn and child. Further prepubescent development is characterized by a nominal weight gain, and it is not until puberty that a significant 10-fold increase in both weight and size occurs [3]. The gland elongates, connective tissue and smooth muscle cells increase in number, and the glandular epithelium takes on its adult form. Figure 6a shows the complicated duct system of the adult seminal vesicle as demonstrated by corrosion casting. Parallel to the differentiation of the glandular parenchyma, the capillary bed supporting the individual glandular portions becomes fully developed (Fig. 6b).

Changes in the ultrastructural organization of the main cells in both vesicular and ampullary glands occur at the onset of puberty, in close association with the onset of secretory activity. Characteristics of active secretory cells include abundant cytoplasmic organelles, such as cisternae of rough endoplasmic reticulum, polyribosomes, small mitochondria, several lipofuscine granules, a well-developed supranuclear Golgi apparatus, and membrane-bound secretory granules in a more apical location. The histological characteristics of the adult seminal vesicle are illustrated in Figure 7. For a detailed description of the adult seminal vesicle and ampulla of the deferent duct in man, see references 2, 18, 21, and 22.

4. Development of the Bulbourethral Glands

At the age of 10 weeks, the bulbourethral glands start their development as outgrowths of the urethral epithelium distal to the prostatic buds. Two epithelial buds grow from the pelvic portion of the urogenital sinus [6]. After the penile urethra has closed, the openings of the bulbourethral glands are located between the membranous and cavernous portions of the male urethra [9]. During the fourth fetal month, the epithelial buds representing the primordium of the excretory duct of the bulbourethral gland become branched. A

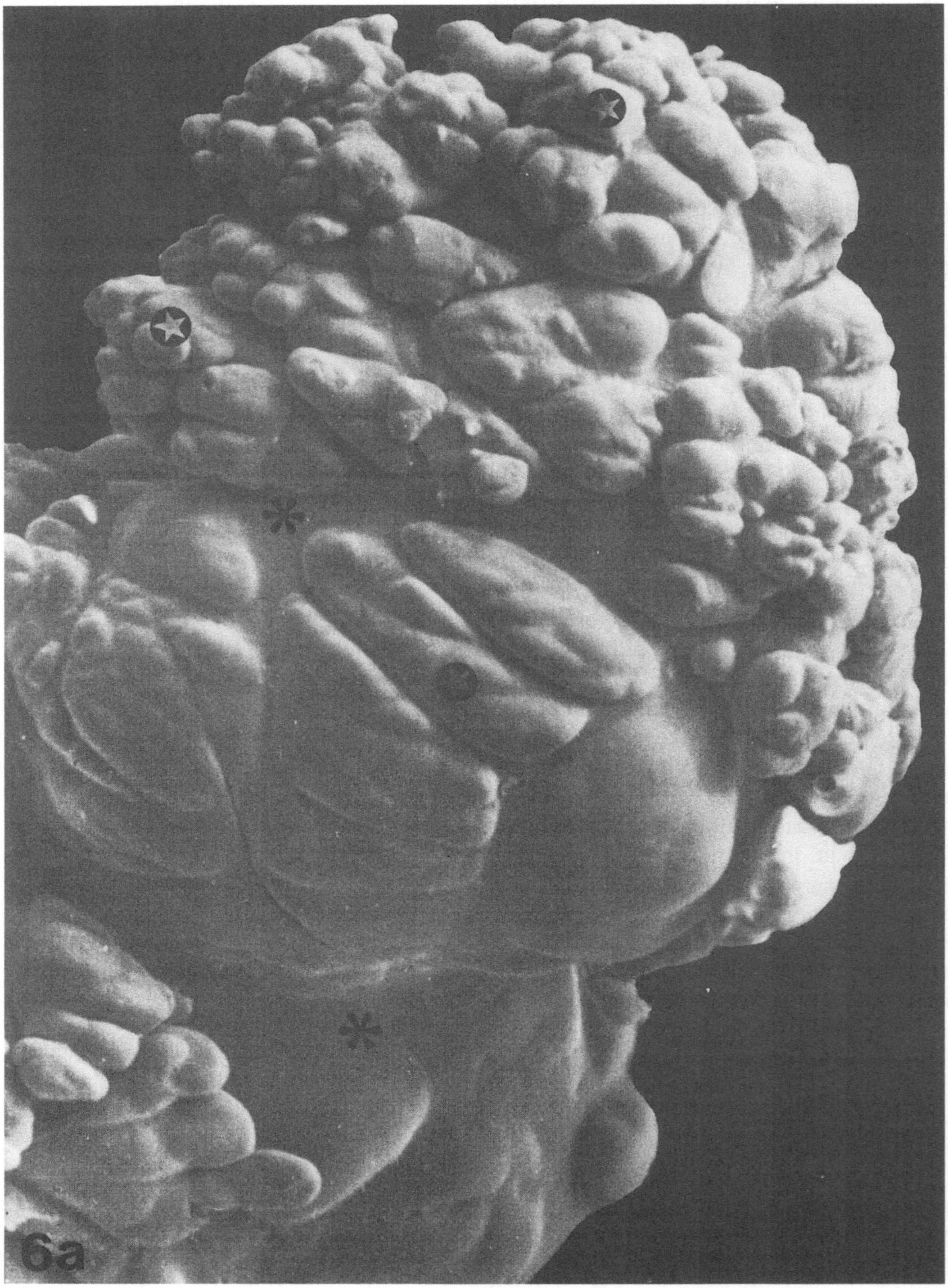

Fig 6 *a* Corrosion cast of the duct system of a human seminal vesicle (age 23 years) * main duct ☆ irregularly branched glands of various diameter *b* Corrosion cast of the capillary system in the human seminal vesicle The capillary bed surrounding the main duct (arrows) is particularly well developed Bars 200 μm

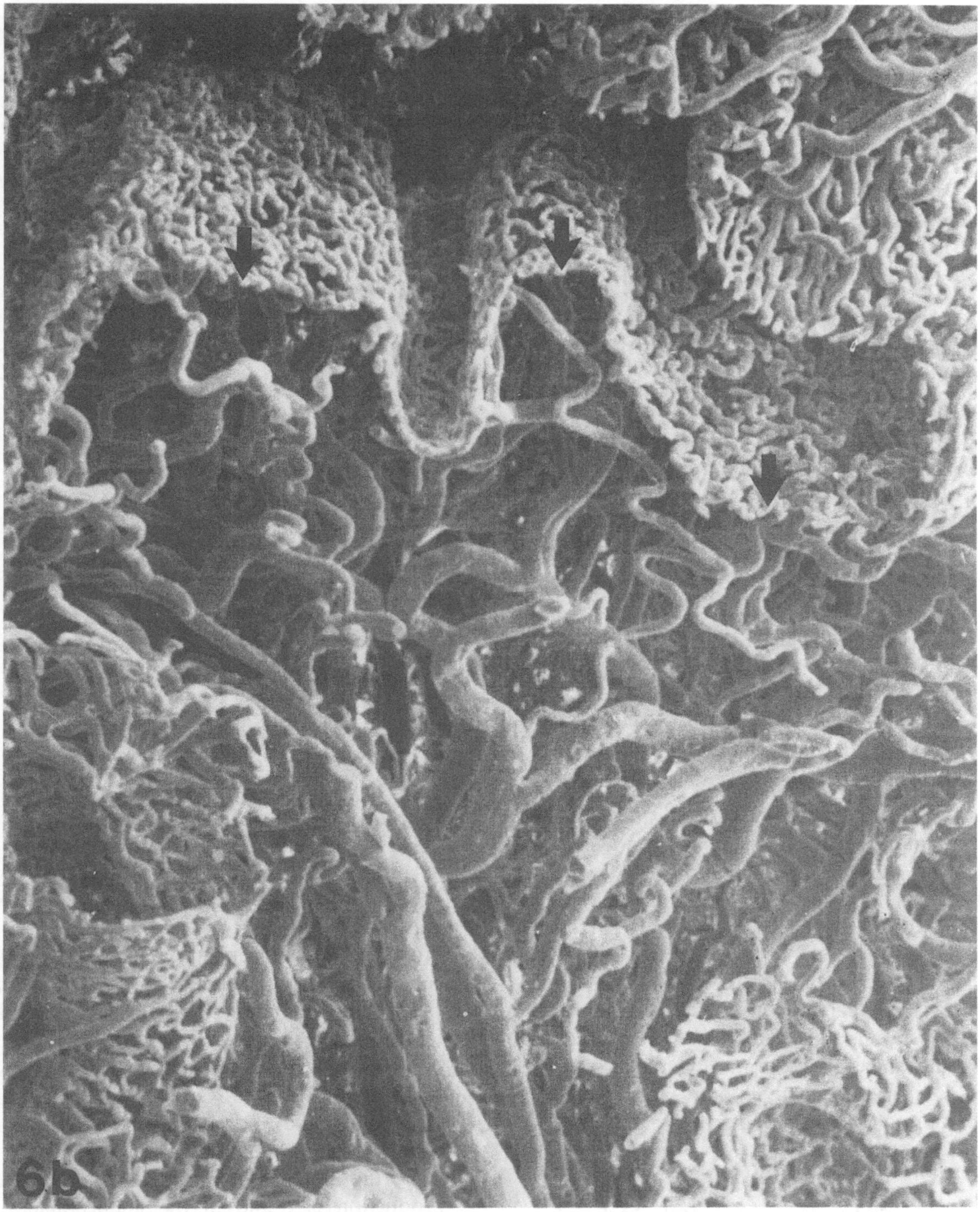
6b

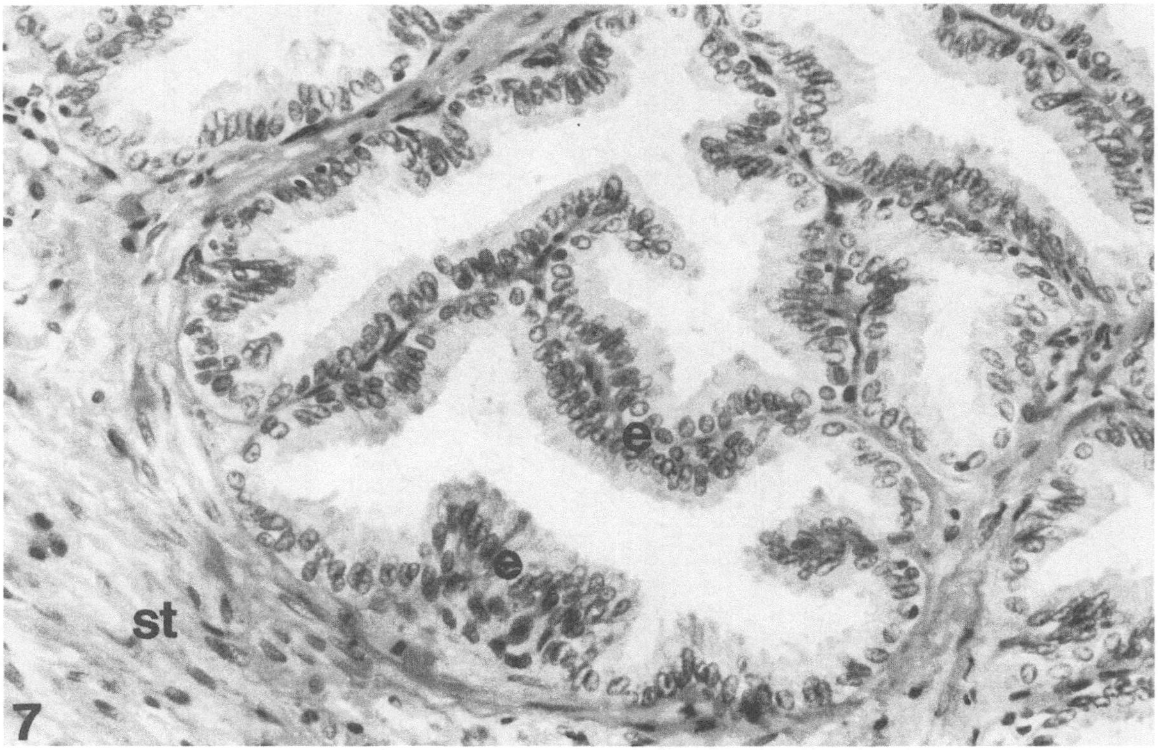

Fig 7 Histological section of the adult seminal vesicle e = epithelium of the glands, st = stroma (×420)

lumen develops within the solid cords. Mucin-containing secretory granules also appear at this time in the supranuclear and apical cytoplasm. The stroma of the bulbourethral glands differentiates from the mesenchymal cells surrounding the epithelial outgrowths. Urethral glands (of Littré) develop during the second half of pregnancy [9]. Beginning with the fifth month, epithelial sprouts of the cavernous urethra are seen. At the same time, primordia of the preputial glands appear as small buds arising from the ectodermal glando-preputial lamella [9].

5. Congenital Malformations of the Male Accessory Sex Glands in the Fetus and Neonate

Normal development of the prostate and seminal vesicles can be impaired, and this is due to various malformations, such as anencephaly and abnormalities of the urogenital tract. Hormonal therapy to the mother during pregnancy may lead to certain malformations of the fetal accessory sex glands [29]. An extreme degree of squamous metaplasia and cyst formation is found in the prostates of anencephalic fetuses [28], and is generally considered to be the result of increased estrogenic stimulation. Mothers of anencephalic fetuses, however, have low blood estriol levels [7], and the concentration of estriol is low in amniotic fluid as well. On the other hand, levels of estrone and estradiol appear relatively high by comparison.

Furthermore, severely diminished androgen production is found in the anencephalic. The disturbances in hormonal equilibrium between androgens and estrogens may be responsible for the extreme metaplastic changes seen in the prostate [24]. The seminal vesicles are generally abnormal in anencephalics as well. The bilateral agenesis, or unilateral agenesis, of all derivatives of the mesonephric ducts has been reported [29]. If seminal vesicles are present, their lumina are usually narrow or slitlike, and the glandular epithelium shows little or no secretory activity.

Malformations of the kidney are frequently associated with malformations or absence of part of the genital tract. The complete absence of both kidneys and ureters in the male is accompanied by bilateral absence or hypoplasia of the vas deferens, epididymis, and seminal vesicles, whereas the testis and ductuli efferentes remain well formed [27]. A recent study [8] demonstrated that men with congenital absence of the vas deferens often have seminal vesicles. Also, in several cases of malformation of the upper urinary tract, various degrees of prostatic immaturity were observed, including diminished proliferation and secretory activity of the epithelium. Hypospadia is sometimes associated with a large distended prostatic utricle. Otherwise, the gland appears to be normally developed [29].

The prune belly syndrome (PBS) has been recognized since 1950 as a triad of absent abdominal wall musculature, undescended te॰ts, and anomalities of the urinary tract. Additional abnormalities affect other organ systems. In some cases fetal urethral obstruction was seen [20,26]. Although distinct obstruction was not always evident, the entire anterior urethra appeared to be narrowed. Such cases were usually associated with hypoplasia of the prostate and dilatation of the prostatic portion of the urethra. Reduction or absence of prostatic epithelium and a lack of smooth muscle cells may also occur. The etiology of prostatic alterations is unknown. Recent studies on PBS [20] suggest that prostatic growth and development are hindered because of destruction or absence of the appropriate primitive mesenchyme and disturbed mesenchymal-epithelial interactions.

6. Concluding Remarks

It has been known for a long time that normal and abnormal development of male accessory sex glands are strongly influenced by androgens and estrogens. During the last few years increasing evidence has been found that steroid hormones are not the only substances that have the capacity to influence the growth and development of the male accessory sex glands. A number of polypeptides that either stimulate or inhibit growth and differentiation have been identified in the prostate [30] and also in other male accessory sex glands in several species. These include basic fibroblast growth factor (bFGF), transforming growth factor-beta 1 (TGF-beta 1), epidermal growth factor (EGF), platelet-derived growth factor (PDGF), insulin-like growth factor 1 (IGF-1), and several less well characterized peptides, such as osteoblast growth factors. In some cases, the cell population, stromal or epithelia, that synthesizes the growth factor or its receptor is known, but it will take much work in the future to fully elucidate the precise role of these polypeptide modulators in the normal and abnormal development of male accessory sex glands.

References

1 Andrews GS The histology of the human foetal and prepubertal prostates J Anat 85 44–54, 1951

2 Aumuller G Prostate gland and seminal vesicles In Handbuch der mikroskopischen Anatomie des Menschen, Vol 7 6 A Oksche, L Vollrath (eds) Berlin Springer, 1979

3 Aumuller G, Riva A Morphology and functions of the human seminal vesicle Andrologia 24 183–196, 1992

4 Brewster SF The development and differentiation of human seminal vesicles J Anat 143 45–55, 1985

5 Burkl W Uber die Entwicklung der Samenblase und der Ampulle des Ductus deferens beim Menschen Z Anat Entw Gesch 117 155–165, 1953

6 Chwalla R Uber die Entwicklung der Harnblase und der primaren Harnrohre des Menschen mit besonderer Berucksichtigung der Art und Weise, in der sich die Ureteren von den Urnierengangen trennen, nebst Bemerkungen uber die Entwicklung der Mullerschen Gange und des Mastdarms Z Anat Entwickl Gesch 83 615–647, 1927

7 Frandsen VA, Stakemann G The site of production of oestrogenic hormones in human pregnancy Hormone excretion in pregnancy with anencephalic foetus Acta Endocrinol (Copenh) 38 383–394, 1961

8 Goldstein M, Schlossber S Men with congenital absence of the vas deferens often have seminal vesicles J Urol 140 85–86, 1991

9 Jirásek JE Normal development of the male accessory glands In Male Accessory Sex Glands E Spring Mills, ESE Hafez (eds) Amsterdam Elsevier/North-Holland Biomedical, 1980, pp 1–16

10 Kellokumpu-Lehtinen P The histochemical localization of acid phophatase in human fetal urethral and prostatic epithelium Invest Urology 435–440, 1980

11 Kellokumpu-Lehtinen P Development of sexual dimorphism in human urogenital sinus complex Biol Neonate 48 157–167, 1985

12 Kellokumpu-Lehtinen P Correlation of embryonic development and adult neoplastic changes of human prostate Eur Urol 16 386–390, 1989

13 Kellokumpu-Lehtinen P, Santti R, Pelliniemie LJ Early cytodifferentiation of human fetal prostate and Leydig cells Anat Rec 194 429–444, 1979

14 Kellokumpu-Lehtinen P, Santti R, Pelliniemie LJ Correlation of early cytodifferentiation of human fetal prostate and Leydig cells Anat Rec 196 263–273, 1980

15 Kellokumpu-Lehtinen P, Santti RS, Pelliniemi LJ Development of human fetal prostate in culture Urol Res 9 89–98, 1981

16 Lowsley DS The development of the human prostate gland with reference to the development of other structures at the neck of the urinary bladder Am J Anat 13 299–349, 1912

17 Moore RA The histology of the newborn and prepubertal prostate gland Anat Rec 66 1–36, 1936

18 Nistal M, Santamaria L, Paniagua R The ampulla of the ductus deferens in man Morphological and ultrastructural aspects J Anat 180 97–104, 1992

19 Pallin G Beitrage zur Anatomie und Embryologie der Prostata und der Samenblasen Arch Anat Phys (Leipzig) 25 135–176, 1901

20 Popek EJ, Tyson RW, Miller GJ, Caldwell SA Prostate development in prune belly syndrome (PBS) and posterior urethral valves (PUV) Etiology of PBS Lower urinary tract obstruction or primary mesenchymal defect? Pediatr Pathol 11 1–29, 1991

21 Riva A, Testa-Riva F, Usai E, Cossu M The ampulla ductus deferentis in man, as viewed by SEM and TEM Arch Androl 8 157–164, 1982

22 Riva A, Usai E, Scarpa R, Cossu M, Lantini MS Fine structure of the accessory glands of the human male genital tract In Development in Ultrastructure of Reproduction Progress in Clinical and Biological Research, Vol 296 PM Motta (ed) New York Alan R Liss, 1989, pp 233–240

23 Stieve H Mannliche Genitalorgane Die Vorsteherdruse Handbuch der mikroskopischen Anatomie des Menschen, VII Berlin Springer, 1930

24 Tapanainen J, Kellokumpu-Lehtinen P, Pelliniemi L, Huhtaniemi I Age-related changes in endogenous steroids of human fetal testis during early and midpregnancy J Clin Endocrinol Metab 52 98–102, 1981

25 Webber MM, Stonington OG Ultrastructural changes in human prepubertal prostatic epithelium grown in vitro Invest Urol 12 389–395, 1975

26 Wigger HJ, Blanc WA The prune belly syndrome Pathol Ann 12 17–37, 1977

27 Willis RA The Borderland of Embryology and Pathology London Betterworth, 1962

28 Zondek LH, Zondek T The human prostate in anencephaly Acta Endocrinol (Copenh) 64 548–557, 1970

29 Zondek LH, Zondek T Congenital malformations of the male accessory sex glands in the fetus and neonate In Male Accessory Sex Glands E Spring Mills, ESE Hafez (eds) Amsterdam Elsevier/North-Holland Biomedical, 1980, pp 17–37

30 Story MT Polypeptide modulators of prostatic growth and development Cancer Surv 11 123–146, 1991

Role of Mesenchymal-Epithelial Interactions in Normal and Abnormal Development of Male Urogenital Glands

GERALD R. CUNHA

1. Introduction

Malignant cells usually fail to express specialized functions of the tissue from which they arise and are frequently undifferentiated. The loss of specialized function in carcinoma cells has been attributed to mutations or other forms of genetic rearrangement that result in the malignant phenotype. It is important to recognize that virtually all of the various features that characterize malignant cells are expressed in normal cells during various phases of normal embryonic development. For example, the invasive properties of tumor cells are shared by the trophoblast and neural crest cells. The ability of tumor cells to metastasize to distance sites is mimicked by primordial germ cells and developing lymphoid cells. High proliferative capacity is certainly not unique to tumor cells. The differentiative capacity of malignant cells is demonstrated by the capability of malignant stem cells to produce differentiated benign tissues [153], and in the case of the embryonal carcinoma, these highly malignant cells have been shown to be able to participate in normal embryonic development with complete loss of the malignant phenotype [131]. Findings of this nature have led to the concept that malignancy represents a caricature of tissue renewal [154] and that ablative therapies might be augmented by differentiation therapy whereby nontoxic differentiation inducers might convert proliferating cells with neoplastic properties to differentiated cells with reduced proliferative potential. Recent studies suggest that differentiation therapy could be applied to prostate cancer, which is one of the most prevalent neoplasms afflicting men, with 120,000 new cases of prostatic adenocarcinoma and 30,000 deaths per year [22]. For the prostate, mesenchyme induces and specifies patterns of normal epithelial development, growth, and differentiation [36], and thus cell-cell interactions may provide the basis for devising new differentiation therapy protocols for prostatic adenocarcinoma. The goal of this review will be to consider the developmental biology of the prostate and other urogenital glands, and to explore the potential for experimental manipulation of differentiation and growth in prostatic carcinomas.

2. Androgen-Dependent Development of the Male Urogenital Tract

All vertebrate embryos display a so-called ambisexual phase of sex differentiation before distinct sex differentiation takes place. During this period the gonads are morphologically undifferentiated. The developing internal genitalia are represented by the Wolffian and Müllerian ducts, mesonephric tubules, and the urogenital sinus (UGS). For each organ rudiment, the timing of sex differentiations is slightly different, with the gonads being the first structures to undergo sex differentiation and the UGS being the last. The male internal genitalia develop principally from two embryonic rudiments: the Wolffian ducts and urogenital sinus. The UGS, whose epithelium is derived from endoderm, develops into

Riva, A., Testa Riva, F., and Motta, P.M., (eds), Ultrastructure of Male Urogenital Glands Prostate, Seminal Vesicles, Urethral, and Bulbourethra Glands © 1994 Kluwer Academic Publishers ISBN 0-7923-2800-0 All rights reserved

the prostate, bulbourethral glands, urethra, and periurethral glands [33]. The Wolffian duct, whose epithelim is mesodermal in origin, develops into the epididymis, ductus deferens, seminal vesicle, and ejaculatory duct. The mesonephric tubules associated with the Wolffican duct develop into the efferent ducts.

Development and growth of male accessory sexual glands are androgen dependent [36,94, 209]. In rodents androgen production by the developing fetal testes begins during the ambisexual period and continues until birth, after which androgen levels fall [51,155,162,206,212]. Ablation of fetal testes during the ambisexual period of sex differentiation inhibits masculine development [94,159]. Similarly, administration of antiandrogens to pregnant females suppresses masculine development of internal and external genitalia [54,139,140]. Postnatally in rodents, the continued development of the prostate, seminal vesicles, and bulbourethral glands is also androgen dependent [28,51,180]. While testosterone is the primary androgen produced by the testis, dihydrotestosterone (DHT) appears to be the active intracellular androgen responsible for development of the prostate and bulbourethral gland as well as postnatal morphogenesis of the seminal vesicle [29,180,210]. The role of testosterone itself in development of the Wolffian duct is unclear, since only testosterone is present initially, but later DHT is produced by the Wolffian duct [180,200, 203–205]. DHT is produced by enzymatic reduction of testosterone by 5α-reductase. This enzyme has been detected in the UGS, Wolffian duct, neonatal seminal vesicle, and external genitalia [103,180,181,201,204,205,209,211]. Inhibition of this enzyme blocks masculinization of the external genitalia and urethra, and partially inhibits prostatic morphogenesis in the rat [83]. Likewise, humans with 5α-reductase deficiency are born with ambiguous but distinctly female external genitalia; prostates are small or undetectable, but Wolffian derivatives are normal [82,84,85]. The development of a rudimentary prostate in the case of 5α-reductase deficiency or in the presence of 5α-reductase inhibitors suggests that the developing prostate may be responsive to exceedingly low levels of DHT or other androgens [83].

Androgens masculinize the developing male genital tract via androgen receptors (ARs) present in fetal urogenital anlage. Androgen receptors are detectable in the mesenchyme of urogenital rudiments during the ambisexual stage, but androgen receptors are not detectable in epithelium of the developing male urogenital tract until later periods [81,135,175,177,192,193]. In the mouse, mesenchymal androgen receptors are present from as early as 14 days of gestation, while epithelial androgen receptors appear in a cranial to caudal sequence beginning in the efferent ducts at 16 days of gestation, followed in the epididymis and ductus deferens at 19 days of gestation, the seminal vesicle epithelium at 1–2 days postnatal, the prostatic epithelium at 4–6 days postnatal, and the bulbourethral gland epithelium at 8 days postnatal [27,175]. Findings in the rat are in agreement with these studies in the mouse [81]. Before epithelial ARs are detectable in the urogenital tract, a wide range of androgen-dependent developmental processes are expressed in these ostensibly androgen receptor-negative epithelia. These include: (a) prevention of programmed cell death in the Wolffian duct, (b) appearance and initial morphogenesis of the seminal vesicle anlagen, (c) emergence and initial branching morphogenesis of ducts of the prostate and bulbourethral gland, and (d) androgen-induced degeneration of male mammary epithelial anlagen. These effects of androgens have been inferred to be due to paracrine interactions between the androgen receptor-positive mesenchyme and the apparently androgen receptor-negative epithelium as described below.

2.1. Prenatal and Postnatal Growth and Development of the Prostate

The prostate arises from solid epithelial outgrowths (prostatic buds) that emerge from the UGS directly below the bladder. Prostatic buds grow into the mesenchyme investing the UGS, elongate, and arborize to form a complex ductal network. For many species prostatic buds arise from different parts of the prostatic urethra, thus giving rise to the various prostatic lobes, each with its distinctive ductal branching pattern [4,72, 92,104,107,109,128,156,190]. In rats and mice, prostatic growth and ductal branching morphogenesis are continuous processes, beginning in late fetal life and terminating in early adulthood.

In the human, prostatic development commences at 10–12 weeks of fetal life when solid prostatic buds emerge from the UGS, elongate, and arborize in the urogenital sinus mesenchyme [96, 107,216]. This period of embryonic prostatic growth is followed after birth in humans by growth quiescence until puberty, when elevating androgen levels promote renewed prostatic growth [14,24]. During periods of prostatic growth, the rate of cell proliferation exceeds the rate of cell death, and there is a net increase in prostatic DNA content [87,88]. When adulthood is reached, prostatic growth ends. However, in man and dogs prostatic growth is reestablished in old age during the pathogenesis of benign prostatic hyperplasia (BPH). After several years of hyperplastic growth, prostatic weight plateaus at an elevated level, where it remains until death. Prostatic doubling times have been computed over the entire course of normal and hyperplastic growth in the human prostate [24]. Two important points arise from thse observations: (a) Actual hyperplastic growth of the human prostate apparently occurs early in the etiology of BPH and is highest in prostates from 30- to 50-year-old men when prostatic doubling time is 4–5 years. (b) BPH generally becomes clinically evident after the period of hyperplastic growth when prostatic doubling times are extremely low [14,24]. The implications of Coffey's studies are that most BPH surgical specimens are obtained from patients during periods when prostatic growth is minimal. Thus, growth-quiescent human surgical BPH tissues may be entirely inappropriate specimens for studying the regulation of prostatic growth.

Even though prostatic growth has been investigated for many years with a variety of biochemical and morphological techniques, only recently has it been shown that DNA synthesis is not homogeneous within the growing prostate but instead is focused at the tips of elongating ducts (Fig. 1) [5,157,191]. This pattern of focally elevated levels of DNA synthesis at the ductal tips is also seen in other glands, such as the mammary gland [16], salivary gland [11,12], and lung [64], and thus represents a basic biological process of ductal growth. Any mechanism of prostatic growth must consider not only the high levels of DNA synthesis at ductal tips, but also the reduced levels of DNA synthesis along the proximal duct. The great differences in DNA synthetic activity along growing prostatic ducts (Fig. 1) cannot be

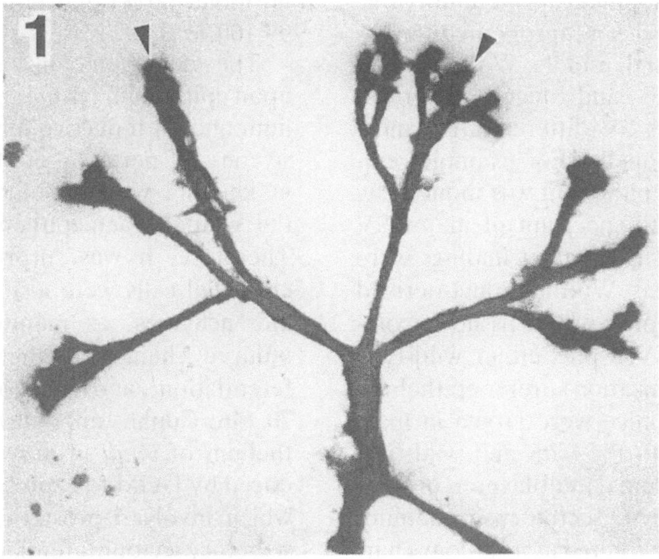

Fig. 1. [^{14}C]-thymidine autoradiogram of whole-mounted ducts from the ventral prostate of a 30-day-old rat. Following microdissection of a single developing duct, the tissue was incubated with [^{14}C]-thymidine and processed autoradiographically as described earlier [191]. Note that the distal tips of this rapidly growing ductal system (arrows) show heavy silver grain density, whereas the proximal regions of the duct exhibit relatively light labeling with [^{14}C]-thymidine (×32)

explained by parallel differences in androgen receptors or DHT production in distal versus proximal ductal regions [157]. On the other hand, paracrine interactions between epithelium and mesenchyme involving growth factors may provide an appropriate mechanistic framework for explaining the heterogeneous nature of DNA synthesis during androgen-dependent prostatic growth.

3. Role of Epithelial-Mesenchymal Interactions in Development of the Male Genital Tract

Mesenchymal-epithelial interactions play a crucial role in masculine urogenital development in that mesenchyme induces and specifies patterns of epithelial morphogenesis, regulates epithelial proliferation, determines epithelial cytodifferentiation, and induces and specifies epithelial functional or biochemical activity. For the fetal prostate, urogenital sinus mesenchyme (UGM) induces ductal morphogenesis, induces the expression of epithelial androgen receptors, regulates epithelial proliferation, and specifies the expression of prostatic secretory proteins [23,32, 35,36,70,176,189,194].

For the seminal vesicle (SV) the mesenchyme (SVM) elicits SV development in the embryonic Wolffian duct [31,76] and can reprogram differentiation of the upper and middle Wolffian duct (prospective epididymis and ductus deferens, respectively) to express SV differentiation morphologically and functionally. For example, embryonic Wolffian duct epithelium was induced by SVM to express the full spectrum of major SV secretory proteins [76]. Equivalent findings were obtained with postnatal Wolffian duct-derived epithelium. For example, when tissue recombinants composed of SVM plus either wild-type or Tfm (testicular feminization) ureter epithelium (URE) from neonatal mice were grown in male hosts for 1 month, both the Tfm and wild-type URE were converted from a multilayered urothelium to a simple columnar secretory epithelium, exhibiting the highly convoluted morphology characteristic of SV (Fig. 2A,B) [39,40]. In SVM + wild-type URE tissue recombinants, these morphological changes in epithelial differentiation culminated in the expression of epithelial androgen receptors and all of the major SV secretory proteins (Fig. 2C) [40]. Conversely, in SVM + Tfm URE recombinants, functional androgen receptors cannot be expressed in the androgen-insensitive Tfm epithelium [73]. Significantly, SVM + Tfm URE recombinants failed to express SV secretory proteins, even though the SVM had induced the development of SV epithelial morphology in the Tfm ureter (Fig. 2C) [39]. This implies that while certain "androgenic" effects (epithelial morphogenesis, proliferation, and change in epithelial cytodifferentiation) are elicited via paracrine influences from the androgen receptor-positive mesenchyme and do not require epithelial androgen receptors, the expression of androgen-dependent secretory proteins requires intraepithelial androgen receptors [40]. Thus, the lack of androgen receptors in Tfm URE absolutely precludes the expression of androgen-dependent SV secretory proteins [39]. These studies, and comparable observations in the developing prostate and embryonic mouse mammary gland, demonstrate that the mesenchyme is the key androgen target tissue during development and that many androgenic effects expressed in the epithelium are evoked via paracrine influences from the mesenchyme, which is the requisite inducer of epithelial development in hormone target and nontarget organs [36,38,66, 99,100,171].

The developmental effects of mesenchyme upon epithelium require both a responsive epithelium and an inductive mesenchyme. The responsiveness of perinatal epithelia described above is in keeping with the undifferentiated nature of the genital tract epithelia during development. Therefore, it was surprising that certain adult epithelial cells were also responsive to inductive mesenchymes, as manifested by mesenchyme-induced changes in their morphology, cytodifferentiation, and functional differentiation [40, 70,146; Cunha, unpublished]. For example, epithelium of *adult* urinary bladder (BLE) was induced by UGM to express prostatic development, which involved prostatic ductal morphogenesis, secretory cytodifferentiation, expression of epithelial androgen receptors, prostate-specific secretory proteins, and androgen dependency for DNA synthesis [37,52,138,189,194]. In analogous fashion, seminal vesicle mesenchyme (SVM) *in-*

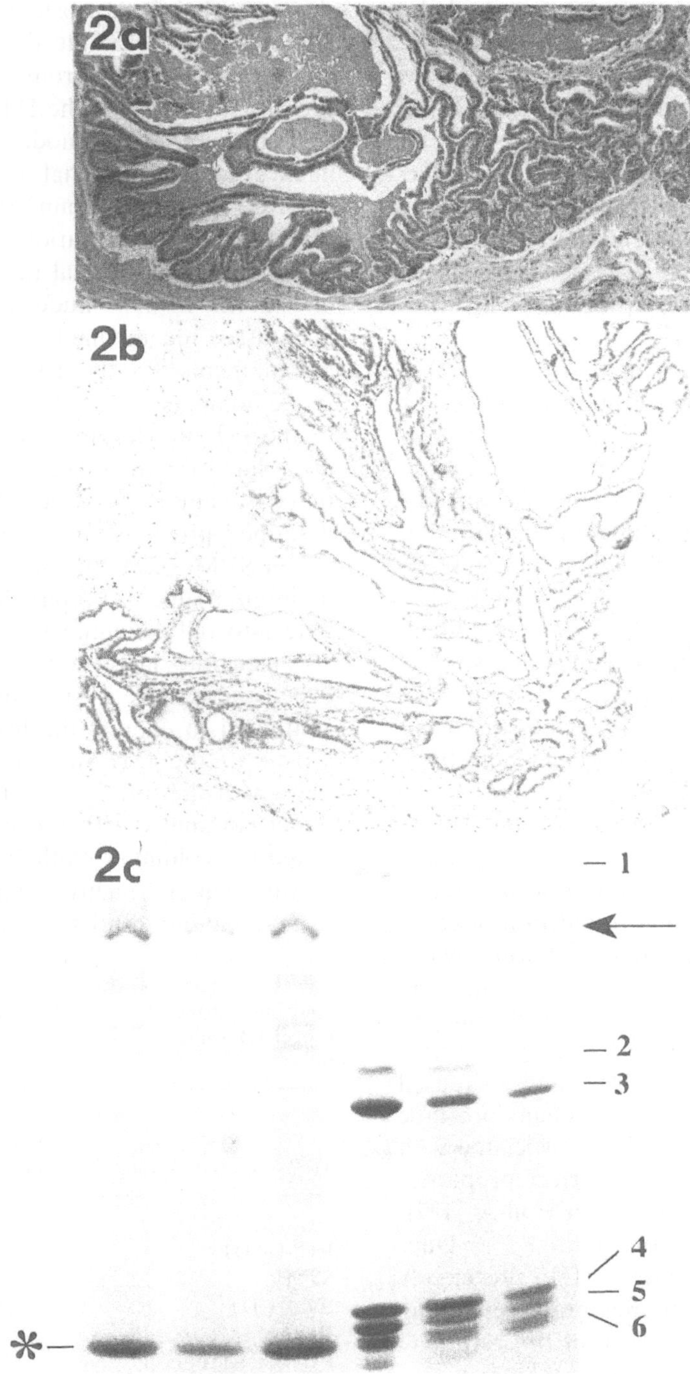

Fig 2 Tissue recombinants composed of rat seminal vesicle mesenchyme associated with either wild type (*A*) or Tfm mouse ureter epithelium (*B*) Note the formation of a complex mucosa lined with a simple columnar epithelium in both types of tissue recombinants (A and B ×80) From Cunha and Young [39] with permission *C* SDS PAGE of secretory proteins from individual tissue recombinants composed of rat SVM plus Tfm mouse URE (lanes 1–3) and rat SVM plus wild type mouse URE (lanes 4–6) Proteins extracted from individual tissue recombinants were separated by SDS PAGE and stained with Coomassie Blue Note the six characteristic mouse SV secretory proteins present when wild type but not Tfm URE was used The arrow denotes albumin and the asterisk denotes globin unavoidable contaminants present in most samples From Cunha and Young [39] with permission

structively induced SV development in epithelia of the adult epididymis [202], adult ductus deferens, and adult ureter [40]. In all of these SV inductions, the adult epithelia were induced to change their original phenotype and to express SV differentiation morphologically and functionally. Moreover, in the case of SV induction from adult epididymal epithelium, the expression of SV secretory proteins was associated with the loss of epididymal secretory proteins [202].

4. Role of Epithelial-Stromal Interactions in Carcinogenesis

The ongoing importance of epithelial-stromal interactions in regulating adult epithelial differentiation raises the possibility that emerging or established carcinomas might also be influenced by their connective tissue environment [30,42, 43,61–63,112]. Disturbances in epithelial-stromal interactions during carcinogenesis have been recognized for many years [196]. Such disturbances are manifested in many ways: gaps in the basal lamina [10], duplication and thickening of the basal lamina [188], uncontrolled growth of tumor stromal fibroblasts in vitro [45], agglutinability of peritumoral fibroblasts with concanavalin A (Con-A) [21,147], abnormal production of collagenase by dermal fibroblasts [9], elevated chondroitin sulfate proteoglycan and hyaluronic acid production [86], stromelysin-3 [8], tenascin [56, 113], a fibroblast-oncofetal antigen [7], stromal growth factor expression [215], and increased laminin expression [57]. In human prostatic adenocarcinomas, the fibroblasts associated with carcinoma cells have abnormal surface properties manifested as agglutinability with Con-A [147]. Stromal-epithelial interactions in the R3327 Dunning prostatic adenocarcinoma (CT) are clearly abnormal, as the basement membrane separating the neoplastic epithelia cells from the "stroma" is frequently discontinuous or excessively reduplicated [213]. An apparent process of micrometastasis has been described in the DT, in which keratin-positive carcinoma cells migrate from the epithelial ducts through gaps in the basement membrane into the stroma [10]. Thus, from several perspectives the "stroma" of the DT is clearly abnormal in comparison to stroma of the normal rodent prostate. These findings encouraged us to examine the effect of certain inductive mesenchymes from the urogenital tract on the differentiation of the DT.

Our experimental model for studying the influence of mesenchymal inductors on the DT involved growing 0.5 mm^3 fragments of the DT in association with various mesenchymes from embryonic and neonatal rat organ rudiments for one month in male nude mouse hosts (Fig. 3). Such tissue recombinants were named as primary recombinants. Grafts of DT alone preserved the stable homogeneous histopathology characteristic of the DT and formed tumors containing small ducts lined by one or more layers of undifferentiated squamous or cuboidal epithelial cells, as described previously [89]. In grafts of UGM + DT or SVM + DT, the mesenchyme induced the undifferentiated DT epithelial cells to differentiate into tall columnar secretory epithelial cells arranged into large cystic ducts [69,71]. In between these more normal ducts were ducts that continued to express the histopathology characteristic of the DT. In fortuitous sections ducts lined with the undifferentiated DT cells were in direct continuity with the more highly differentiated tall columnar epithelial cells (Fig. 4), suggesting that the highly differentiated cells arose from the undifferentiated DT epithelial cells. The

Table 1 Secretory cytodifferentiation of Dunning tumor epithelium grown in combination with mesenchyme from the urogenital sinus, seminal vesicle, bulbourethral gland, or bladder

Tissues grafted	No grafts	Secretory cytodifferentiation	Proportion of responding (%)
UGM	28	0	0[a]
UGM + DT	80	70	88[b]
SVM	22	0	0[a]
SVM + DT	60	50	83[b]
BUG-M	10	0	0[a]
BUG-M + DT	17	14	82[b]
BLM	16	0	0[a]
BLM + DT	27	0	0[b]

[a] Control grafts of mesenchyme only were recovered as undifferentiated fibromuscular tissues
[b] Unresponsive recombinations showed original DT histology
DT = Dunning tumor, UGM = urogenital sinus, SVM = seminal vesicle, BUGM = bulbourethral gland, BLM = bladder

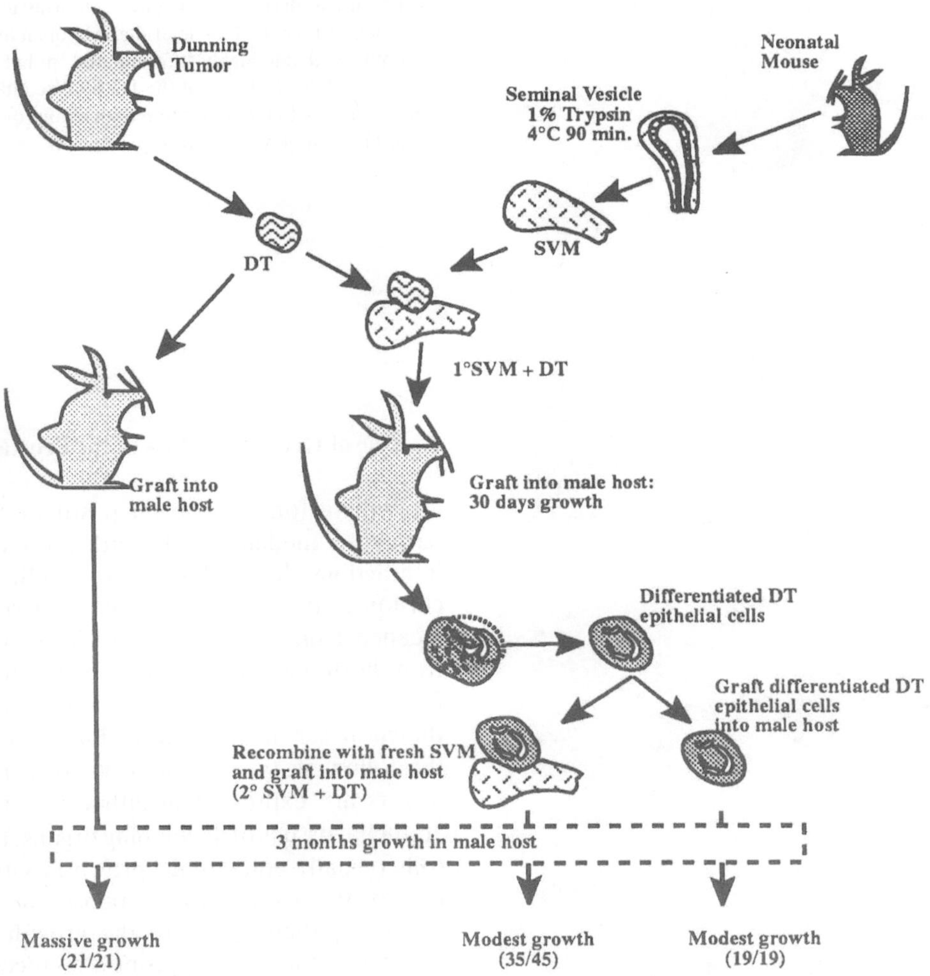

Fig 3 Experimental protocol for analyzing the effect of inductive mesenchyme on differentiation and growth of the Dunning prostatic adenocarcinoma SVM = seminal vesicle mesenchyme, DT = Dunning tumor

effects of UGM and SVM were shared with mesenchymes from other genital tract organs but not with that of the urinary bladder (Table 1).

These mesenchyme-induced changes in DT histodifferentiation were associated with changes in neoplastic growth [69]. When SVM-induced differentiated DT cells were tested for their ability to grow as tumors (see Fig. 3 for experimental protocol), tumorigenesis was dramatically reduced. For example, when the large fluid-filled ducts of primary SVM + DT recombinants were grafted to new male hosts or combined with fresh SVM to form secondary SVM + DT recombinants, overall growth was modest during a 3 month period, and the differentiated DT epithelium was maintained (Fig. 5). In contrast, grafts of the DT fully overgrew the host's kidney forming a single large tumor mass weighting 5–7 g. The reduction in growth rate and reduction, if not loss, in tumorigenesis of the SVM-induced DT epithelial cells was associated with a sevenfold reduction in ^{3}H-thymidine labelling index [69]. While this model of mesenchyme-induced differentiation therapy is interesting, the crucial issues will be to determine the paracrine mediators of these cell-cell interactions that are capable of regulating both normal and neoplastic prostatic development. Growth factors are likely candidates.

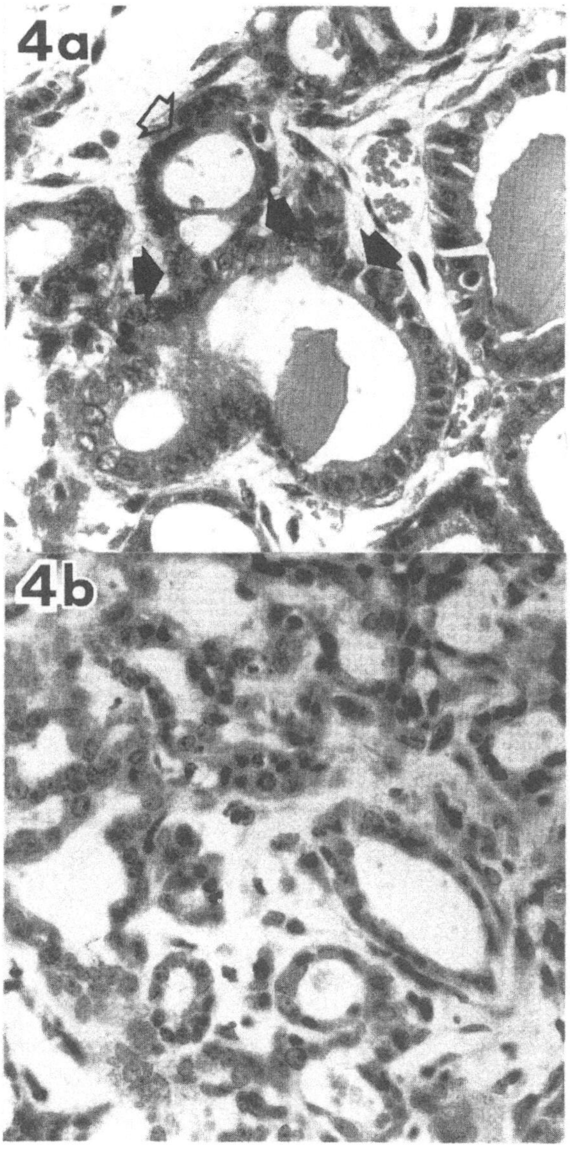

Fig 4 A A tissue recombinant composed of neonatal rat seminal vesicle mesenchyme plus Dunning tumor (DT) grown for 1 month as described in Figure 3, showing undifferentiated epithelial cells characteristic of the DT (open arrow) in direct continuity with tall, highly differentiated epithelial cells (closed arrows) (×250) *B* Graft of the DT alone contains only small tubules lined with undifferentiated squamous or cuboidal cells From Hayashi et al [71], with permission

5. Role of Growth Factors in the Prostate

Growth factors have been postulated to be the paracrine mediators of epithelial-mesenchymal interactions [67,74,110,141,142,149]. This conclusion is based on many types of observations gleaned from a variety of model systems, some from hormone target organs. The role of growth factors as autocrine/paracrine mediators of epithelial-mesenchymal interactions is based upon the following types of observations: (a) Growth factors are expressed in either mesenchymal or epithelial tissues of developing organs. (b) Isolated cells (usually epithelium) grown in vitro respond to growth factors. (c) Responses of mesenchymal or epithelial cells to the growth factor are mediated through appropriate receptors. (d) Neutralizing antibodies to a growth factor or its receptor block biological effects. (e) Overexpression of a growth factor in transgenic mice perturbs growth and development. In the prostate, polypeptide growth factors have been implicated in

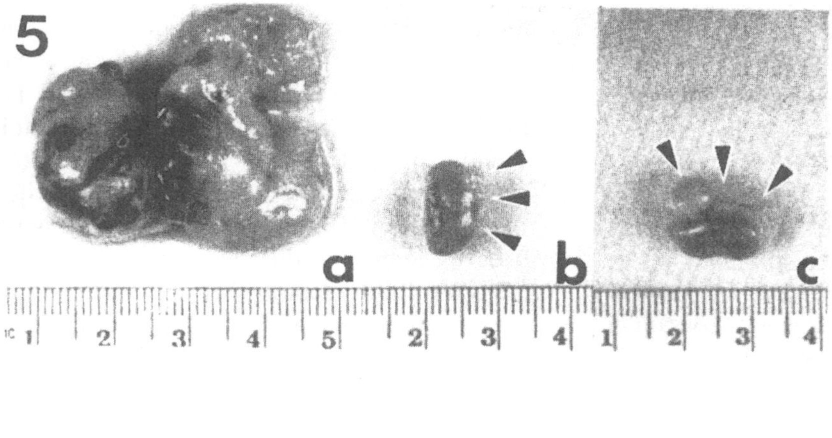

Fig 5 Gross appearance of grafts grown for 3 months under renal capsule Three grafts each of 2°SVM + DT recombinants (*B*) and of differentiated DT epithelial cells derived from 1°SVM + DT recombinants (*C*) (see text and Fig 3 for abbreviations and protocol) have grown modestly Note that the three grafts of the parental DT have grown into a single tumorous mass that obscures the host's kidney (*A*) (×32) From Hayashi and Cunha [69], with permission

benign and malignant growth, and have been suggested to be possible mediators of epithelial-stromal interactions [123,185,197,198]. Examination of the literature relevant to prostatic growth raises the troubling paradox that *trophic* growth factors generally have been investigated in the growth-quiescent adult rat prostate. For example, of the dozens of studies of growth factors in the rat prostate, only the report of Mansson et al. [117] has utilized prostates from young rats (6–8 weeks). They find that heparin-binding growth factors (HBGFs) are expressed at highest levels in these growing prostates, and thereafter HBGFs declined to undetectable levels at 35 weeks when prostatic growth was nil [117]. All the remaining studies dealing with growth factors in the prostate have used growth-quiescent adult prostates as the source of experimental tissue. The biology of growth factors in the adult prostate is unclear and is a troubling paradox, requiring further critical examination. Moreover, the extensive proliferation achieved by adult prostatic epithelial cells cultured in vitro is in stark contrast to their growth quiescence in vivo. Our firm belief is that the role of growth factors in the prostate *must* be investigated during periods of actual prostatic growth so that in vitro models truly mimic in vivo events. Examination of prostatic growth must also take into consideration the specific temporal/spatial parameters of growth observed in the prostate. A key feature of prostatic growth is that DNA synthesis does not occur homogeneously throughout the gland but is concentrated on the tips (Fig. 1) of the elongating prostatic ducts [5,157,191]. Thus, to truly understand prostatic growth the proposed mechanism must provide an explanation for the extremely high level of DNA synthesis in prostatic ductal tips as well as the rapid falloff in DNA synthesis proximally along the duct. None of the published studies address these issues and thus it is difficult to assess the role of growth factors in the prostate from a biological perspective.

Growth factors from 6 major families have been described in the prostate: insulinlike growth factors, platelet derived growth factor, nerve growth factor, epidermal growth factor, transforming growth factor-betas (TGFβ), and heparin-binding growth factors. In virtually all cases, it is difficult to relate growth factors to the biology of cell-cell interactions, prostatic ductal morphogenesis, epithelial growth, cytodifferentiation, functional expression, or neoplasia because in almost all cases the growth-quiescent adult prostate has been utilized.

5.1. Insulin and Insulinlike Growth Factors (IGF)

Insulin is known to have a spectrum of metabolic effects and to stimulate the growth and proliferation of a variety of cells in vitro [77,187]. It can act directly through its own high affinity receptor [6,187] or through low affinity binding to the IGF-I receptor [44,160,161,187]. Receptors for insulin have been reported for the ventral prostate [18] whose epithelial cells proliferate in vitro in response to insulin [17,126]. IGF-I gene expression has been reported in regenerating rat prostate (predominantly in the mesenchymal cells) and in the Dunning R-3327 tumor and some of its variants [123]. IGF-I or IGF-II receptors have not been described in the prostate, but have been inferred from dose-response studies [123].

5.2. Nerve Growth Factor (NGF)

NGF is known to be present in prostatic tissue [68,179]. Its role is unknown, but its expression in the prostate may relate to the presence of autonomic ganglia (the pelvic plexus) located adjacent to the prostatic capsule. Djakiew et al. have shown that human prostatic stromal cells produce an NGF-like protein that stimulates proliferation of a prostatic epithelial cell line [49,50].

5.3. Platelet-Derived Growth Factor (PDGF)

McKeehan reports in a recent review unpublished observations indicating that prostatic epithelial cells are unresponsive to PDGF, whereas growth of prostatic stromal cells is stimulated by PDGF [123]. The PC-3 and DU-145 human prostatic carcinoma cell lines produce PDGF, which has been suggested to play a paracrine role in organizing the stromal matrix of these malignant cells [182]. Thus, the roles of PDGF, NGF, insulin, and IGFs are poorly understood in the prostate and require further attention in the future.

5.4. Epidermal Growth Factor and Transforming Growth Factor-Alpha (TGFα)

Epidermal growth factor (EGF) has been detected in rat and human prostatic and seminal fluid [55,65,79,90,98,151]; in extracts of human, mouse, rat, and guinea pig prostate [55,78,91, 166,167,173]; and in conditioned medium from DU-145 human prostatic carcinoma cells [26]. The probable epithelial origin of EGF is supported by immunocytochemical staining of normal and neoplastic prostatic epithelial cells [60, 179] and the fact that it is secreted into prostatic fluids. The presence of EGF mRNA in the guinea pig prostate [166] and EGF secretion by DU-145 cells [26] further supports the idea that EGF is synthesized and secreted by prostatic epithelium. In the mouse prostate, EGF levels are androgen dependent [78]. EGF is clearly a mitogen for prostatic epithelial cells in vitro [19,20,53,125, 126,144,145,150,195], and EGF receptors have been detected in normal rat prostatic epithelial cells and in epithelial cells of human BPH and prostatic adenocarcinomas [41,53,59,80,108,114, 184,199]. Several reports demonstrate that androgens downregulate EGF receptors in the prostate [59,184,199], although in LNCAP prostatic carcinoma cells androgen increased EGF receptor levels [133,172]. While responsiveness to EGF in vitro means that EGF is a possible mitogen for prostatic epithelium, there is no evidence that prostate-produced EGF functions as a mitogen for any cells in the prostate in vivo.

TGFα is a member of the EGF family, having considerable structural homology to EGF [46] and, thus, mimics the actions of EGF. TGFα has significant, although limited, sequence homology with EGF [119]. For this reason, TGFα interacts with the EGF receptor, but not with EGF antibodies [120]. TGFα was initially thought to be only produced by transformed cells, but is now known to be present in rapidly growing normal tissues [25,105,158,169,183]. TGFα is expressed by several human prostatic carcinoma lines [97, 207] and appears to function as an autocrine growth stimulator of prostatic carcinoma cells [80, 97,111,207]. As yet there are no reports of TGFα expression in the normal prostate. However, overexpression of TGFα in transgenic mice results in carcinoma of the mammary gland, and hyperplasia and dysplasia of the anterior prostate (also known as the coagulating gland) [170]. Therefore, TGFα has been postulated to be a growth stimulator that may be critical in the cell proliferation associated with prostatic carcinogenesis.

5.5. Heparin-Binding Growth Factors

Heparin-binding growth factors believed to be acidic and/or basic fibroblast growth factors (FGF) have been isolated from normal and neoplastic human prostatic tissue as well as from normal and cancerous rat prostate [75,93,116,121,122,136, 137,143–145,185]. Story and colleagues have suggested that basic FGF is produced by prostatic stromal cells [185,186], whose growth may be controlled by this factor [178]. Basic-FGF levels are increased in human BPH [132,185], and thus a role for basic FGF has been postulated for the development of human BPH. However, this conclusion is difficult to accept since most surgical BPH specimens come from elderly patients whose hyperplastic prostates are probably growth quiescent [24]. In addition, Katz et al. have shown that while basic FGF is androgen inducible in castrated rats, the induction of basic FGF transcripts occurs after the peak of DNA synthetic activity [95]. Additionally, there is the problem of how FGF is secreted, given the fact that it lacks a signal peptide [3].

Responsiveness to heparin-binding growth factors observed in vitro is presumably via appropriate receptors. Prostatic epithelial cells as well as a variety of fibroblasts express receptors for the heparin-binding growth factors (acidic and basic FGF) and proliferate in response to these growth factors [13,124,125,127,152]. Moreover, transgenic mice expressing Int-2, a member of the FGF family, have hyperplastic prostates [134]. Thus, evidence demonstrates the production of basic and acidic FGF, the expression of FGF receptors, responsiveness to FGFs in vitro, as well as a possible involvement of FGFs in BPH. While these findings can be incorporated into a reasonable mechanistic scenario, it is disturbing that induction of basic FGF mRNA by androgen occurs after the peak of DNA synthesis in the prostate [95]. In addition, neutralizing antibodies to basic

FGF (anti-β-FGF) fail to block development of the prostate. Infusion of a specific neutralizing antibody to basic FGF into grafts of embryonic rat genital tracts growing as transplants under the renal capsule had been shown to inhibit growth and differentiation in transplants of rat embryos [106]. In similar experiments this antibody also inhibited epididymal development in grafts of the urogenital ridge, but prostatic ductal morphogenesis and growth occurred normally in cotransplanted urogenital sinuses (UGS) [1]. Control UGSs treated by in vivo infusion with normal rabbit serum (NRS) and UGSs treated with anti-β-FGF had virtually identical DNA contents of 26.6 ± 4.9 mg and 24.0 ± 4.5 mg, respectively. At 2 weeks of treatment with NRS or anti-β-FGF, prostatic buds formed, elongated, and differentiated into ducts with lumina in both cases [34]. Nonethelss, current information on the FGFs in the prostate certainly merits further examination, particularly of new biologically meaningful models.

Keratinocyte growth factor (KGF) is a recently discovered member of the FGF family and has been implicated in prostatic growth [214]. KGF is produced by various fibroblasts and has a high degree of specificity for epithelial cells [118]. KGF has been cloned and sequenced [15,58], and specific neutralizing antibodies are available. The receptor for KGF has been characterized, cloned, and sequenced [15,129] and is normally expressed only on epithelial cells. Recently, KGF has been identified in the human and rat prostate [185,214] and has been shown to play an important role in androgen-dependent development of the neonatal mouse SV [2].

The neonatal mouse SV rudiment is a particularly versatile model to study the role of growth factors in androgen-dependent growth, morphogenesis, and differentiation because normal SV development is elicited in vitro by androgens under serum-free conditions [180]. Neonatal mouse SVs undergo growth and branching morphogenesis when grown in serum-free medium (containing EGF, BSA, insulin, transferrin, cholera toxin) containing either testosterone or dihydrotestosterone (T or DHT). In the absence of T or DHT, SV development does not proceed. This simplified culture system has provided the opportunity to examine the effects of exogenous growth factors or their neutralizing antibodies on growth and development. By using a sensitive reverse-transcription/polymerase chain reaction assay, mRNA encoding KGF was detected in neonatal mouse SVs [2]. A neutralizing monoclonal antibody to KGF (anti-KGF) inhibited androgen-stimulated growth (total DNA content) by 50% after 6 days in culture. This overall inhibition was due to decreased epithelial growth; the mesenchymal layer was not affected. The extent of epithelial branching morphogenesis was quantified by image analysis. The anti-KGF inhibited epithelial branching by 65% after 6 days of culture. These data demonstrate that KGF is present during the time of active SV morphogenesis and that it functions as an important mediator of androgen-stimulated SV development [2]. Thus, androgens act on mesenchyme to elicit synthesis and secretion of KGF (and probably other paracrine factors), which regulates epithelial growth and morphogenesis.

Two other members of the heparin-binding growth factor family, which merit further study, are the product of the Int-2 oncogene and hepatocyte growth factor. Transgenic mice expressing Int-2 have greatly enlarged hyperplastic prostates and develop mammary cancer [134]. Hepatocyte growth factor has been shown to be expressed in the prostate [168].

5.6. Transforming Growth Factor-Beta (TGFβ)

Transforming growth factor-beta (TGFβ) is primarily a growth inhibitor that is antagonistic to growth factors such as TGFα or FGF. Three mammalian isoforms of TGFβ have been identified and termed *TGFβ1*, *TGFβ2*, and *TGFβ3* [47,48,115,130]. TGFβ has been detected in normal and neoplastic prostatic tissue [101,148,174, 208]. In the normal rat prostate and in the PC-82 human prostatic tumor line, levels of TGFβ are downregulated by androgen [101,102] and are expressed at high levels during prostatic regression following androgen deprivation. Both normal and malignant prostatic tissue have TGFβ receptors and generally respond to TGFβ through reduction in proliferation [102,124,174,208]. These observations imply that TGFβ may be a critical growth inhibitor in the prostate and may be a key player in mesenchymal-epithelial interac-

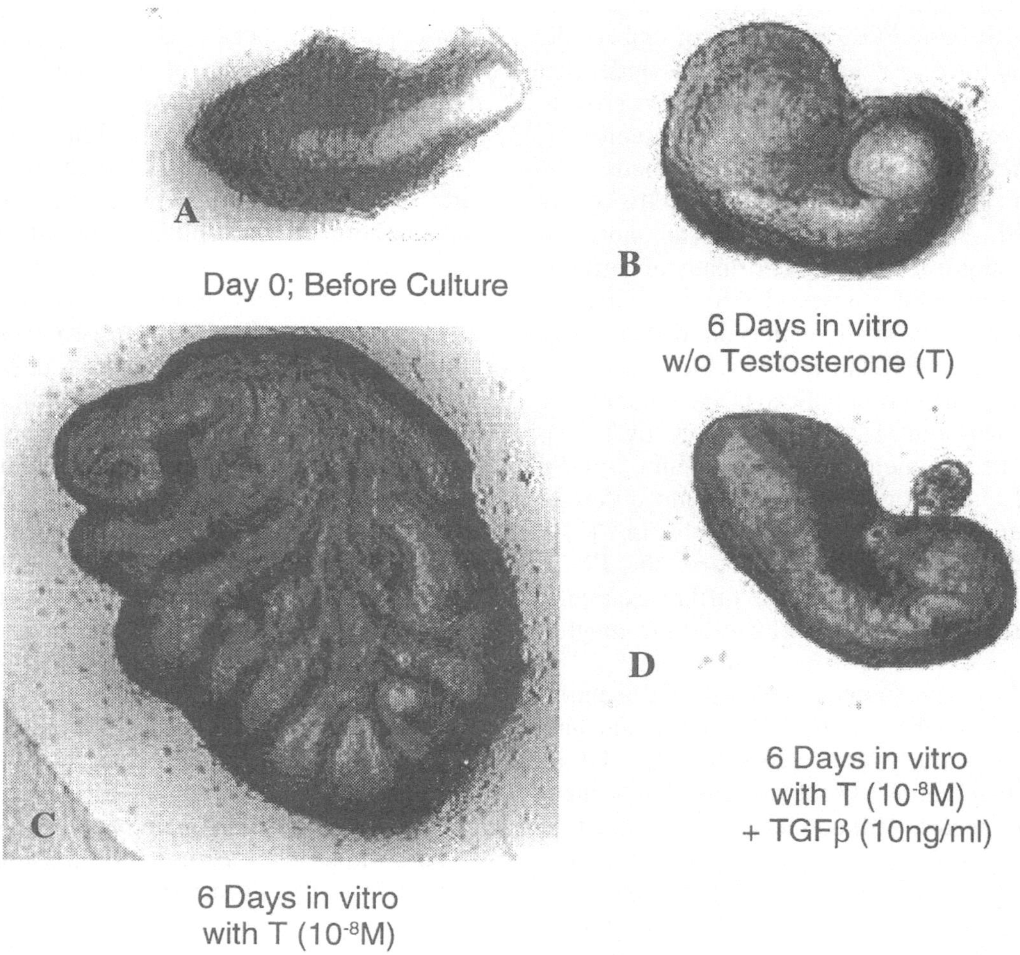

Fig 6 Anterior prostate (AP) rudiments from newborn Fisher 344 rats were cultured for 6 days in vitro on Millipore filter rats in serum-free medium [Ham's F12 DMEM (1 1)] supplemented with insulin (10 μg/ml) and transferrin (10 μg/ml) *A* AP before culture *B* AP cultured without testosterone (T) does not grow or undergo branching morphogenesis *C* AP grown in the presence of T (10^{-8} M) has exhibited considerable epithelial growth and branching morphogenesis *D* AP grown in the presence of T (10^{-8} M) plus TGFβ (10 ng/ml) shows complete inhibition of epithelial development (×32)

tions that regulate normal and abnormal prostatic growth and differentation. TGFβ may be specifically required to control the actions of other growth factors such as TGFα, FGF, or KGF. Unfortunately, the literature on TGFβs in the prostate does not address the biological parameters of actual prostatic growth as it occurs in vivo. To study this issue a serum-free system has been recently developed for growing explants of neonatal rat anterior prostate (AP). At birth the rat AP is a simple, unbranched epithelial bud surrounded by mesenchyme (Fig. 6). These AP rudiments exhibit growth and extensive ductal branching morphogenesis comparable to that in vivo when grown with testosterone or dihydrotestosterone. The trophic effect of androgens can be blocked in a dose-dependent manner by addition of TGFβ to the medium (Fig. 6). The cardinal feature of this model is that it mimics the androgen-induced growth and morphogenesis that occur in vivo and, thus, provides an appropriate and highly relevant biological context for studying prostatic growth.

Finally, Rowley has shown that a substance

called urogenital sinus inhibitory factor (UGIF) isolated from UGM-conditioned medium reversibly inhibits proliferation of a variety of tumor cell lines, stimulates protein synthesis, and alters phenotypic morphology of NBT-II bladder tumor cells [163,165]. UGIF (which is not TGFβ) is heat and acid stable, is neutralized in reducing conditions, and is stable to dialysis with 1 M acetic acid, freezing, and lyophilization [164]. While Rowley's studies are certainly intriguing, it is troubling that the inhibitory activity derived from UGM-conditioned medium contrasts so markedly with the trophic effects of UGM on epithelial morphogenesis, growth, cytodifferentiation, and functional differentiation in vivo [36]. Thus, the physiological relevance of Rowley's findings to normal prostatic growth and development remains to be elucidated.

6. Concluding Remarks

While significant progress has been made on the role of growth factors in the male urogenital tract, there has been little advance in the biology of growth factor action in androgen target organs in vivo, and consequently, the physiological roles of growth factors are generally unknown. Future progress in this area will require innovative new model systems that faithfully mimic processes occurring in vivo. For the prostate, it is important to recognize that androgen-dependent growth does not occur homogeneously throughout the gland, but instead has a very specific temporal/spatial signature. This fact largely abrogates the value of whole organ extracts for obtaining biologically relevant data. Finally, validity of earlier in vitro models, particularly the use of adult epithelial cells, must be questioned since in vivo these cells normally are growth quiescent. Whereas the cataloging of growth factor expression, the in vitro response to growth factors, and the expression of growth factor receptors are central to elucidating the role of growth factors in the male urogenital tract, it is now timely to focus attention on the in vivo biological relevance of growth factors in the growing or developing male urogenital tract.

7. Acknowledgments

This work was supported by NIH grants DK32157, CA05388, CA49996, and HD11979.

References

1 Alarid ET, Cunha GR, Young P, Nicoll CS Evidence for a possible organ- and sex-specific role of bFGF in the development of the fetal mammalian reproductive tract Endocrinology 129 2148–2154, 1991
2 Alarid ET, Rubin JS, Young P, Chedid M, Ron D, Aaronson SA, Cunha GR Keratinocyte growth factor functions in epithelial induction during seminal vesicle development Proc Natl Acad Sci USA 91 1074–1078, 1994
3 Amalric F, Baldin V, Bosc-Bierne I, Bugler B, Couderc B, Guyader M, Patry V, Prats H, Roman AM, Bouche G Nuclear translocation of basic fibroblast growth factor Ann NY Acad Sci 638 127–138, 1991
4 Aumuller G Morphologic and regulatory aspects of prostatic function Anat Embryol (Berl) 179 519–531, 1989
5 Banerjee PP, Banerjee S, Sprando RL, Zirkin BR Regional cellular heterogeneity and DNA synthetic activity in rat ventral prostate during postnatal development Biol Reprod 45 773–782, 1991
6 Barnes D, Sato G Methods for growth of cultured cells in serum-free medium Anal Biochem 102 255–270, 1980
7 Bartal AH, Lichtig C, Cardo CC, Feit C, Robinson E, Hirshaut Y Monoclonal antibody defining fibroblasts appearing in fetal and neoplastic tissues J Natl Cancer Inst 76 415–421, 1986
8 Basset P, Bellocq JP, Wolf C, Stoll I, Hutin P, Limacher JM, Podhajcer OL, Chenard MP, Rio MC, Chambon P A novel metalloproteinase gene specifically expressed in stromal cells of breast carcinomas Nature 348 699–704, 1990
9 Bauer EA, Gordon JM, Reddick ME, Eisen AZ Quantitation and immunocytochemical localization of human skin collagenase in basal cell carcinoma J Invest Dermatol 69 363–367, 1977
10 Beckman WC, Camps JL, Weissman RM, Kaufman SL, Sanofsky SJ, Reddick RL, Siegal GP The epithelial origin of a stromal cell population in adenocarcinoma of the rat prostate Am J Pathol 128 555–565, 1987
11 Bernfield MR, Banerjee SD, Cohn RH Dependence of salivary epithelial morphology and branching morphogenesis upon acid mucopolysaccharide-protein (proteoglycan) at the epithelial surface J Cell Biol 52 674–689, 1972
12 Bernfield MR, Cohn RH, Banerjee SD Glycosaminoglycans and epithelial organ formation Am Zool 13 1067–1083, 1973
13 Berns EMJJ, Schuurmans AIG, Bolt J, Lamb DJ, Foekens JA, Mulder E Antiproliferative effects of

suramin on androgen responsive tumour cells Eur J Cancer 26 470–474, 1990
14 Berry SJ, Coffey DS, Walsh PC, Ewing LL The development of human benign prostatic hyperplasia with age J Urol 132 474–479, 1984
15 Bottaro DP, Rubin JS, Ron D, Finch PW, Florio C, Aaronson SA Characterization of the receptor for keratinocyte growth factor Evidence for multiple fibroblast growth factor receptors J Biol Chem 265 12767–12770, 1990
16 Bresciani F Topography of DNA synthesis in the mammary gland of the C3H mouse and its control by ovarian hormones An autoradiographic study Cell Tissue Kinet 1 51–63, 1968
17 Buchanan LJ, Riches AC Proliferative responses of rat ventral prostate Effects of variations in organ culture media and methodology Prostate 8 63–74, 1986
18 Carmena MJ, Fernandez-Moreno MD, Prieto JC Characterization of insulin receptors in isolated epithelial cells of rat ventral prostate Effect of fasting Cell Biochem Function 4 19–24, 1986
19 Chapronıere DM, McKeehan WL Serial culture of single adult human prostatic epithelial cells in serum-free medium containing low calcium and a new growth factor from bovine brain Cancer Res 46 819–824, 1986
20 Chapronıere DM, Webber MM Dexamethasone and retinyl acetate similarly inhibit and stimulate EGF- or insulin-induced proliferation of prostatic epithelium J Cell Physiol 122 249–253, 1985
21 Chaudhuri S, Koprowska I, Rowinski J Different agglutinability of fibroblasts underlying various precursor lesions of human uterine cervical carcinoma Cancer Res 35 2350–2354, 1975
22 Chiarodo A National Cancer Institute Roundtable on Prostate Cancer Future research directions Cancer Res 51 2498–2505 1991
23 Chung LWK, Cunha GR Stromal-epithelial interactions II Regulation of prostatic growth by embryonic urogenital sinus mesenchyme Prostate 4 503–511, 1983
24 Coffey DS, Berry SJ, Ewing LL An overview of current concepts in the study of benign prostatic hyperplasia In Benign Prostatic Hyperplasia CH Rodgers, DS Coffey, GR Cunha, JT Grayhack, JF Hinman, R Horton (eds) Washington, D C U S Government Printing Office, 1987, pp 1–14
25 Coffey RJ, Derynck R, Wilcox JN, Bringman TS, Goustin AS, Moses HL, Pittelkow MR Production and auto-induction of transforming growth factor-α in human keratinocytes Nature 328 817–820, 1987
26 Connolly JM, Rose DP Secretion of epidermal growth factor and related polypeptides by the DU 145 human prostate cancer cell line Prostate 15 177–186, 1989
27 Cooke PS, Young P, Cunha GR Androgen receptor expression in developing male reproductive organs Endocrinology 128 2867–2873, 1991
28 Cooke PS, Young PF, Cunha GR Androgen dependence of growth and epithelial morphogenesis in neonatal mouse bulbourethral glands Endocrinology 121 2153–2160, 1987
29 Cooke PS, Young PF, Cunha GR A new model system for studying androgen-induced growth and morphogenesis in vitro The bulbourethral gland Endocrinology 121 2161–2170, 1987
30 Cooper M, Pinkus H Intrauterine transplantation of rat basal cell carcinoma A model for reconversion of malignant to benign growth Cancer Res 37 2544–2552, 1977
31 Cunha GR Epithelio-mesenchymal interactions in primordial gland structures which become responsive to androgenic stimulation Anat Rec 172 179–196, 1972
32 Cunha GR Epithelial-stromal interactions in development of the urogenital tract Int Rev Cytol 47 137–194, 1976
33 Cunha GR Development of the male urogenital tract In Urologic Endocrinology J Rajfer (ed) Philadelphia WB Saunders, 1986, pp 6–16
34 Cunha GR, Alarid ET, Turner T, Donjacour AA, Bountin EL, Foster BA Normal and abnormal development of the male urogenital tract Role of androgens, mesenchymal-epithelial interactions and growth factors J Androl 13 465–475, 1992
35 Cunha GR, Chung LWK, Shannon JM, Taguchi O, Fujii H Hormone-induced morphogenesis and growth Role of mesenchymal-epithelial interactions Recent Prog Horm Res 39 559–598, 1983
36 Cunha GR, Donjacour AA, Cooke PS, Mee S, Bigsby RM, Higgins SJ, Sugimura Y The endocrinology and developmental biology of the prostate Endocr Rev 8 338–363, 1987
37 Cunha GR, Fujii H, Neubauer BL, Shannon JM, Sawyer LM, Reese BA Epithelial-mesenchymal interactions in prostatic development I Morphological observations of prostatic induction by urogenital sinus mesenchyme in epithelium of the adult rodent urinary bladder J Cell Biol 96 1662–1670, 1983
38 Cunha GR, Shannon JM, Taguchi O, Fujii H, Chung LWK Epithelial-mesenchymal interactions in hormone-induced development In Epithelial-Mesenchymal Interactions in Development RH Sawyer, JF Fallon (eds) New York Praeger Scientific, 1983, pp 51–74
39 Cunha GR, Young P Inability of Tfm (testicular feminization) epithelial cells to express androgen-dependent seminal vesicle secretory proteins in chimeric tissue recombinants Endocrinology 128 3293–3298, 1991
40 Cunha GR, Young P, Higgins SJ, Cooke PS Neonatal seminal vesicle mesenchyme induces a new morphological and functional phenotype in the epithelia of adult ureter and ductus deferens Development 111 145–158, 1991
41 Davies P, Eaton CL Binding of epidermal growth factor by human normal, hypertropic, and carcinomatous prostate Prostate 14 123–132, 1989
42 De Cosse J, Gossens CL, Kuzma JF Breast cancer Induction of differentiation by embryonic tissue Science 181 1057–1058, 1973
43 De Cosse JJ, Gossens CL, Kuzma JF, Unsworth BR Embryonic inductive tissues that cause histological differentiation of murine mammary carcinoma in vitro J Natl Cancer Inst 54 913–921, 1975

44 De Pablo F, Scott LA, Roth J Insulin and insulin-like growth factor I in early development Peptides, receptors and biological events Endocr Rev 11 558–577, 1990

45 Delinassios JG, Kottaridis SD, Garas J Uncontrolled growth of tumour stromal fibroblasts in vitro Expl Cell Biol 51 201–209, 1983

46 Derynck R Transforming growth factor-α Structure and biological activities J Cell Biochem 32 293–304, 1986

47 Derynck R, Jarrett JA, Chen EY, Eaton DH, Bell JR, Assoian RK, Roberts AB, Sporn MB, Goeddel DV Human transforming growth factor-β complementary DNA sequencing and expression in normal and transformed cells Nature 316 701–705, 1985

48 Derynck R, Linquist PB, Lee A, Wen D, Tamm J, Graycar JL, Rhee L, Mason AJ, Miller DA, Coffey RJ, Moses HL, Chen EY A new type of transforming growth factor-β, TGFβ3 EMBO J 7 3737–3743, 1988

49 Djakiew D, Delsite R, Pflug B, Wrathall J Regulation of growth by a nerve growth factor-like protein which modulates paracrine interactions between a neoplastic epithelial cell line and stromal cells of the human prostate Cancer Res 51 3304–3310, 1991

50 Djakiew D, Tarkington M, Lynch J Paracrine stimulation of polarized secretion from monolayers of a neoplastic prostatic epithelial cell line by prostatic stromal cell proteins Cancer Res 50 1966–1974, 1990

51 Donjacour AA, Cunha GR The effect of androgen deprivation on branching morphogenesis in the mouse prostate Dev Biol 128 1–14, 1988

52 Donjacour AA, Cunha GR, Higgins SF Detection of specific prostatic proteins in an epithelium that lacks androgen receptors Endocrinology 122(Suppl) 502, 1988

53 Eaton CL, Davies P, Phillips ME Growth factor involvement and oncogene expression in prostatic tumours J Steroid Biochem 30 341–345, 1988

54 Elger W, Graf KJ, Steinback H, Neumann F Hormonal control of sexual development Adv Biosci 13 41–69, 1974

55 Elson SD, Browne CA, Thorburn GD Identification of epidermal growth factor-like activity in human male reproductive tissues and fluids J Clin Endocrinol Metab 58 589–597, 1984

56 Erikson HP, Bourdon MA Tenascin An extracellular matrix protein prominent in specialized embryonic tissues and tumors Annu Rev Cell Biol 5 71–92, 1989

57 Faber M, Wewer UM, Berthelsen JG, Liotta LA, Albrechtsen R Laminin production by human endometrial stromal cells relates to the cyclic and pathologic state of the endometrium Am J Pathol 124 384–398, 1986

58 Finch PW, Rubin JS, Miki T, Ron D, Aaronson SA Human KGF is FGF-related with properties of a paracrine effector of epithelial cell growth Science 245 752–755, 1989

59 Fiorelli G, DeBellis A, Longo A, Natali A, Constantini A, Serio M Epidermal growth factor receptors in human hyperplastic prostate tissue and their modulation by chronic treatment with a gonadotropin-releasing hormone analog J Clin Endocrin Metab 68 740–743, 1989

60 Fowler JE, Lau JLT, Ghosh L, Mills SE, Mounzer A Epidermal growth factor and prostatic carcinoma An immunohistochemical study J Urol 139 857–861, 1988

61 Fujii H, Cunha GR, Norman JT The induction of adenocarcinomatous differentiation in neoplastic bladder epithelium by an embryonic prostatic inductor J Urol 128 858–861, 1982

62 Fukamachi H, Mizuno T, Kim YS Morphogenesis of human colon cancer cells with fetal rat mesenchymes in organ culture Experientia 42 312–315, 1986

63 Fukamachi I, Mizuno T, Kim YS Gland formation of human colon cancer cells combined with foetal rat mesenchyme in organ culture An ultrastructural study J Cell Sci 87 615–621, 1987

64 Goldin GV, Wessells NK Mammalian lung development The possible role of cell proliferation in the formation of supernumerary tracheal buds in branching morphogenesis J Exp Zool 208 337–346, 1979

65 Gregory H, Willshire IR, Kavanagh JP, Blacklock NJ, Chowdury S, Richards RC Urogastrone-epidermal growth factor concentrations in prostatic fluid of normal individuals and patients with benign prostatic hypertrophy Clin Sci 70 359–363, 1986

66 Haffen K, Kedinger M, Simon-Assmann P Mesenchyme-dependent differentiation of epithelial progenitor cells in the gut J Pediatr Gastroenterol Nutr 6 14–23, 1987

67 Han VK, D'Ercole AJ Lund PK Cellular localization of somatomedin (insulin-like growth factor) messenger RNA in the human fetus Science 236 193–197, 1987

68 Harper GP, Barde YA, Burnstock G, Carstairs JR, Dennison ME, Suda K, Vernon CA Guinea pig prostate is a rich source of nerve growth factor Nature 279 160–162, 1979

69 Hayashi N, Cunha GR Mesenchyme-induced changes in neoplastic characteristics of the Dunning prostatic adenocarcinoma Cancer Res 51 4934–4930, 1991

70 Hayashi N, Cunha GR, Parker M Permissive and instructive induction of adult rodent prostatic epithelium by heterotypic urogenital sinus mesenchyme Epithel Cell Biol 2 66–78, 1993

71 Hayashi N, Cunha GR, Wong YC Influence of male genital tract mesenchymes on differentiation of Dunning prostatic adenocarcinoma Cancer Res 50 4747–4754, 1990

72 Hayashi N, Sugimura Y, Kawamura J, Donjacour AA, Cunha GR Morphological and functional heterogeneity in the rat prostatic gland Biol Reprod 45 308–321, 1991

73 He WW, Kumar MV, Tindall DJ A frameshift mutation in the androgen receptor gene causes complete androgen insensitivity in the testicular-feminized mouse Nucleic Acids Res 19 2373–2378, 1991

74 Heine UI, Munoa EF, Flanders KC, Ellingsworth LR, Lam H-YP, Thompson NL, Roberts AB, Sporn MB Role of transforming growth factor-β in the development of the mouse embryo J Cell Biol 105 2861–2876, 1987

75 Hierowski MT, McDonald MW, Dunn L, Sullivan JW The partial dependency of human prostatic growth factor

on steroid hormones in stimulating thymidine incorporation into DNA J Urol 138 909–912, 1987

76 Higgins SJ, Young P, Cunha GR Induction of functional cytodifferentiation in the epithelium of tissue recombinants II Instructive induction of Wolffian duct epithelia by neonatal seminal vesicle mesenchyme Development 106 235–250, 1989

77 Hill DJ, Milner RDG Insulin as a growth factor Pediatr Res 19 879–886, 1985

78 Hiramatsu M, Kashimata M, Minami N, Sato A, Murayama M, Minami N Androgenic regulation of epidermal growth factor in the mouse ventral prostate Biochem Int 17 311–317, 1988

79 Hirata Y, Uchihashi M, Hazama M, Fujita T Epidermal growth factor in human seminal plasma Horm Metab Res 19 35–37, 1987

80 Hofer DR, Sherwood ER, Bromberg WD, Mendelsohn J, Lee C, Kozlowski JM Autonomous growth of androgen-independent human prostatic carcinoma cells Role of transforming growth factor alpha Cancer Res 51 2780–2785, 1991

81 Husmann DA, McPhaul M, Wilson JD Androgen receptor expression in the developing rat prostate is not altered by castration, flutamide, or suppression of the adrenal axis Endocrinology 128 1902–1906, 1991

82 Imperato-McGinley J 5α reductase deficiency in man Prog Cancer Res Ther 31 491–496, 1984

83 Imperato-McGinley J, Binienda Z, Arthur A, Minenberg DT, Vaughan ED, Quimby FW The development of a male pseudohermaphroditic rat using an inhibitor of the enzyme 5α-reductase Endocrinology 116 807–812, 1985

84 Imperato-McGinley J, Guerrero L, Gautier T, Peterson RE Steroid 5α-reductase deficiency in man An inherited form of pseudohermaphroditism Science 186 1213–1215, 1974

85 Imperato-McGinley J, Peterson RE, Gautier T Primary and secondary 5α-reductase deficiency In Sexual Differentiation Basic and Clinical Aspects M Serio, M Zanisi, M Motta, L Martini (eds) 1984, pp 233–245

86 Iozzo RV, Sampson PM, Schmitt GK Neoplastic modulation of extracellular matrix Stimulation of chondroitin sulfate proteoglycan and hyaluronic acid synthesis in co-cultures of human colon carcinoma and smooth muscle cells J Cell Biochem 39 355–378, 1989

87 Isaacs JT Antagonistic effect of androgen on prostatic cell death Prostate 5 545–557, 1984

88 Isaacs JT Control of cell proliferation and cell death in the normal and neoplastic prostate A stem cell model In Benign Prostatic Hyperplasia CH Rodgers, DS Coffey, G Cunha, JT Grayhack, F Hinman Jr, R Horton (eds) Washington D C U S Government Printing Office, 1987, pp 85–94

89 Isaacs JT Development and characteristics of the available animal model systems for the study of prostatic cancer In Current Concepts and Approaches to the Study of Prostate Cancer DS Coffey, N Bruchovsky, WW Gardner Jr, MI Resnick, JP Karr (ed) New York Alan R Liss, 1987, pp 513–576

90 Jacobs SC, Story MT Exocrine secretion of epidermal growth factory by the rat prostate Effect of adrenergic agents, cholinergic agents and vasoactive intestinal peptide Prostate 13 79–87, 1988

91 Jacobs SC, Story MT, Sasse J, Lawson RK Characterization of growth factors derived from the rat ventral prostate J Urol 139 1106–1110, 1988

92 Jesik CJ, Holland JM, Lee C An anatomic and histologic study of the rat prostate Prostate 3 81–97, 1982

93 Jinno H, Ueda K, Otaguro K, Kato T, Ito J, Tanaka R Prostate growth factor in the extracts of benign prostatic hypertrophy Partial purification and physicochemical characterization Eur Urol 12 41–48, 1986

94 Jost A Problems of fetal endocrinology The gonadal and hypophyseal hormones Recent Prog Horm Res 8 379–418, 1953

95 Katz AE, Benson MC, Wise GJ, Olsson CA, Bandyk MG, Sawczuk IS, Tomashefsky P, Buttyan R Gene activity during the early phase of androgen-stimulated rat prostate regrowth Cancer Res 49 5889–5894, 1989

96 Kellokumpu-Lehtonen P, Santti R, Pelliniemi LJ Correlation of early cytodifferentiation of the human fetal prostate and Leydig cells Anat Rec 196 263–273, 1980

97 Kim JH, Sherwood ER, Sutkowski DM, Lee C, Kozlowski JM Inhibition of prostatic tumor cell proliferation by suramin Alterations in TGF alpha-mediated autocrine growth regulation and cell cycle distribution J Urol 146 171–176, 1991

98 Kishi H, Ishibe T, Usui T, Miyachi Y Epidermal growth factor (EGF) in seminal plasma and prostatic gland A radioreceptor assay Arch Androl 20 243–249, 1988

99 Kollar EJ the development of the integument Spatial, temporal and phylogenetic factors Am Zool 12 125–135, 1972

100 Kratochwil K Tissue combination and organ culture studies in the development of the embryonic mammary gland In Developmental Biology A Comprehensive Synthesis RBL Gwatkin (ed) New York Plenum Press, 1987, pp 315–334

101 Kyprianou N, Isaacs JT Expression of transforming growth factor β in the rat ventral prostate during castration-induced programmed cell death Mol Endocrinol 3 1515–1522, 1989

102 Kyprianou N, Martikainen P, Davis L, English HF, Issacs JT Programmed cell death as a new target for prostatic cancer therapy In Prostate Cancer Cell and Molecular Mechanisms in Diagnosis and Treatment JT Isaacs (ed) Cold Spring Harbor, NY Cold Spring Harbor Laboratory Press, 1991, pp 265–278

103 Lasnizki I, Franklin HR The influence of serum on uptake, conversion and action of testesterone in rat prostate glands in organ culture J Endocrinol 54 333–342, 1972

104 Lee C, Sensibar JA, Dudek SM, Hiipakka RA, Liao S Prostatic ductal system in rats Regional variation in morphological and functional activities Biol Reprod 43 1079–1086, 1990

105 Lee DC, Rochford RM, Todaro GJ, Villareal LP Developmental expression of rat transforming

growth factor-α mRNA Mol Cell Biol 5 3644–3646, 1985

106 Liu LM, Nicoll CS Evidence for a role of basic fibroblast growth factor in rat embryonic growth and differentiation Endocrinology 123 2027–2031, 1988

107 Lowsley OS The development of the human prostate gland with reference to the development of other structures at the neck of the urinary bladder Am J Anat 13 299–349, 1912

108 Lubrano C, Petrangeli E, Catizone A, Santonati A, Concolino G, Rombola N, Frati L, Di Silverio F, Sciarra F Epidermal growth factor binding and steroid receptor content in human benign prostatic hyperplasia J Steroid Biochem 34 499–504, 1989

109 Lung B, Cunha GR Development of seminal vesicles and coagulating glands in neonatal mice 1 The morphogenetic effects of various hormonal conditions Anat Rec 199 73–88, 1981

110 Lyons KM, Hogan BLM TGF-β-like genes in mammalian development In Genetics of Pattern Formation and Growth Control AP Mahowald (ed) New York Wiley-Liss, 1990, pp 137–156

111 MacDonald A, Chisholm GD, Habib FK Production and response of a human prostatic cancer line to transforming growth factor-like molecules Br J Cancer 62 579–584, 1990

112 Mackenzie J, Dabelsteen E, Roed-Peterson B A method for studying epithelial-mesenchymal interactions in human oral mucosal lesions Scand J Dent Res 87 234–243, 1979

113 Mackie EJ, Chiquet-Ehrismann R, Pearson CA, Inaguma Y Tenascin is a stromal marker for epithelial malignancy in the mammary gland Proc Natl Acad Sci USA 84 4621–4625, 1987

114 Maddy SQ, Chisholm GD, Hawkins RA, Habib FK Localization of epidermal growth factor receptors in the human prostate by biochemical and immunocytochemical methods J Endocrinology 113 147–153, 1987

115 Madisen L, Webb NR, Rose TM, Marquardt H, Ikeda T, Twardzik D, Seyedin S, Purchio AF Transforming growth factor-β2, cDNA cloning and sequence analysis DNA 7 1–8, 1988

116 Maehama S, Li D, Nanri H, Leykam JF, Deuel TF Purification and partial characterization of prostate-derived growth factor Proc Natl Acad Sci USA 83 8162–8166, 1986

117 Mansson PE, Adams P, Kan M, McKeehan WL Heparin-binding growth factor gene expression and receptor characteristics in normal rat prostate and two transplantable rat prostate tumors Cancer Res 49 2485–2494, 1989

118 Marchese C, Rubin J, Ron D, Faggioni A, Torrisi MR, Messina A, Frati L, Aaronson SA Human keratinocyte growth factor activity on proliferation and differentiation of human keratinocytes Differentiation response distin guishes KGF from EGF family J Cell Physiol 144 326–332, 1990

119 Marquardt H, Hunkapiller MW, Hood LE, Todaro G Rat transforming growth factor type 1 Structure and relation to epidermal growth factor Science 223 1079–1082, 1984

120 Massague J Transforming growth factor-α A model for membrane anchored growth factors J Biol Chem 265 21393–21396, 1990

121 Matuo Y, Nishi N, Matsui S, Sandberg AA, Isaacs JT, Wada F Heparin binding affinity of rat prostatic growth factor in normal and cancerous prostates Partial purification and characterization of rat prostatic growth factor in the Dunning tumor Cancer Res 47 188–192, 1987

122 Matuo Y, Nishi N, Wada F Growth factors in the prostate Arch Androl 19 193–210, 1987

123 McKeehan WL Growth factor receptors and prostate cell growth In Prostate Cancer Cell and Molecular Mechanisms in Diagnosis and Treatment JT Isaacs (ed) Cold Spring Harbor, NY Cold Spring Harbor Laboratory Press, 1991, pp 165–176

124 McKeehan WL, Adams PS Heparin-binding growth factor/prostatropin attenuates inhibition of rat prostate tumor epithelial cell growth by transforming growth factor type beta In Vitro Cell Dev Biol 24 243–246, 1988

125 McKeehan WL, Adams PS, Fast D Different hormonal requirements for androgen-independent growth of normal and tumor epithelial cells from rat prostate In Vitro Cell Dev Biol 23 147–152, 1987

126 McKeehan WL, Adams PS, Rosser MP Direct mitogenic effects of insulin, epidermal growth factor, glucocorticoid, cholera toxin, unknown pituitary factors and possibly prolactin, but not androgen, on normal rat prostate epithelial cells in serum-free, primary cell culture Cancer Res 44 1988–2010, 1984

127 McKeehan WL, Crabb JW Isolation and characterization of different molecular and chromatographic forms of heparin-binding growth factor 1 from bovine brain Anal Biochem 164 563–569, 1987

128 McNeal JE The prostate gland Morphology and pathobiology Monogr Urolo 4 3–37, 1983

129 Miki T, Fleming TP, Bottaro DP, Rubin JS, Ron D, Aaronson SA Expression cDNA cloning of the KGF receptor by creation of a transforming autocrine loop Science 251 72–75, 1991

130 Miller DA, Lee A, Pelton RW, Chen EY, Moses HL, Derynck R Murine transforming growth factor B2 cDNA sequence and expression in adult tissues and embryos Mol Endocrinol 3 1108–1114, 1989

131 Mintz B Genetic mosaicism and in vivo analyses of neoplasia and differentiation In Cell Differentiation and Neoplasia G Saunders (ed) New York Raven Press, 1987, pp 27–56

132 Mori HM, Maki K, Oishi M, Jaye K, Igarashi O, Hatanaka M Increased expression of genes for basic fibroblast growth factor and transforming growth factor type β2 in human benign prostatic hyperplasia Prostate 16 71–80, 1990

133 Mulder E, van Loon D, de Boer W, Schuurmans AL, Bolt J, Voorhorst MM, Kuiper GG, Brinkmann AO Mechanisms of androgen action Recent observations on the domain structure of androgen receptors and the

induction of EGF receptors by androgens in prostate tumor cells J Steroid Biochem 32 151–156, 1989
134 Muller JW Lee FS, Dickson C, Peters G, Pattengale P, Leder P The *int*-2 gene product acs as an epithelial growth factor in transgenic mice EMBO J 9 907–913, 1990
135 Murakami R Autoradiographic studies of the localization of androgen-binding cells in the genital tubercles of fetal rats J Anat 151 209–219, 1987
136 Mydlo JH, Bulbul MA, Richon VM, Heston WD, Fair WR Heparin-binding growth factor isolated from human prostatic extracts Prostate 12 343–355, 1988
137 Mydlo JH, Michaeli J, Heston WD, Fair WR Expression of basic fibroblast growth factor mRNA in benign prostatic hyperplasia and prostatic carcinoma Prostate 13 241–247 1988
138 Neubauer BL, Chung LWK, McCormick KA, Taguchi O, Thompson TC, Cunha GR Epithelial-mesenchymal interactions in prostatic development II Biochemical observations of prostatic induction by urogenital sinus mesenchyme in epithelium of the adult rodent urinary bladder J Cell Biol 96 1671–1676, 1983
139 Neumann F, Elger W, Steinbeck H Antiandrogens and reproductive development Philos Trans R Soc Lond [Biol] 259 179–184, 1970
140 Neumann F Graf KJ, Elger W Hormone-induced disturbances in sexual differentiation Adv Biosci 13 71–101, 1974
141 Nilsen-Hamilton M Growth factor signaling in early mammalian development In Growth Factors in Mammalian Development IY Rosenblum, S Heyner (eds) Boca Raton, FL CRC Press, 1989, pp 135–166
142 Nilsen-Hamilton M Transforming growth factor-β and its actions on cellular growth and differentiation Curr Top Dev Biol 24 95–136, 1990
143 Nishi M Matuo Y Muguruma Y Yoshitake Y Nishikawa K Wada F A human prostatic growth factor (hPGF) Partial purification and characterization Biochem Biophys Res Commun 132 1103–1109, 1985
144 Nishi N, Matuo Y, Kunitomi K, Takenaka I, Usami M, Kotake T, Wada F Comparative analysis of growth factors in normal and pathologic human prostates Prostate 13 39–48, 1988
145 Nishi N, Matuo Y, Nakamoto T, Wada F Proliferation of epithelial cells derived from rat dorsolateral prostate in serum-free primary cell culture and their response to androgen In Vitro Cell Dev Biol 24 778–786, 1988
146 Norman JT, Cunha GR, Sugimura Y The induction of new ductal growth in adult prostatic epithelium in response to an embryonic prostatic inductor Prostate 8 209–220, 1986
147 Oishi K, Romijn JC, Schroeder FH The surface character of separated prostatic cells and cultured fibroblasts of prostatic tissue as determined by concanavalin-a hemadsorption Prostate 2 11–21, 1981
148 Pai LH, Gallo MG, FitzGerald DJ, Pastan I Antitumor activity of a transforming growth factor alpha-Pseudomonas exotoxin fusion protein (TGF-alpha-PE40) Cancer Res 51 2808–2812, 1991
149 Partanen AM Epidermal growth factor and transforming growth factor-α in the development of epithelial-mesenchymal organs of the mouse Curr Top Dev Biol 24 31–55, 1990
150 Peehl DM, Stamey TA Serum-free growth of adult human prostatic epithelial cells In Vitro Cell Dev Biol 22 82–90, 1986
151 Pesonen K, Viinikka L, Koskimies A, Banks AA, Nicholson M, Perheentupa J Size heterogeneity of epidermal growth factor in human body fluids Life Sci 40 2489–2494, 1987
152 Pienta KJ, Isaacs WB, Vindivich D, Coffey DS The effects of basic fibroblast growth factor and suramin on cell motility and growth of rat prostate cancer cells J Urol 145 199–202, 1991
153 Pierce G The benign cells of malignant tumors In Developmental Aspects of Carcinogenesis and Immunity T King (ed) New York Academic Press, 1974, pp 3–22
154 Pierce G, Cox W Neoplasms as caricatures of tissue renewal In Cell Differentiation and Neoplasia G Saunders (ed) New York Raven Press, 1978, pp 57–66
155 Pointis G, Latreille MT, Cedard L Gonado-pituitary relationships in the fetal mouse at various times during sexual differentiation J Endocrinol 86 483–488, 1980
156 Price D, Williams-Ashman HG The accessory reproductive glands of mammals In Sex and Internal Secretions, 3rd ed WC Young (ed) Baltimore, MD Williams and Wilkins, 1961, pp 366–448
157 Prins GS, Cooke PS, Birch L, Donjacour AA, Yalcinkaya TM, Siiteri PK, Cunha GR Androgen receptor expression and 5α-reductase activity along the proximal-distal axis of the rat prostatic duct Endocrinology 130 3066–3073, 1992
158 Rappolee DA, Brenner CA, Schultz R, Mark D, Werb Z Developmental expression of PDGF, TGF-alpha, and TGF-β genes in preimplantation mouse embryos Science 241 1823–1825, 1988
159 Raynaud A, Frilley M Destruction de cerveau des embryos de souris au trezieme jour de la gestation, par irradiation au moyen des rayons X Compt Rend Soc Biol 141 658–662, 1947
160 Rechler MM, Podskalny JM, Nissley SP Interaction of multiplication-stimulating activity with chick embryo fibroblasts demonstrates a growth receptor Nature 259 134–136, 1976
161 Rechler MM, Podskalny JM, Nissley SP Characterization of the binding of multiplication-stimulating activity to a receptor for growth polypeptides in chick embryo fibroblasts J Biol Chem 252 3898–3910, 1977
162 Resko JA Androgen secretion by the fetal and neonatal rhesus monkey Endocrinology 87 6803–6807, 1978
163 Rowley DR Urogenital sinus derived growth inhibitory factor In Molecular and Cellular Biology of Prostate Cancer DS Coffey, RB Smith, DJ Tindall, JP Karr (eds) New York Plenum Press, 1990
164 Rowley DR Characterization of a fetal urogenital sinus mesenchymal cell line of U4F Secretion of a negative growth regulatory activty In Vitro Cell Dev Biol 28 29–38, 1992

165 Rowley DR, Tindall DJ Responses of NBT-II bladder carcinoma cells to conditioned medium from normal fetal urogenital sinus Cancer Res 47 2955–2960, 1987
166 Rubin JS, Bradshaw RA Isolation and partial amino acid sequence analysis of nerve growth factor from the guinea pig prostate J Neurosci Res 6 451–464, 1981
167 Rubin JS, Bradshaw RA In Methods for Preparation of Media, Supplements and Substrate for Serum Free Animal Cell Culture DW Barnes, DA Sirbasku, GH Sata (eds) New York Alan R Liss, 1984, p 139
168 Rubin JS, Chan AM-L, Bottaro DP, Burgess WH, Taylor WG, Cech AC, Hirschfield DW, Wong J, Miki T, Finch PW, Aaronson SA A broad-spectrum human lung fibroblast-derived mitogen is a variant of hepatocyte growth factor Proc Natl Acad Sci USA 88 415–419, 1991
169 Samsoonder J, Kobrin MS, Kudlow JE α-Transforming growth factor secreted by untransformed bovine anterior pituitary cells in culture J Biol Chem 261 14408–14413, 1986
170 Sandgren EP, Luetteke NC, Palmiter RD, Brinster RL, Lee DC Overexpression of TGFα in transgenic mice Induction of epithelial hyperplasia, pancreatic metaplasia, and carcinoma of the breast Cell 61 1121–1135, 1990
171 Sawyer RH The role of epithelial-mesenchymal interactions in regulating gene expression during avian scale morphogenesis In Epithelial-Mesenchymal Interactions in Development RH Sawyer, JF Fallon (eds) New York Praeger, 1983, pp 115–146
172 Schuurmans ALG, Bolt J, Mulder E Androgens stimulate both growth rate and epidermal growth factor receptor activity of the human prostate tumor cell LNCaP Prostate 12 55–63, 1988
173 Shaikh N, Lai L, McLoughlin J, Clark D, Williams G Quantitative analysis of epidermal growth factor in human benign prostatic hyperplasia and prostatic carcinoma and its prognstic significance Anticancer Res 10 873–874, 1990
174 Shain SA, Lin AL, Koger JD, Karaganis AG Rat prostate cancer cells contain functional receptors for transforming growth factor-beta Endocrinology 126 818–825, 1990
175 Shannon JM, Cunha GR Autoradiographic localization of androgen binding in the developing mouse prostate Prostate 4 367–373, 1983
176 Shannon JM, Cunha GR Characterization of androgen binding and deoxyribonucleic acid synthesis in prostate-like structures induced in testicular feminized (Tfm/Y) mice Biol Reprod 31 175–183, 1984
177 Shannon JM, Pitelka DR The influence of cell shape on the induction of functional differentiation in mouse mammary cells in vitro In Vitro 17 1016–1028, 1981
178 Sherwood ER, Fong C-J, Lee C, Kozlowski JM Basic fibroblast growth factor A potential mediator of stromal growth in the human prostate Endocrinology 130 2955–2963, 1992
179 Shikata H, Utsumi N, Hiramatsu M, Minami N, Nemoto N, Shikata T Immunohistochemical localization of nerve growth factor and epidermal growth factor in guinea pig prostate gland Histochemistry 80 411–413, 1983
180 Shima H, Tsuji M, Young PF, Cunha GR Postnatal growth of mouse seminal vesicle is dependent on 5α-dihydrotestosterone Endocrinology 127 3222–3233, 1990
181 Siiteri PK, Wilson JD Testosterone formation and metabolism during male sexual differentiation in the human embryo J Clin Endocrinol Metab 38 113–125, 1974
182 Sitaras NM, Sariban E, Bravo M, Pantiazis P, Antoniades HN Constitutive production of platelet-derived growth factor-like proteins by human prostate carcinoma cell lines Cancer Res 49 1930–1935, 1988
183 Skinner MK, Takacs K, Coffey RJ Transforming growth factor-α gene expression and action in the seminiferous tubule Peritubular cell-Sertoli cell interactions Endocrinology 124 845–854, 1989
184 St Arnaud R, Poyet P, Walder P, Labrie F Androgens modulate epidermal growth factor receptor levels in the rat ventral prostate Mol Cell Endocrinol 56 21–27, 1988
185 Story MT Polypeptide modulators of prostatic growth and development In Prostate Cancer Cell and Molecular Mechanisms in Diagnosis and Treatment JT Isaacs (ed) Cold Spring Harbor NY Cold Spring Harbol Laboratory Press, 1991, pp 123–146
186 Story MT, Livingston B, Baeten L, Swartz SJ, Jacobs SC, Begun FP, Lawson RK Cultured human prostate-derived fibroblasts produce a factor that stimulates their growth with properties indistinguishable from basic fibroblast growth factor Prostate 15 355–365, 1989
187 Straus DS Growth stimulatory actions of insulin in vitro and in vivo Endocr Rev 5 356–369, 1984
188 Sugar J Ultrastructural and histochemical changes during the development of cancer in various human organs In Tissue Interactions in Carcinogenesis D Tarin (ed) London Academic Press 1972, pp 127–159
189 Sugimura Y, Cunha GR, Bigsby RM Androgenic induction of deoxyribonucleic acid synthesis in prostatic glands induced in the urothelium of testicular feminized (Tfm/y) mice Prostate 9 217–225, 1986
190 Sugimura Y, Cunha GR, Donjacour AA Morphogenesis of ductal networks in the mouse prostate Biol Reprod 34 961–971, 1986
191 Sugimura Y, Cunha GR, Donjacour AA, Bigsby RM, Brody JR Whole-mount autoradiography study of DNA synthetic activity during postnatal development and androgen-induced regeneration in the mouse prostate Biol Reprod 34 985–995, 1986
192 Takeda H, Chang C Immunohistochemical and in situ hybridization analysis of androgen receptor expression during the development of the mouse prostate gland J Endocrinol 129 83–89, 1991
193 Takeda H, Mizuno T, Lasnitzki I Autoradiographic studies of androgen-binding sites in the rat urogenital sinus and postnatal prostate J Endocrinol 104 87–92, 1985
194 Takeda H, Suematsu N, Mizuno T Transcription of prostatic steriod binding protein (PSBP) gene is induced

by epithelial-mesenchymal interaction Development 110 273–282, 1990

195 Taketa S, Nishi N, Takasuga H, Okutani T, Takenaka I, Wada F Differences in growth requirements between epithelial and stromal cells derived from rat ventral prostate in serum-free primary culture Prostate 17 207–218, 1990

196 Tarin D Morphological studies on the mechanism of carcinogenesis In Tissue Interactions in Carcinogenesis D Tarin (ed) London Academic Press, 1972, pp 227–289

197 Tenniswood M Role of epithelial-stromal interactions in the control of gene expression in the prostate An hypothesis Prostate 9 375–385, 1986

198 Thompson TC Growth factors and oncogenes in prostate cancer Cancer Cells 11 345–354, 1990

199 Traish AM, Wotiz HH Prostatic epidermal growth factor receptors and their regulation by androgens Endocrinology 121 1461–1467, 1987

200 Tsuji M, Shima H, Cunha GR Morphogenetic and proliferative effects of testosterone and insulin on the neonatal mouse seminal vesicle in vitro Endocrinology 129 2289–2297, 1991

201 Tsuji M, Shima H, Cunha GR Morphogenetic and proliferative effects of testosterone and insulin on the neonatal mouse seminal vesicle in vitro Endocrinology 129 2289–2297, 1991

202 Turner T, Young P, Cunha GR Seminal vesicle induction of adult mouse epididymal epithelium by newborn mouse and rat seminal vesicle mesenchyme (abstract) J Cell Biol 109 69, 1989

203 Weniger J-P, Zeis A Developpment du canal de Wolff d'embryon de Souris cultive in vitro en presence de dihydrotestosterone C R Acad Sci III 271 2367–2369, 1970

204 Weniger J-P, Zeis A Transformation de la testosterone en dihydrotestosterone par les canaux de Wolff de l embryon de Souris C R Acad Sci III 271 1307–1310, 1970

205 Weniger J-P, Zeis A Metabolisme de la testosterone par les testicule et canaus de Wolff de l'embryon de Souris J Steroid Biochem 3 749–754, 1971

206 Weniger J-P, Zeis A Sur la secretion precoce de testosterone par le testicule embryonnaire de souris C R Acad Sci III 275 1431–1433, 1972

207 Wilding G, Valvarius E, Knabbe C, Gelmann EP The role of transforming growth factor alpha in human prostate cancer cell growth Prostate 15 1–12, 1989

208 Wilding G, Zugmeier G, Knabbe C, Flanders K, Gelmann E Differential effects of transforming growth factor-β on human prostate cancer cells in vitro Mol Cell Endocrinol 62 79–87, 1989

209 Wilson J, George F, Griffin J The hormonal control of sexual development Science 211 1278–1284, 1981

210 Wilson JD, Griffin JE, Leshin M, George FW Role of gonadal hormones in development of the sexual phenotypes Hum Genet 58 78–84, 1981

211 Wilson JD, Lasnitzki I Dihydrotestosterone formation in fetal tissues of the rabbit and rat Endocrinology 89 659–668, 1971

212 Winter JSD, Faiman C, Reyes F Sexual endocrinology of fetal and perinatal life In Mechanisms of Sex Differentiation in Animals and Man CR Austin, RG Edwards (eds) New York Academic Press, 1981, pp 205–254

213 Wong YC, Cunha GR, Hayashi N Effects of mesenchyme of embryonic urogenital sinus and neonatal seminal vesicle on the cytodifferentiation of the Dunning tumor Ultrastructural study Acta Anat 143 139–150, 1992

214 Yan G, Fukabori Y, Nikolaropoulos S, Wang F, McKeehan WL Heparin-binding kerationcyte growth factor is a candidate stromal to epithelial cell andromedin Mol Endocrinol 6 2123–2128, 1992

215 Yee D, Paik S, Lebovic GS, Marcus RR, Favoni RE, Cullen KJ, Lippman ME, Rosen N Analysis of insulin-like growth factor I gene expression in malignancy Evidence for a paracrine role in human breast cancer Mol Endocrinol 3 509–517, 1989

216 Zondek T, Zondek LH The fetal and neonatal prostate In Normal and Abnormal Growth of the Prostate M Goland (ed) Springfield, IL Charles C Thomas, 1975, pp 5–27

CHAPTER 3

Epithelium of the Distal Portion of the Human Spermatic Pathway: Seminal Vesicle, Ampulla Ductus Deferentis, and Ejaculatory Duct

ALESSANDRO RIVA & GERHARD AUMÜLLER

1. Introduction

Confirming early findings [76,77,83], histochemical and ultrastructural investigations have shown that the seminal vesicle [4,62,66,68,69], ampulla ductus deferentis [4,5,17,63,67,74], and ejaculatory duct [16,70,71] possess an identical epithelium, consisting of principal (secretory) and basal cells. This represents the lining of the human genital tract from the beginning of the ampulla to the opening of the ejaculatory duct into the prostatic urethra.

The physiology and morphology (from embryology to gross anatomy) of all tissue components of the three organs involved have been the object of a recent review [6]. This chapter will describe in more detail the fine structure of the epithelium by combining transmission and scanning electron microscopic (TEM and SEM) findings, and particularly by the use of the newly introduced techniques [23,25,39,46,54,71,78,79] that allow the three-dimensional visualization of external and internal cell surfaces. It must be noted to this regard that the only SEM data presently available on the epithelium are those obtained by conventional methods and, therefore, concerning solely the luminal surface [6,58,59,63,65,71].

2. General Features of the Epithelium

In SEM, even at low magnification (Figs. 1 and 2) the epithelium seen from the lumen shows an outline more irregular and indented than that observed in the homologous organs of rat [33], guinea pig [87], rabbit [37,48], hamster [14], cat [47], dog [49], and monkey [51]. This is due to the conical projections (Figs. 5–7) of the secretory (principal) cells that protrude into the lumen, and it is more evident in less aged subjects [62,81]. The authors [86] who have quantified, at the light microscope level, the early changes occurring in seminal vesicle epithelium report, in fact, that cuboidal cells, which are less than 50% in men under 51 years, become the great majority (98%) over the age of 71. This change seems to be an androgen-dependent phenomenon, since severe flattening of principal cells has been observed even under SEM in the seminal vesicle of laboratory animals subjected to castration [87,89]. Moreover, this has been shown to occur [6] also in patients treated with antiandrogens.

Even the pattern of the mucosa in toto in man seems to be more intricate than that observed in most animals. In specimens treated with the method for removing the epithelium from the stroma [54], a typical honeycombed configuration is seen (Fig. 3). On the other hand, with the techniques that remove the connective tissue and basal lamina (Fig. 4), the diverticula of the organs look like outpocketings, similar to those seen in simple tubular glands, such as the glands of Littré of the male urethra. At variance with the latter, however, the stromal surface of the epithelium shows clearly the basal outlines of cells (Fig. 4).

Riva, A., Testa Riva, F., and Motta, P.M., (eds.), Ultrastructure of Male Urogenital Glands: Prostate, Seminal Vesicles, Urethral, and Bulbourethral Glands.

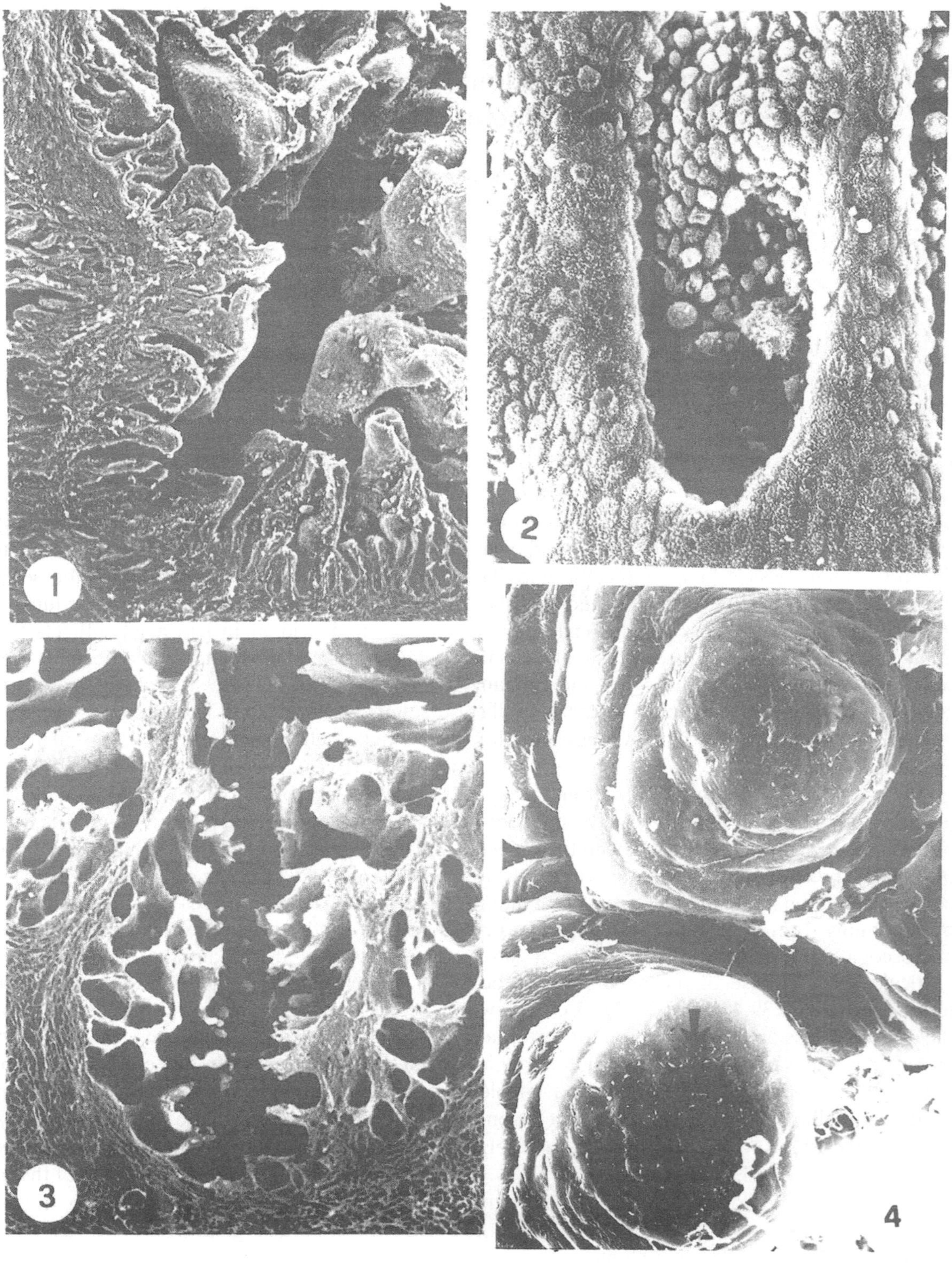

Fig. 1. General view of a fractured seminal vesicle showing infoldings of the mucosa (×65).
Fig. 2. Portion of the epithelium seen from the lumen. The apexes of principal cells are more prominent within the diverticulum than on the surface of the folds (×700).
Fig. 3. Method for the removal of the epithelium from the stroma. Note the honeycombed pattern of the mucosa (×110).
Fig. 4. Diverticula of the mucosa seen from their stromal surface following removal of the connective tissue and digestion of the basal lamina. Note (arrow) the polygonal areas representing the basal outlines of cells (×1150).

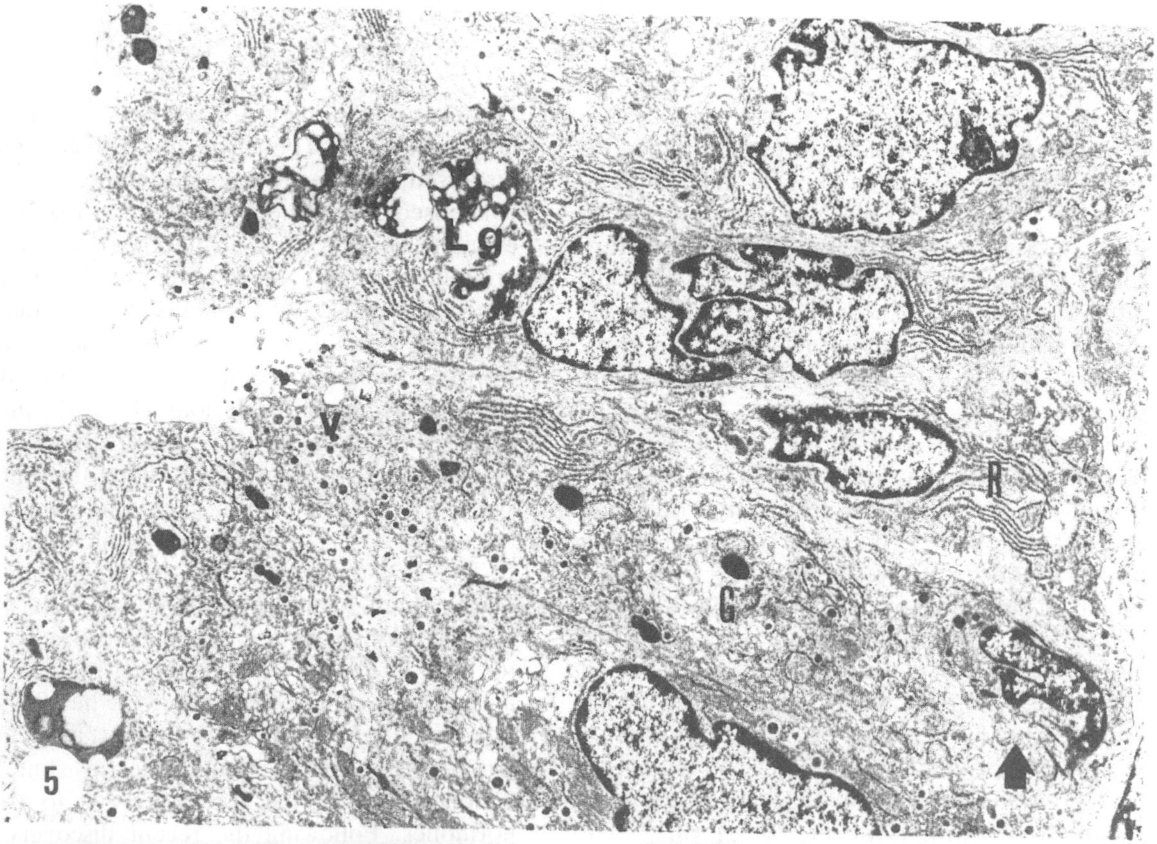

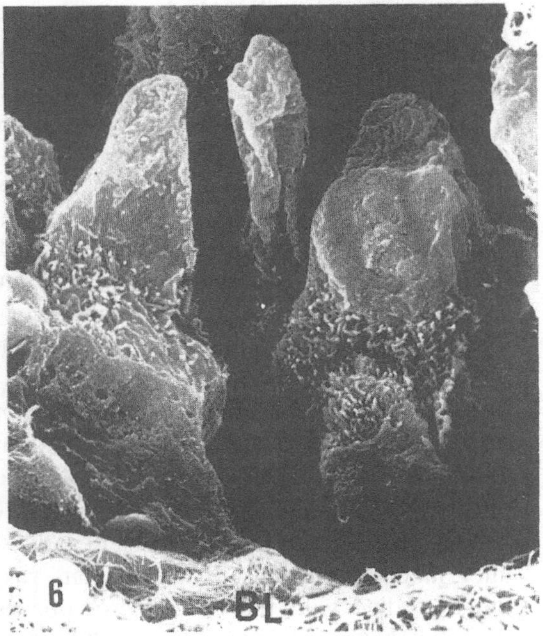

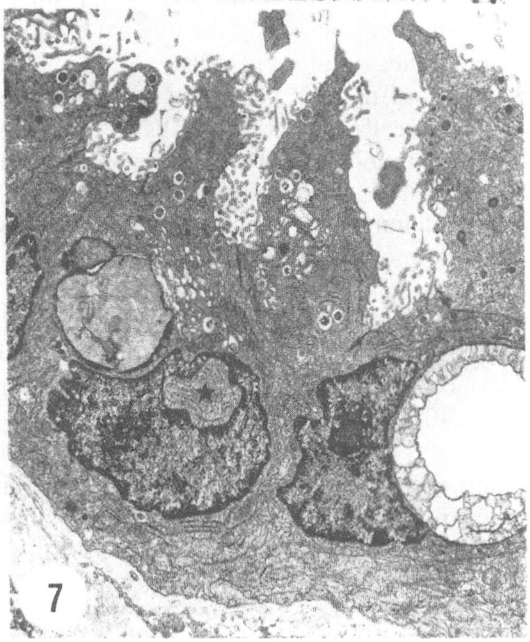

Fig. 5. TEM survey of the epithelium. The principal cells exhibit secretory vacuoles (v), elements of the RER (R), and prominent Golgi areas (G). Indented nuclei, dense bodies, and large lipofuscin granules (Lg) are also evident. A small triangular basal cell is seen on the right lower corner (arrow) (×7000).

Fig. 6. Epithelial cells seen from their lateral aspect after removal of adjacent cells. The arrow indicates the zone, possibly corresponding to the junctional complexes. BL = basal lamina (×4500).

Fig. 7. TEM image corresponding to Figure 6. The nucleus in the center exhibits a pseudoinclusion (*). Note the presence of two large lipofuscin granules (Lg) (×4100).

3. Principal Secretory Cells

As already noted the principal secretory cells vary in shape from low cuboidal, or even flattened, to columnar (Fig. 5). Even though some authors [4,18,19] maintain that the extremes are evidence for the presence of two distinct kinds of secretory cells, we believe that they represent, instead, different stages of cell activity. There are, in fact, [6,16,65] all intermediate forms, while their ultrastructural and histochemical features are basically the same.

The luminal surface (see Figs. 5, 6, 7, and 21) of principal cells may be rather smooth or bear irregular microvillosities, which are often branched and twisted. A few cells, more frequently in the proximal portion of the ampulla, bear stereocilia similar in structure to those present in the other segments of the vas. Occasionally ciliated cells are also observed. Just beneath the lumen, lateral cell membranes are joined by complexes, which usually consist of a *zonula occludens* followed by a *zonula adhaerens*. True desmosomes are rarely seen both in the junctional complex and elsewhere. There are, however, [4,62] small filamentous densities along the inner side of parallel membranes of adjacent cells.

Toward the cell base, and particularly where principal cells contact basal cells (see Fig. 22), cell interdigitations are sometimes observed. In the areas where basal cells are absent, the basal plasmalemma of principal cells is dotted by hemidesmosomelike structures.

Although the detachment of adjacent cells from each other seems here to be more difficult than in other human epithelia, the lateral cell surfaces can be visualized even in SEM (Fig. 6). Beneath the conical projections, which at their base may be covered by microvillosities (Fig. 6), there is a smooth band, possibly corresponding to the area occupied by the junctional complexes (Fig. 6). Below it, cell surfaces are usually devoid of plications. In some instances, however, there are a number of horizontally oriented processes (see Fig. 24) that likely correspond to the digitations seen in TEM (see Fig. 22) between the principal and basal cells. It may be noteworthy to recall that these processes seem to be different from those observed in other human exocrine glands [72].

3.1. Nuclei of Principal Cells

Nuclei are rather large and are located at variable heights (Fig. 5). The chromatin, which is mostly dispersed or arranged in small clumps, tends to be condensed along the inner side of the nuclear envelope (Figs. 5, 7, 9, 10, and 21). Nuclear pores are numerous and are clearly marked at TEM by zones free of heterochromatin (Figs. 5 and 10). They are evident at SEM in specimens treated with the osmium maceration method (Fig. 8). In some cases, pseudoinclusions (Fig. 7), that is, cytoplasmic invaginations encircled by a double membrane, are observed. Besides the nucleoli (Fig. 10), which are often large and prominent, the nuclei may show two kinds of inclusions.

The first is represented by the ubiquitous nuclear bodies [84] or sphaeridia [11] that have been described in the seminal vesicle as well [62,88]. As recently reviewed [9], these nuclear bodies were extensively studied in the 1970s and were found to be most abundant in hyperactive cells, including tumors, lectin stimulated lymphocytes, and tissues responsive to steroid hormones. Following the recent discovery that human autoantibodies, specific for nuclear antigens, bind to some nuclear bodies, new interest in their functional significance has been aroused [9].

The second kind of inclusions (Figs. 9 and 10), first reported in this epithelium by our group [16,65,67], is very similar to that described in TEM in the principal cells of the human epididymis [30,32] and *vas deferens* [12,29,55]. These inclusions, which consist of spherical globules of dense material (Figs. 9 and 10), may occur singly or in clusters (up to more than 30 in one section of a nucleus) and are sometimes limited by a single membrane. They have been detected in approximately one third of the nuclei examined and are constantly surrounded by an area of rarefied nucleoplasm. Their diameter ranges from 0.4 to 2.5 μm. The nuclear globules present in the scrotal and inguinal portions of the human vas have been studied with the light microscope as well [26,40,84]. According to Gilmour [26] these inclusions are androgen-dependent structures, since they appear after the onset of puberty. They are devoid of nucleic acid and contain a basic protein [40]. Chakraborty et al. [12], after having studied in detail their fine structure, distribution, and

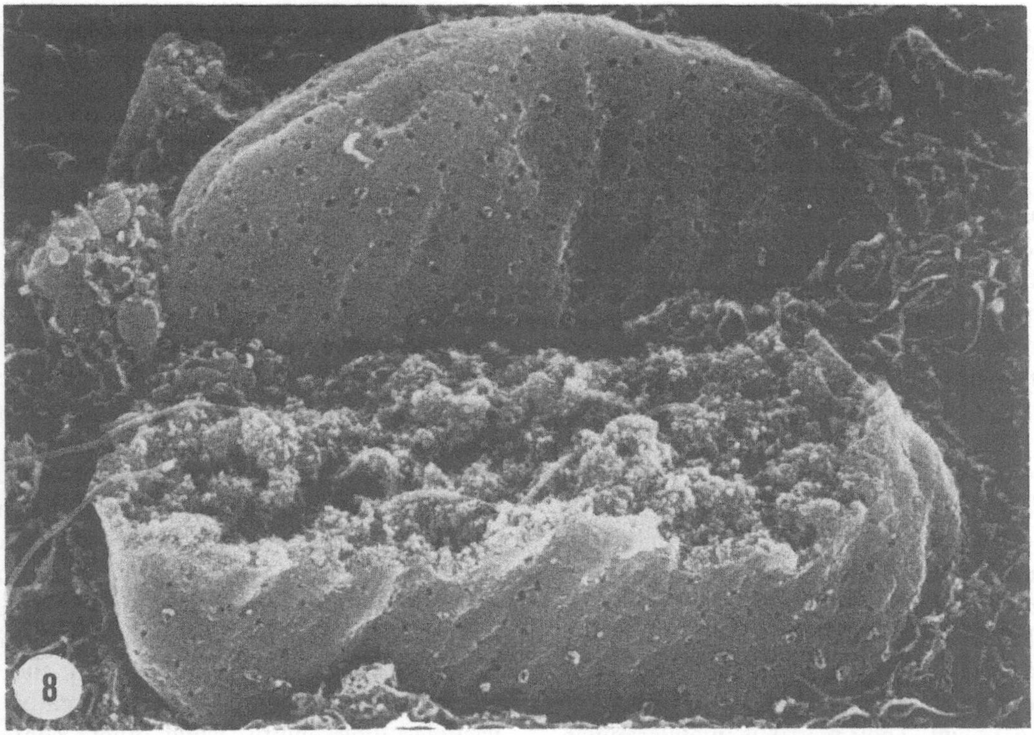

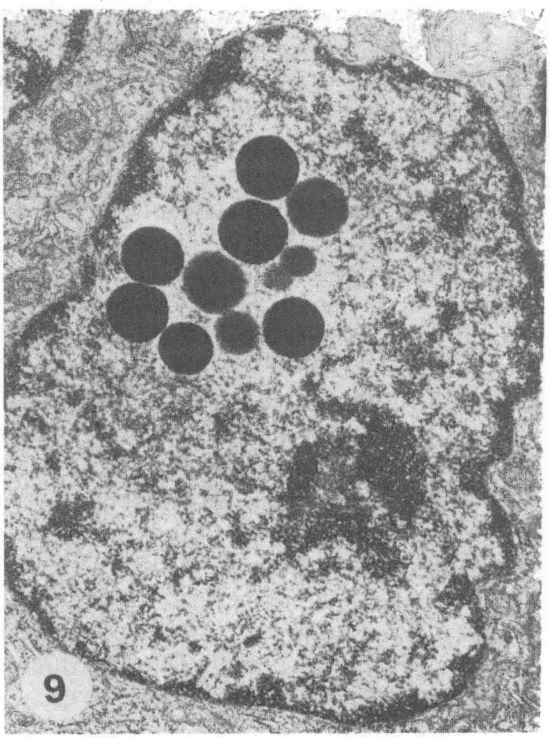

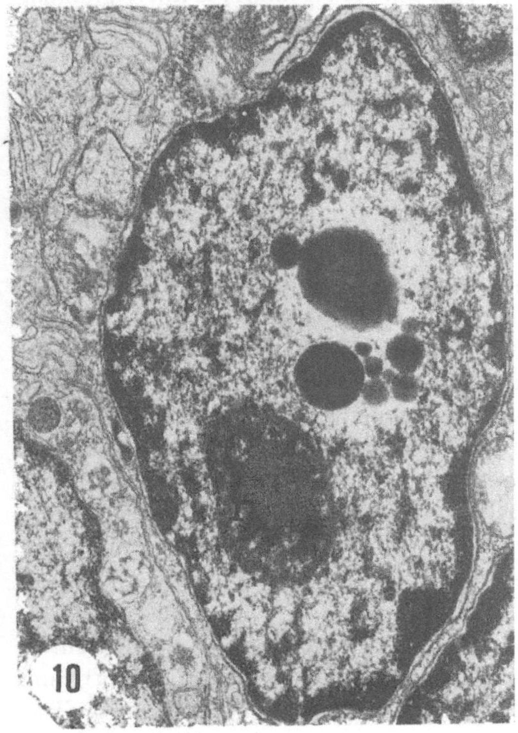

Fig 8 Nuclei of principal cells seen in a specimen treated with the osmium maceration method Numerous pores are evident on the nuclear surface The nucleus on the lower side which is fractured shows its content (×13 000)

Fig 9 Section of the nucleus showing several globular inclusions encircled by an area of rarefied nucleoplasm (×8000)

Fig 10 Besides nuclear inclusions of various size a prominent nucleolus (n) is seen (×13 000)

formation in the nuclei of the principal cells of the human vas, were unable to decide wether they are of cytoplasmic or intranuclear origin. It must be noted, however, that similar androgen-dependent globular inclusions, present in nuclei of the epididymis of the garden dormouse, were found [27] to be of cytoplasmic origin. On the basis of results obtained in TEM by electron energy loss spectroscopy, it was concluded that these inclusions are made [27] of protein crosslinked by disulphur bonds and contain iron, magnesium, and phosphorus.

3.2. Cytoplasmic Organelles of Principal Cells

Mitochondria are numerous, particularly in basal and perinuclear zones. They are usually spherical or ovoidal, with an average length of 0.7 μm and a width of 0.2 μm. There are, however, some elongated mitochondria, reaching a length of more than 3.5 μm. Their matrix is finely granular and of a rather low density (Fig. 14). While mitochondrial granules are rarely seen, there are sometimes, bandlike structures [4,16] located within the matrix among the *cristae*. Mitochondria, as seen in specimens treated with the osmium maceration method (Figs. 11 and 13), have cristae that are partly tubular and partly of the platelike type (Fig. 13). This is at variance with results obtained with the same method in rats [38], in which nearly all mitochondria have tubular cristae. Very frequently mitochondria are wrapped around by cisternal profiles of the rough endoplasmic reticulum (RER; Figs. 11, 13, and 14).

The RER is abundant in these cells, which also contain numerous free ribosomes. In its most typical form, the RER consists of stacks of three to five elogated *cisternae* with a clear content and is located not only around the nucleus but in apical regions as well (Fig. 5). In these areas concentric layers of parallel cisternae are seen. In other instances they are curved and short, and may show different degrees of dilatation. In SEM also (Fig. 12), the cisternae of the RER are clearly distinguishable due to the presence of granular ribosomes on their outer surfaces. In many cases (Figs. 12 and 14) at the boundary between the RER and the smooth elements of the Golgi apparatus, there are small spherical vesicles. According to Aumüller [2,4] the distribution and shape of RER seem to be dependent on cell functional activity.

The Golgi apparatus is often prominent (Figs. 5, 11, and 14) and exhibits an oval or rounded outline. It consists (Fig. 14) of vesicles, vacuoles, and stacks of parallel cisternae. On the *cis* (convex) face of the latter, small vesicles, seemingly originating from degranulated RER elements, are seen. Newly formed secretory vacuoles of various size and density are, instead, present on their *trans* (concave) aspect. In SEM specimens, the tubular components (Fig. 12) of the Golgi apparatus also become evident.

Secretory vacuoles represent the distinctive feature of principal cells and, as results even from morphometric studies [20], they tend to accumulate in the apical regions (Fig. 15). They have a diameter of 0.04–0.3 μm and contain a globular mass of dense material that rarely fills them completely. The interval (*halo*) between the dense core and the vacuolar wall varies greatly. Some vacuoles look empty, while others contain ill-defined fragmented material. The morphology of secretory vacuoles looks basically the same in SEM specimens treated with the osmium maceration technique, since they appear as membrane-bounded vesicles containing a globular mass (Fig. 16).

On the basis of findings obtained in seminal vesicles of rat, Brandes [8] put forward the hypothesis that the smallest among the secretory vacuoles, frequently observed just beneath the luminal plasmalemma, represent a second kind of secretory material. This assumption has been recently substantiated in the same animal in specimens postfixed with the osmium-ferrocyanide mixture [35] by Clermont et al. [13]. These authors showed that the small secretory vacuoles differed morphologically from the large ones and no intermediate forms were present. They also postulated a different mechanism of formation by the Golgi apparatus for the two kinds of vacuoles.

Even though, in the absence of cytochemical findings at the TEM level, we cannot exclude the presence of different kinds of secretory vacuoles, our morphological results in human tissues seem to be at variance with those obtained in rat. In our specimens, including those postfixed with the Karnovsky mixture [35], large or small secretory vacuoles exhibit the same morphological characters, while no clear differences are seen in their

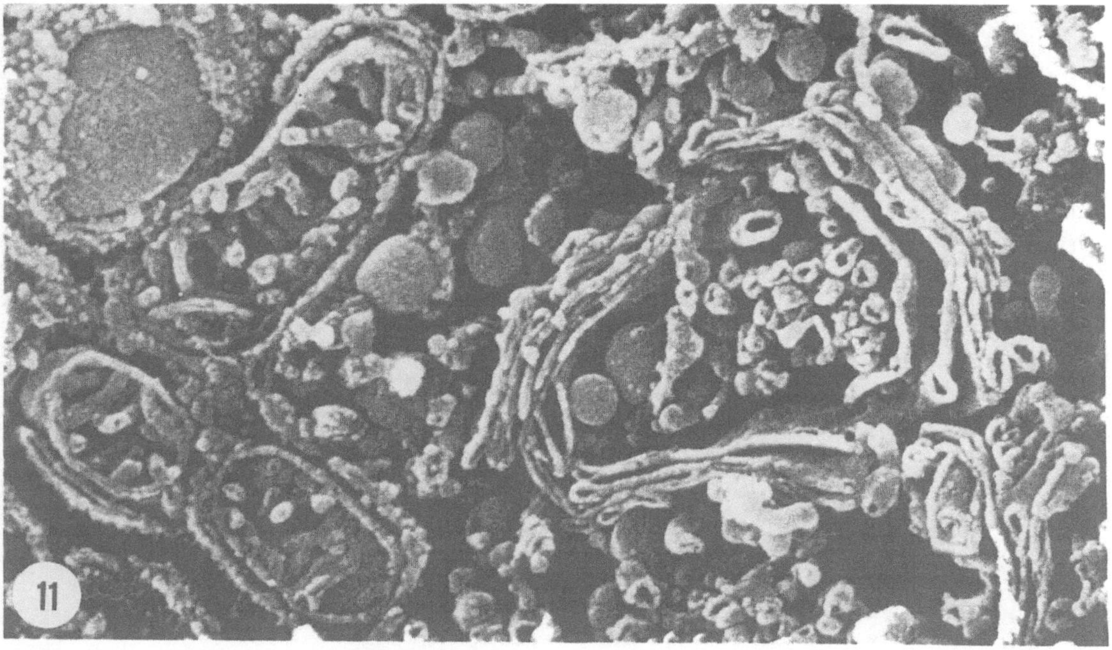

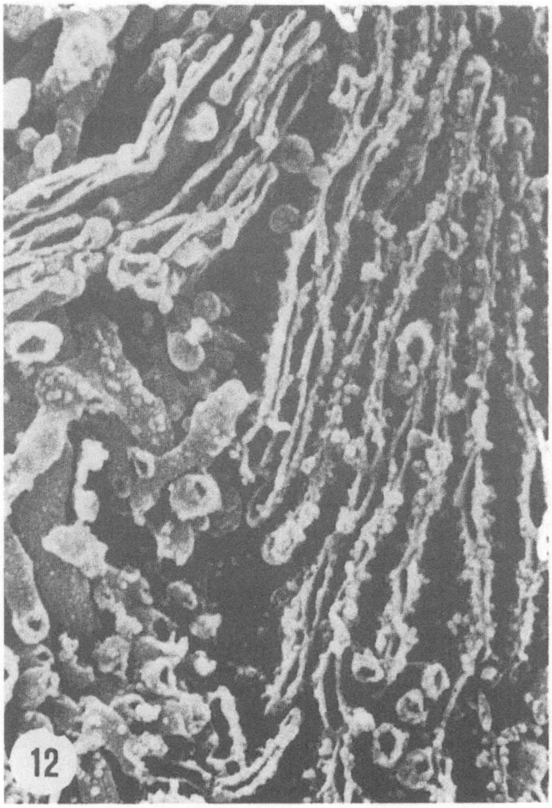

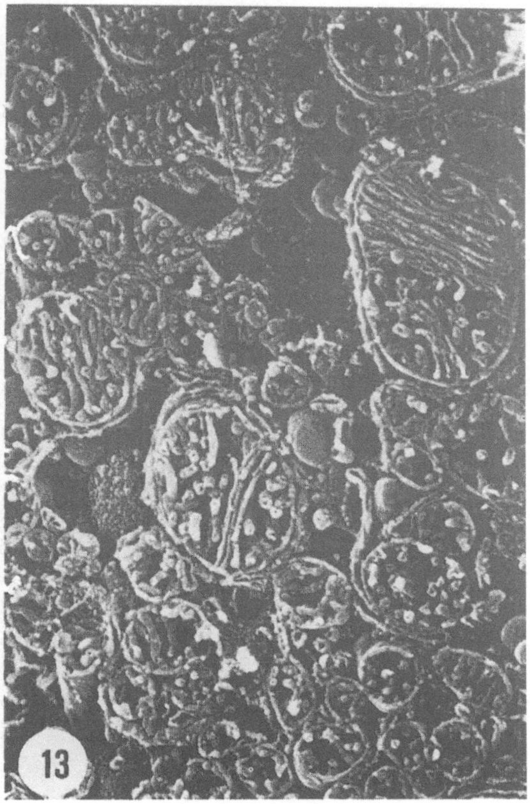

Figures 11–13 are all from osmium macerated specimens

Fig 11 Golgi region of a principal cell Globular masses, some of which representing unsectioned vacuoles are seen on the *cis* and *trans* aspects of the cisternae Note also that the four mitochondria seen on the left side (including the unsectioned one) are encircled by elements of the RER (×50,000)

Fig 12 Detail of the cytoplasm of the principal cells at the boundary between the elements of the RER (right) and those of the Golgi apparatus (left) Note that the latter consists not only of cisternae but also of twisted tubules (*) vesicles (×25,000)

Fig 13 Mitochondria of a principal cell Note that some mitochondria besides the tubular ones, exhibit cristae of the platelike type (×20,000)

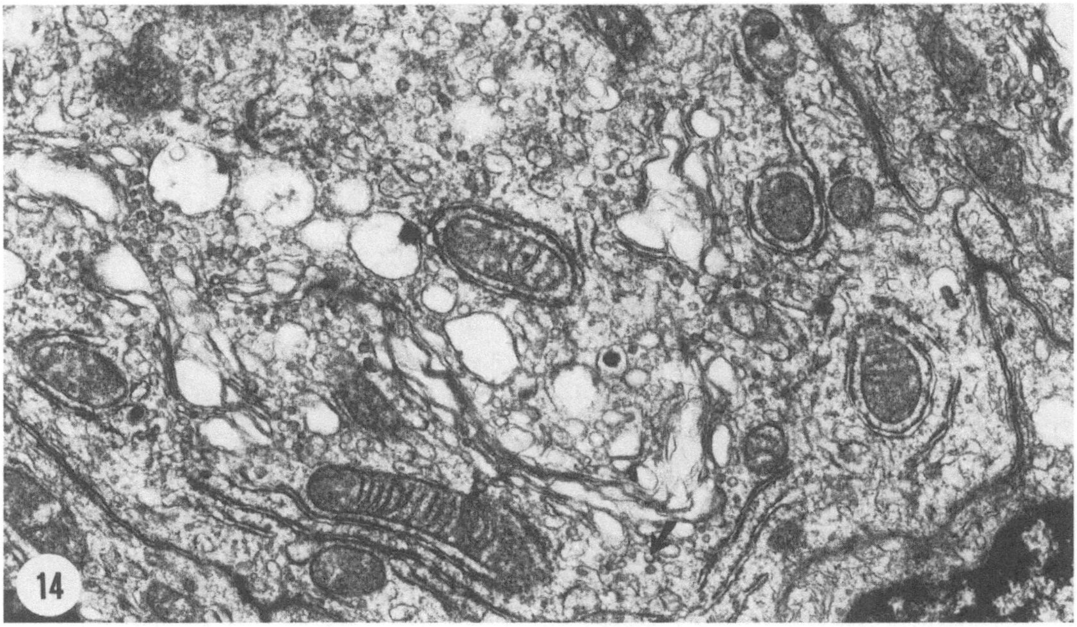

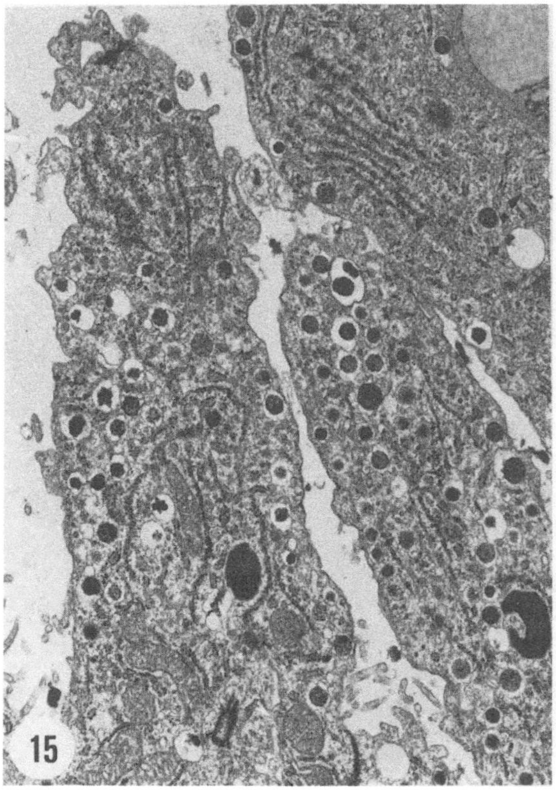

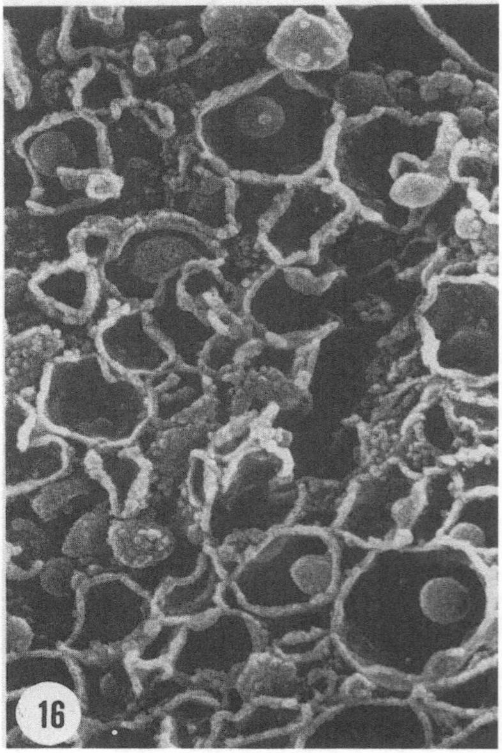

Fig 14 Golgi region of a principal cell Newly formed secretory vacuoles of different size and density are seen on the *trans* aspect of the cisternae Note also the presence of small vesicles (arrow) on the *cis* side that seem to originate from degranulated elements of the RER (×30 000)

Fig 15 Apical portions of principal cells filled with secretory vacuoles of different size (×10 000)

Fig 16 Sectioned secretory vacuoles seen in an osmium macerated specimen Note the spherical bodies that correspond to the dense cores seen in TEM (×27 000)

pattern of formation in the Golgi apparatus. Moreover, even the authors [28], who have demonstrated by electron immunocytochemistry a specific secretory protein (SVA) in the dense core of secretory vacuoles of human seminal vesicles, failed to mention the presence of two distinct populations of secretory vacuoles.

Besides the secretory vacuoles, the cytoplasm contains two kinds of inclusions. The first consists of electron-lucent lipid droplets [16], which are seen in the basal region. These homogeneous droplets are small and do not show any acid phophatase activity. The second is represented by bodies of various density that, in showing different degrees of acid phophatase reactivity, are related to lysosomes [3,66]. The larger inclusions of this second kind, which correspond to the lipofuscin (lipopigment) granules seen with the light microscope, are pleomorphic and composite in structure (Figs. 5, 7, 21, and 22). Sometimes they appear as the result of the fusion of several small- and medium-sized bodies and exhibit a honeycombed configuration (Figs. 5 and 21).

Since only seldom were we able to detect sperm remnants inside [65], we cannot fully support Exner's [24] statement that all lipopigment granules result from the ingestion of sperms. They may derive from autophagic vacuoles [53] or from reabsorbed secretory material, as demonstrated in human ejaculatory duct [6] and hamster seminal vesicles [42]. It must be recalled, however [41], that lipofuscinlike granules are also formed from spermatozoa phagocytosed by macrophages in sperm granuloma and by mouse macrophages cultured in the presence of spermatozoa. In any case, lipopigment granules must have a specific functional role, since in man [86] they appear after the onset of puberty and are absent in eunuchs [85] and in cases in which the ejaculatory duct [7] is absent. Furthermore, these lipopigments are considered by pathologists to be an important cue for distinguishing, in aspiration studies [36] and needle biopsies (80), cells from seminal vesicles and related organs from those originating from prostate gland.

3.3. Spermatophagy by Principal Cells

Spermatozoa (Figs. 17–19) are occasionally seen in man, within the *lumina* of the *ampulla* [50,65, 67], seminal vesicles [6,56–59,64,71], and ejaculatory duct [16,70,71]. Phagocytosis of sperms by principal cells also is noted (Figs. 18–20). Sperms [50,63,65] were first seen in SEM, which allows the survey of large fields and does not require the mincing of tissues into small pieces. This may explain why studies performed exclusively with TEM [2,4,53,62] failed to report the presence of spermatozoa. In fact, we were able to demonstrate spermiophagy in TEM [64,65] only after a search on areas previously selected by SEM.

Segments of engulfed sperms are usually enclosed in membrane-bounded vacuoles of various size within the cytoplasm of principal cells (Fig. 20). The surrounding cytoplasm exhibit bundles of filaments and, in most cases, lysosomelike dense bodies. In advanced stages of digestion, the vacuole is no more discernible and the sperm remnants are surrounded by a dense and fibrous cytoplasm rich in microtubules [65]. As a whole, the process of spermatophagy observed in man [65] strongly recalls that originally described in TEM in the terminal region of the vas deferens of the rat [15] and subsequently seen in a variety of mammals [47–50,52,60,61]. In SEM the heads of sperms undergoing phagocytosis usually look abnormal due to the presence of morphological alterations of various degrees [65].

Phagocytosis by epithelial cells may start from every portion of the spermatozoon, so that a sperm tail or a sperm head may protrude from the epithelium. In other instances, the first ingestion seems to occur at the intermediate region of the tail. In general (Fig. 19) the surface of principal cells that engulf spermatozoa [6,52,65] appear less endowed with microvilli than that of cells not involved in the process.

In other portions of the genital tract [31,52,57, 73], and particularly in the tail of the epididymis [82], spermatophagy is carried out by intraepithelial macrophages. Despite the fact that the presence of these intraepithelial macrophages has been demonstrated in almost the entire length of the male reproductive tract and accessory glands in a variety of animal species [52], we have been unable to find such cells in the organs studied, nor were they detected by immunocytochemical markers [21]. There are, instead, numerous intraepithelial lymphocytes (Fig. 21), which may be part of the so-called mucosa associated lymphoid

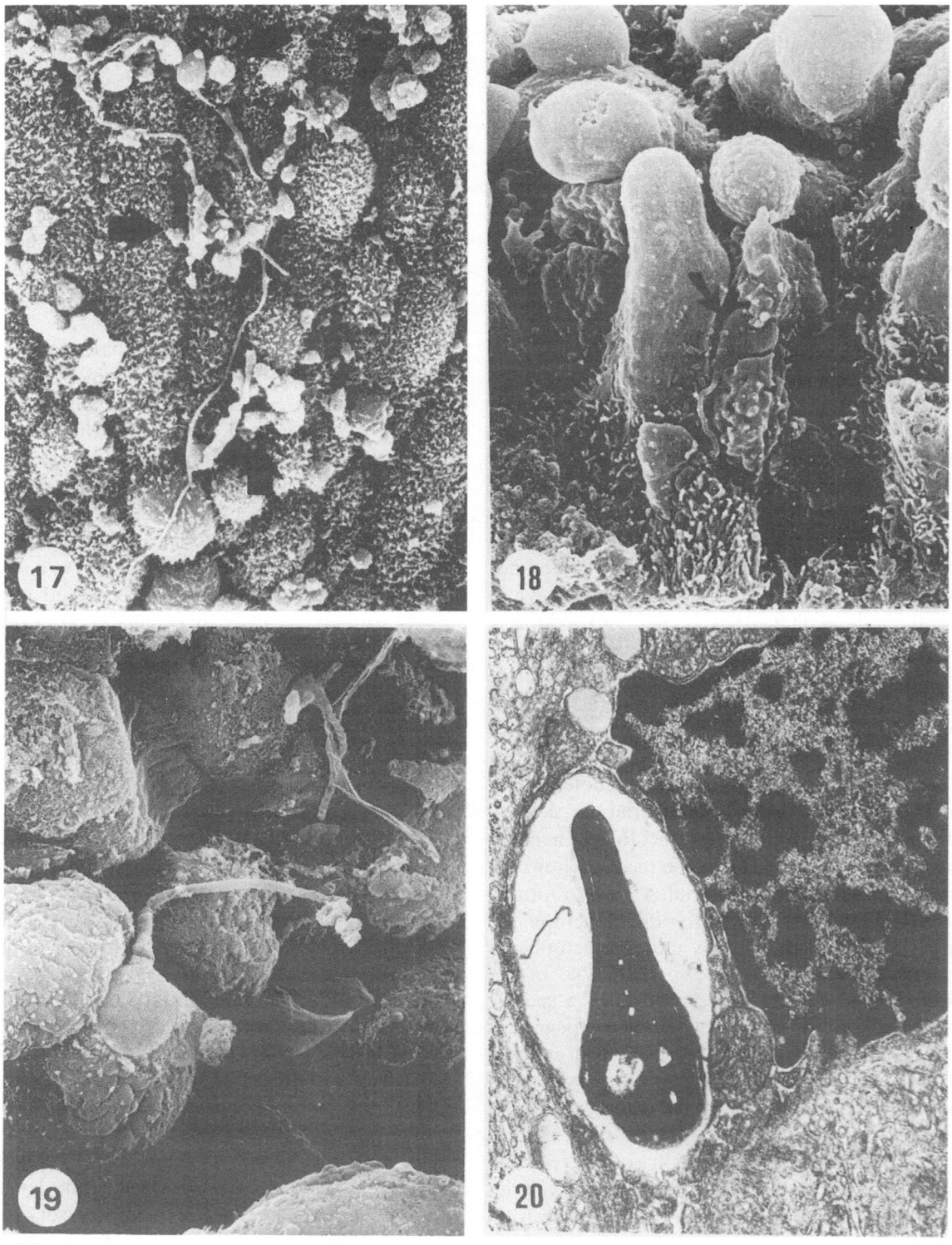

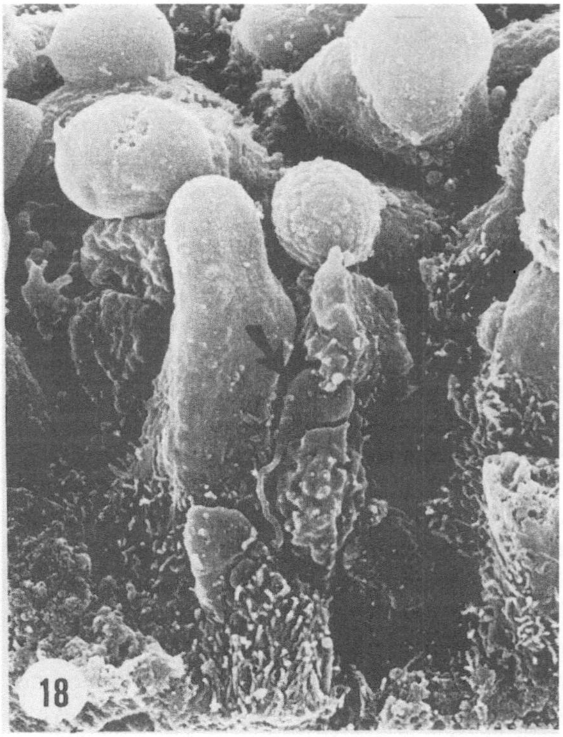

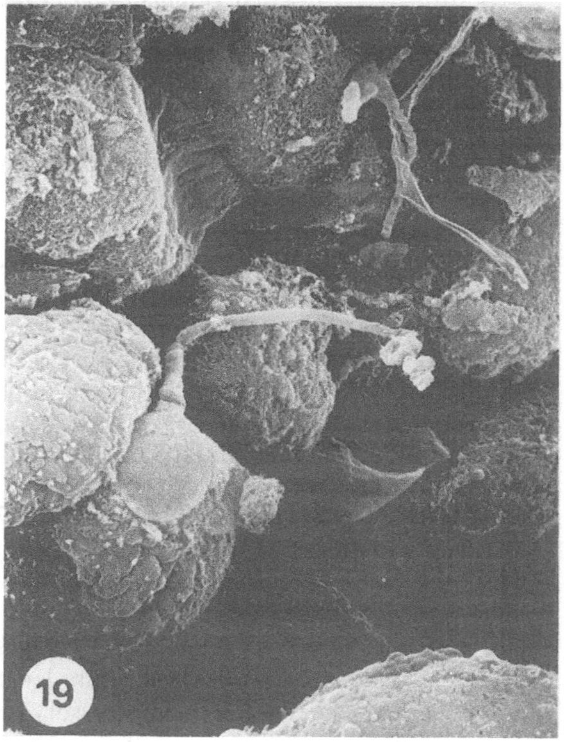

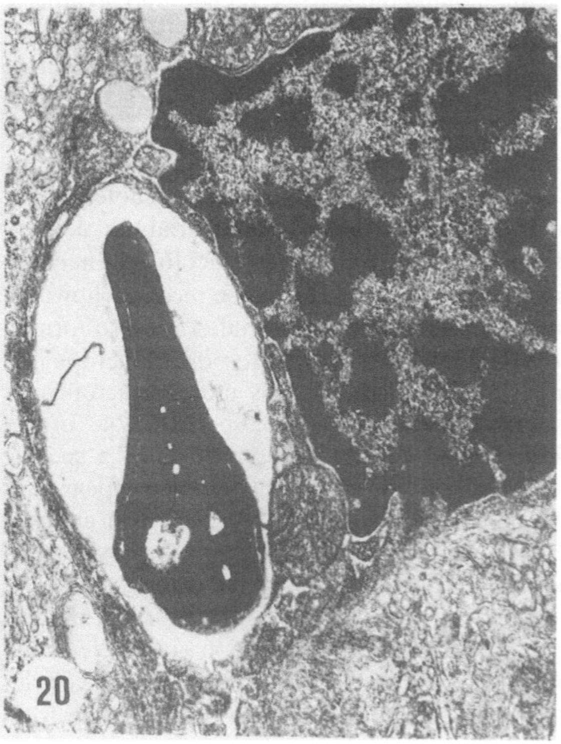

Fig 17 Several sperms (arrows) are seen on the surface of principal cells (×1800)

Fig 18 A sperm (arrow) probably undergoing phagocytosis is seen among the apexes of principal cells (×3800)

Fig 19 Sperm segments adhere to the rather smooth surface of the apexes of the principal cells (×5400)

Fig 20 A large vacuole containing the head of an ingested sperm is seen in the cytoplasm of a principal cell (×15 000)

tissue that has been demonstrated by immunocytochemical methods in the seminal vesicle [21] and other human male accessory glands [45].

Though it is now established [1,44,75] that human seminal vesicles are not reservoirs for unejaculated sperms, light microscopists long ago described [43,76,83] the presence of spermatozoa in their cavities. According to Stieve [76] the longer the period of sexual rest, the larger is the number of sperm that accumulate in the seminal vesicles. The study of split ejaculates [22,44,65] has shown that the last fraction, which consists mainly of seminal vesicle secretions, still contains a number of spermatozoa. On the other hand, numerous sperms are normally present in the ampulla of monkey vas deferens [60,61], and this may happen in humans as well [44]. The first ejaculates after vasectomy [1] in fact contain spermatozoa that were probably stored in the *ampulla* [34]. Morover, in the absence of a sphincter muscle [5] around the opening of the seminal vesicles into the ampulla, sperms may easily migrate into the former.

4. Basal Cells

Basal cells form a discontinuous layer at the base of principal cells and never reach the lumen. They are usually flattened, with a width of 8–12 μm and a height of about 2 μm, but trigonal or cuboidal cells are occasionally seen. Some basal cells, however, have their long axis oriented at an oblique angle to the basal lamina (Figs. 5 and 22), so that they rest only partially upon it. The cytoplasm is devoid of secretory granules and usually looks more dense and compact than that of principal cells. Cytoplasmic organelles are scanty and consist of a few small mitochondria, elements of RER and of Golgi apparatus, and small lipopigment granules. There are also filaments (Figs. 22 and 23), which are often arranged in bundles and tend to accumulate in the perinuclear region (Fig. 23). The plasma membrane may be sinuous due to the presence of processes that interlock with those much more numerous ones originating from principal cells (Figs. 22 and 24). On its basal aspect the plasmalemma may show focal hemidesmosome like densities.

The functional significance of basal cells is still obscure. Histochemically they differ from the myoepithelial cells of human exocrine glands, because at the light microscopical level they are unreactive to actin. Their role as reserve cells is also unclear, since even though in man [10] they decrease in number between birth and 18 years, in castrated animals subjected to testosterone treatment [4] mitoses and labelled nuclei are nearly exclusively seen in principal cells.

5. Concluding Remarks

Results reported here clearly show the high secretory activity of the epithelium and the many peculiarities of its cytoarchitecture in man. Comparative studies have provided a great deal of information useful for gaining a better understanding of the physiological role of male accessory glands. They have uncovered evidence [41], however, that each species exhibits its own characteristics and that, especially from a biochemical point of view, the contributions of different glands to the formation of seminal plasma vary greatly.

Despite this, the great ease of using laboratory animals for ultrastructural investigation has led researchers to extrapolate to man data obtained in rodents. It is probably for this reason that most modern textbooks of histology [71] still consider the ampulla, seminal vesicle, and ejaculatory ducts as distinct organs, all endowed with a different epithelial lining. Paradoxically, as mentioned above, the fact that these organs have an identical epithelium was known to the histologists of the last century [77]. An additional finding that was documented by early microscopists [76] and successively forgotten, is the presence of sperm and their phagocytosis by principal cells. It is due to the introduction of SEM, which allows visualization of fields much wider than those observed in TEM, that this phenomenon has been rediscovered in humans. However, due to the practical impossibility of obtaining a suitable number of specimens from young normal subjects, the extent of sperm phagocytosis and its physiological role have still to be determined.

This chapter reports some of the first results ever published on human tissues studied in high resolution SEM by the use of maceration techniques. There are still some interpretation prob-

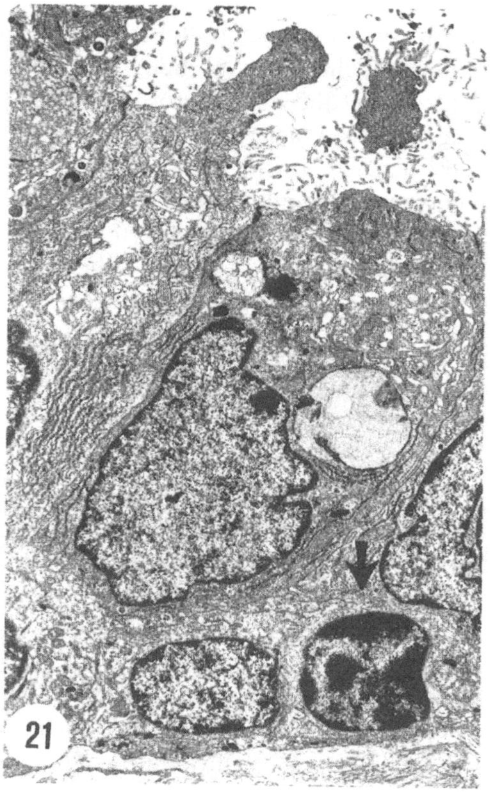

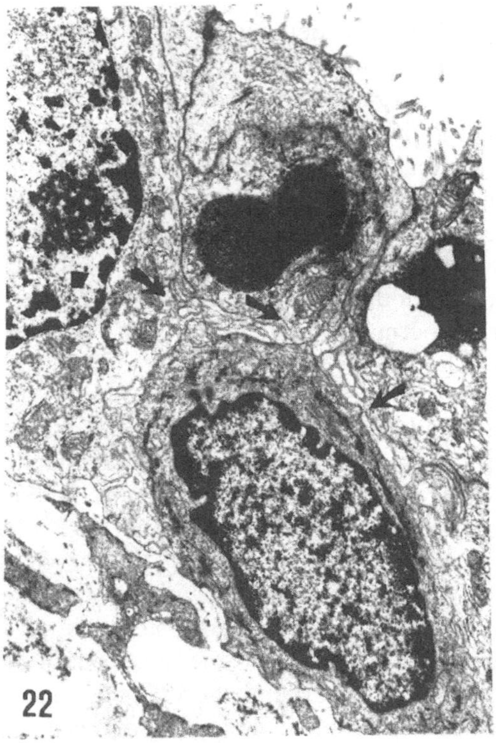

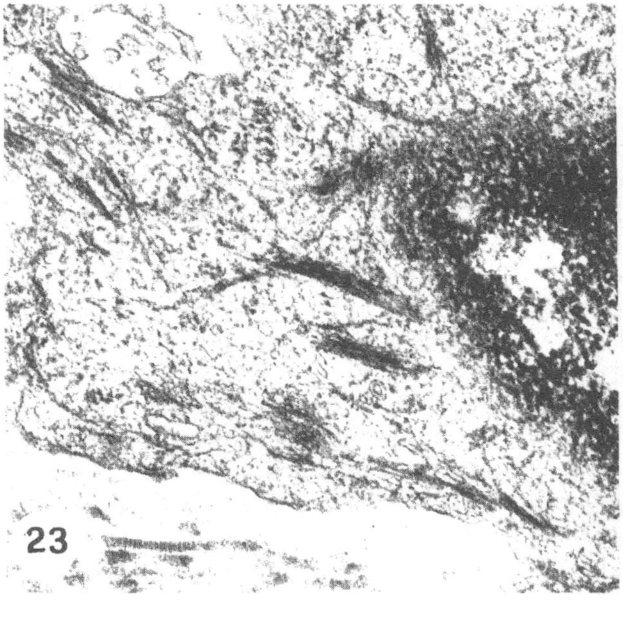

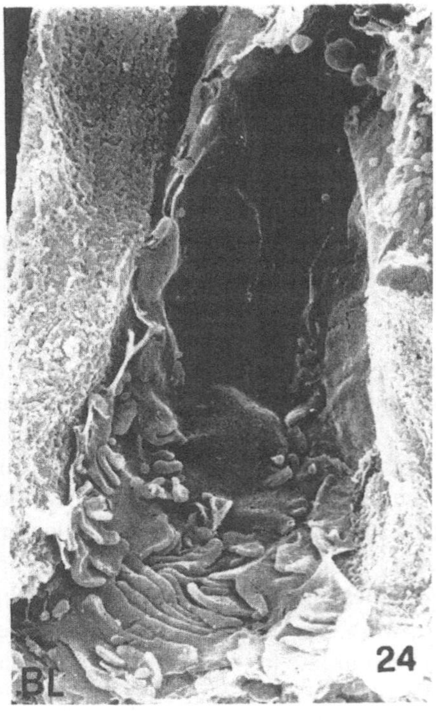

Fig 21 A lymphocyte (arrow) and a cuboidal basal cell are present on the basal aspect of the epithelium (×3000)

Fig 22 Note that the basal cell exhibit an axis oriented obliquely to the basal lamina The arrows indicate some cellular interdigitations (×7500)

Fig 23 Detail of the filamentous cytoplasm of a basal cell (×50,000)

Fig 24 Lateral view of a principal cell exposed from the basal lamina to the lumen Note that the folds seen basally have an horizontal orientation (×6500)

lems, depending on the relevant novelty of the methods and the possible presence of artifacts. Nevertheless, especially when combined with TEM findings, SEM results seem to provide a better knowledge of the cytology of epithelial cells.

It must be remarked, finally, that ultrastructural investigations on human male accessory glands depend on specimens obtained at surgery from patients undergoing operation for retropubic prostatectomy or cancer of the bladder, diseases that, as a rule, occur in the last decades of human life. Moreover, at least in recent years, patients are often subjected to x-rays or treatment with antineoplastic durgs, which may affect the fine morphology of cells and organelles. Thus, among the 63 cases collected over a period of almost 30 years, we have focused our attention on 11 specimens from subjects under the age of 50. They looked histologically normal and, at least in the 6 mounths preceding surgery, they had not been subjected to x-rays or drug treatment.

6. Acknowledgments

This work was supported by the Consiglio Nazionale delle Ricerche (C.N.R.) and the Ministero dell'Università e della Ricerca Scientifica e Tecnologica (M.U.R.S.T.). We are indebted to Professor E. Usai and Drs. R. Scarpa and R. Migliari of the Clinic of Urology of the University of Cagliari for furnishing us with the specimens studied. Thanks are also due to Dr. Terenzio Congiu for his criticism and editorial help. Skillful technical assistance was provided by Mrs. Silvana Bernardini-Foddis and Mr. Alessandro Cadau.

References

1 Arvis G La vasectomie et les tecniques de blocage de l'excretion deferentielle Leurs consequences In Andrologie, Vol 1 G Arvis (ed) Paris Maloine, 1987, pp 344–360
2 Aumuller G Zur funktionellen Morphologie der Blashendruse Heidelberg Habilitationsschrift, 1973
3 Aumuller G Lipopigment fine structure in human seminal vesicle Virchows Arch B Cell Pathol 24 79–85, 1977
4 Aumuller G Seminal vesicle In Prostate Gland and Seminal Vesicles Handbuch der Mikroskopischen Anatomie des Menschen, Vol 7 6 A Oksche, L Vollrath (eds) Berlin Springer, 1979, pp 183–355
5 Aumuller G, Bruhl B Uber den Bau der Ampulla Ductus deferentis des Menschen Verh Anat Gesel 71 561–564, 1977
6 Aumuller G, Riva A Morphology and function of the human seminal vesicle Andrologia 24 183–196, 1992
7 Brack E Aplasie des Ductus deferens bei normalen Hoden Z Urol 15 232–236, 1921
8 Brandes D Fine structure and cytochemistry of male sex accessory organs In Male Accessory Sex Organs Structure and Function in Mammals D Brandes (ed) New York Academic Press, 1974, pp 17–113
9 Brasch K, Ochs RL Nuclear bodies (NBs) A newly "rediscovered" organelle Exp Cell Res 202 211–223, 1992
10 Brewster SF The development and differentiation of human seminal vesicles J Anat 143 45–55, 1985
11 Buttner DW, Horstmann E Das Sphaeridion, eine weitere Differenzierung des Karyoplasma Z Zellforsch 77 589–605, 1967
12 Chakraborty J, Nelson L, Jhunjhunwala J, Young M, Kropp K Intranuclear inclusion bodies in epithelial cells of human vas deferens Arch Androl 2 1–12, 1979
13 Clermont Y, Rambourg A, Hermo L Segregation of secretory material in all elements of the Golgi apparatus in principal cells of the rat seminal vesicle Anat Rec 232 349–358, 1992
14 Chow PH Scanning electron microscopical study of the seminal vesicle, coagulating gland, ampullary gland and ventral prostate in the golden hamster Acta Anat 133 269–273, 1983
15 Cooper TG, Hamilton DM Phagocytosis of spermatozoa in the terminal region and gland of the vas deferens of the rat Am J Anat 150 247–268, 1978
16 Cossu M, Marcello MF, Usai E, Testa-Riva F, Riva A Fine structure of the epithelium of the human ejaculatory duct Acta Anat 116 225–233, 1983
17 Cossu M, Usai E, Sirigu P, Riva A Histochemical demonstration of glucose-6-phosphate dehydrogenase, D-sorbitol dehydrogenase and alkaline phosphatase in human ampulla ductus deferentis Fertil Steril 29 557–559, 1978
18 Dadoune JP Functional morphology of the seminal vesicle In Seminal Vesicle and Fertility C Bollack, A Clavert (eds) Basel Karger, 1985, pp 18–35
19 De Kretser DM, Temple-Smith PD, Kerr JB Anatomical and functional aspects of the male reproductive organs In Disturbances in Male Fertility K Bandhauer, J Frick (eds) Berlin Springer, 1982, pp 82–97
20 Diaz G, Cossu M, Riva A Quantitative ultrastructural approach to the study of the spatial relationship among the cell organelles I Cytological organization of human exocrine epithelia J Electr Microsc Tech 7 167–175, 1982
21 El Demiry MMI, James K Lymphocyte subsets and macrophages in the male genital tract in health and dis-

ease A monoclonal antibody-based study Eur Urol 14 226–235, 1988
22 Eliasson R, Lindholmer C Distribution and properties of spermatozoa in different fractions of split ejaculates Fertil Steril 23 252–256, 1972
23 Evan AP, Dail WG, Damrose D, Palmer C Scanning electron microscopy of cell surfaces following removal of extracellular materials Anat Rec 185 433–447, 1976
24 Exner S reported by Stieve [75], 1904
25 Gattone V, Conforti J A method for obtainig lateral surfaces of renal tubular cells for scanning electron microscopy J Electr Microsc Tech 2 283–284, 1985
26 Gilmour JR Intranuclear inclusions in the epithelium of the human male genital tract Lancet 1 373–375, 1937
27 Hawkes F Rzepka J, Gontrand G Presence of intranuclear inclusions in the principal cells of the epididymis of the garden dormouse *Eliomys quercinus* L J Submicrosc Cytol Pathol 20 471–476, 1988
28 Herr JC Spell DR, Conklin DJ, Flickinger CJ Electron microscopy immunolocalization of seminal vesicle specific antigens in human seminal vesicle Biol Reprod 40 333–342 1989
29 Hofter AP The ultrastructure of the ductus deferens in man Biol Reprod 14 425–443, 1976
30 Holstein AF Morphologische Studien am Nebenhoden des Menschen In Zwanglose Abhandlungen aus dem Gebiet den normalen und pathologischen Anatomie W Bargmann, W Doerr (eds) Stuttgart G Thieme, 1969, pp 1–91
31 Holstein AF Spermatophagy in the seminiferous tubules and excurrent ducts of the testis in rhesus monkey and in man Andrologia 10 331–352, 1978
32 Horstman E, Richter R, Roosen-Runge E Zur Elektronen Mikroskopie der Kerneinschlusse im menschlichen Nebenhodenepithel Z Zellforsch 69 69–79, 1966
33 Hucker H, Aumuller G Internal surface and fine structure of the rat seminal vesicle Acta Anat 94 336–342, 1976
34 Hudson B Burger HG The physiology and function of the testis In Human Reproductive Physiology RP Shearman (ed) Oxford Blackwell, 1972, pp 91–337
35 Karnovsky MJ Use of ferrocyanide-reduced osmium tetroxide in electron microscopy Proceedings of the 11th Meeting of the American Society of Cell Biology New Orleans, abstr 284, 1971, p 146
36 Koivuiniemi A, Tyrkko J Seminal vesicle epithelium in fine needle aspiration biopsies of the prostate as pitfall in the cytologic diagnosis of carcinoma Acta Cytol 20 116–119, 1976
37 Kunkelmann H, Kuhnel W Zur Morphologie der Ampulla Ductus deferentis von Kaninchen Transmissions- und rasterelektronenmikroskopische Untersuchungen Acta Anat 118 1–12, 1984
38 Lea PJ, Hollemberg MJ Mitochondrial structure revealed by high resolution scanning electron microscopy Am J Anat 184 245–257, 1989
39 Low FN, McClugage SG Jr Microdissection by ultrasonication Scanning electron microscopy of the epithelial basal lamina of the alimentary canal in the rat Am J Anat 16 137–147, 1984
40 Mac Donald J Some cytochemical characteristics of certain intranuclear inclusion bodies in the epithelium of the human vas deferens Anat Rec 106 327–343, 1950
41 Mann T, Lutwak-Mann C Male Reproductive Function and Semen Themes and Trends in Physiology, Biochemistry and Investigative Andrology Berlin Springer, 1981
42 Mata LR, Maunsbach AB Absorption of secretory protein by the epithelium of hamster seminal vesicle as studied by electron microscope autoradiography Biol Cell 46 65–74, 1982
43 Mathis J Uber die Bedeutung der Blaschendrusen (Samenblasen) Wien Klin Wochenschr 56 205–206, 1943
44 Mawhinney MG, Tarry WE Male accessory sex organs and androgen action in infertility in the male LI Lipshultz, SS Howards (eds) St Louis, MO CV Mosby, 1991, pp 124–154
45 Migliari R, Riva A, Lantini MS, Melis M, Usai E Diffuse lymphoid tissue associated with the human bulbourethral gland An immunologic characterization J Androl 13 337–341, 1992
46 Miller BS, Woods RI, Bohlen HG, Evan AP A new morphological procedure of viewing microvessels A scanning electron microscopic study of the vasculature of small intestine Anat Rec 203 493–503, 1982
47 Murakami M, Nishida T, Iwanaga S, Shiromoto M Scanning and transmission electron microscopic evidence of epithelial phagocytosis of spermatozoa in the terminal region of the vas deferens of the cat Experienta 40 958–960, 1984
48 Murakami M, Nishida T, Shiromoto M, Inokuchi T Phyagocytosis of spermatozoa and latex beads by epithelial cells of the ampulla vasis deferentis of the rabbit A combined SEM and TEM study Arch Histol Jpn 48 269–277, 1985
49 Murakami M Nishida T, Shiromoto M, Inokuchi T Scanning and transmission electron microscopic study of the ampullary region of the dog vas deferens with special reference to epithelial phagocytosis of spermatozoa and latex beads Anat Anz 162 289–296, 1986
50 Murakami M, Sugita A, Hamasaki M The vas deferens in man and monkey Spermiophagy in its ampulla In Atlas of Human Reproduction by Scanning Electron Microscopy ESE Hafez, P Kenemans (eds) Lancaster, UK MTP, 1982, pp 187–195
51 Murakami M, Sugita A, Shimada T, Yoshimura T Scanning electron microscope observation of the seminal vesicle in the Japanese monkey with special reference to intraluminal spermiophagy by macrophages Arch Histol Jpn 41 275–283, 1978
52 Murakami M, Yokoyama R SEM observation of the male reproductive tract with special reference to epithelial phagocytosis In Developments in Ultrastructure of Reproduction Progress in Clinical and Biological Research, Vol 296 PM Motta (ed) New York Alan R Liss, 1989, pp 207–214
53 Nistal M, Santamaria L, Paniagua R The ampulla of ductus deferens in man Morphological and ultrastructural aspects J Anat 180 97–106, 1992
54 Ohtani O, Ushiki T, Taguki T, Kikuta A Collagen fibril-

lar networks as skeletal framworks A demonstration by cell maceration/scanning electron microscope method Arch Histol Cytol 51 249–261, 1988
55 Orlandini GE The fine structure of the vas deferens epithelium of man Verh Anat Gesel 68 213–218, 1974
56 Orlandini GE, Holstein AF La differenziazione e la progressione degli spermatozoi nell'uomo Arch Ital Anat Embriol S91 11–39, 1986
57 Orlandini GE, Holstein AF Fate of human germ cells after spermiation In Development in Ultrastructure of Reproduction Progress in Clinical and Biological Research, Vol 296 PM Motta (ed) New York Alan R Liss, 1989, pp 215–220
58 Orlandini GE, Gulisano M, Pacini P Studio al MES delle vescichette seminali umane Arch Ital Anat Embriol 85 163–177, 1980
59 Orlandini GE, Pacini P, Gulisano M SEM of human vas deferens and seminal vesicle In Three Dimensional Anatomy of Cell and Tissue Surface DJ Allen, PM Motta, LJA DiDio (eds) New York Elsevier, 1981, pp 299–310
60 Ramos AS Ultrastructural variations and phagocytosis of spermatozoa in the epithelium of the monkey vas deferens Biol Rep 20 61A, 1979
61 Ramos AS Morphologic variations along the length of the monkey vas deferens Arch Androl 3 187–196, 1979
62 Riva A Fine structure of human seminal vesicle epithelium J Anat 102 71–86, 1977
63 Riva A, Cossu M, Testa-Riva F A scanning and transmission electron microscope study of the human ampulla ductus deferentis J Anat 129 858–860A, 1979
64 Riva A, Cossu M, Testa-Riva F, Usai E Spermiofagia nelle cellule epiteliali dell'ampolla deferenziale e delle vescicole seminali umane Studio al microscopio elettronico a trasmissione e scansione Arch Ital Anat Embriol S84 148A, 1979
65 Riva A, Cossu M, Usai E, Testa-Riva F Spermatophagy by epithelial cells of the seminal vesicle and of the ampulla ductus deferentis in man A scanning and transmission EM study In Oligozoospermia Recent Progress in Andrology G Fraiese, ESE Hafez, E Conti, A Fabrini (eds) New York Raven Press, 1981, pp 45–53
66 Riva A, Stockwell RA A histochemical study of human seminal vesicle epithelium J Anat 104 153–262, 1969
67 Riva A Testa-Riva F, Usai E, Cossu M The ampulla ductus deferentis in man, as viewed by SEM and TEM Arch Androl 8 157–164, 1982
68 Riva A, Usai E Histochemical demonstration of sorbitol dehydrogenase (ketose reductase) in human seminal vesicle epithelium Fertil Steril 21 341–343, 1970
69 Riva A, Usai E, Cossu M, Scarpa R, Testa-Riva F Anatomia ultrastrutturale delle ghiandole annesse all apparato genitale dell uomo In Attualita in Andrologia R Giorgino, G Abbaticchio (eds) Bologna Monduzzi 1985 pp 1–12
70 Riva A, Usai E, Pinna A, Lantini MS Scarpa R Marchisio AM Testa-Riva F L epitelio dei dotti eiaculatori del l uomo Studio al microscopio elettronico a trasmissione ed a scansione In Atti 3° Congr naz Soc it Androl Roma Gelmini 1982 pp 129–132
71 Riva A, Usai E, Scarpa R, Cossu M, Lantini MS Fine structure of the accessory glands of the human male genital tract In Developments in Ultrastructure of Reproduction Progress in Clinical and Biological Research, Vol 296 PM Motta (ed) New York Alan R Liss, 1989, pp 233–240
72 Riva A, Zaccheo D, Testa-Riva F A SEM study of human parotid and submandibular glands Proceedings of the XI International Congress on Electron Microscopy, Kyoto, 1986, pp 2863–2864
73 Roosen-Runge EC, Holstein AF The human rete testis Cell Tissue Res 189 409–433, 1978
74 Sirigu P, Cossu M, Usai E Rilievi istochimici sull' epitelio dell'ampolla deferenziale umana Boll Soc Ital Biol Sper 55 2477–2482, 1979
75 Spring Mills E The seminal vesicles In Male Accessory Glands E Spring-Mills, ESE Hafez (eds) Amsterdam Elsevier, 1979, pp 63–77
76 Stieve H Mannliche Genitalorgane In Handbuch der Mikroskopischen Anatomie des Menschen, Vol 7 2 W v Mollendorf (ed) Berlin Springer, 1930, pp 1–399
77 Szymonowicz L Lehrbuch der Histologie und der mikroskopischen Anatomie Wurzburg Kabitzsch, 1900
78 Takahashi-Iwanaga H, Fujita S Application of an NaOH maceration method to a scanning electron microscopic observation of Ito cells in the rat liver Arch Histol Jpn 49 349–357, 1986
79 Tanaka K, Mitsushima A A preparation method for observing intracellular structures by scanning electron microscopy J Microsc (Oxford) 133 213–222, 1984
80 Trainer TD Testis and excretory duct system In Histology for Pathologists SS Sternberg (ed) New York Raven Press, 1992, pp 731–747
81 Vitali-Mazza L Le modificazioni strutturali delle vescichette seminali nelle varie eta' Riv Anat Patol 11 739–761, 1956
82 Wang YF, Holstein AF Intraepithelial lymphocytes and macrophages in human epididymis Cell Tissue Res 233 517–521, 1983
83 Watzka M Zur Kenntnis der menschlichen Samenblase Z Mikrosk Anat Forsch 54 396–418, 1943
84 Weber AF Frommer SP Nuclear bodies Their prevalence, location and ultrastructure in the calf Science 141 912–913, 1963
85 Wendler D Histologisch-histochemische Befunde an der Schleimhaut des ductus deferens (pars funicularis) beim geschlechtsreifen Mann Acta Histochem 31 48–69, 1968
86 Wittstock G, Kirchner Y Zur Biomorphose der Samenblase unter besonderer Berucksichtigung der chronischen Spermatocystitis Virch Arch 351 12–20, 1970
87 Wong YC Surface features of epithelium of the seminal vesicle in young adult and old guinea pigs and after castration Acta Anat 116 257–264, 1983
88 Zaccheo D, Riva A Studio ultrastrutturale di inclusioni nucleari nelle vescichette seminali dell'uomo Acc naz Lincei Rend Cl Sc fis mat nat XLIII 1967, pp 582–585
89 Zecchi S, Pacini P, Orlandini G Vas deferens and seminal vesicles epithelium after castration A SEM study Andrologia 14 143–149 1982

CHAPTER 4

Secretion and Endocytosis in the Seminal Vesicles

LUCINDA R. MATA

1. Introduction

The seminal vesicles are accessory glands of the male genital tract that contribute their secretions to the seminal plasma and whose structure and function depend mainly on androgens. Although the seminal vesicles have often been overlooked and considered as redundant in reproduction, it is now recognized that their secretions assist in a number of ways to ensure fertility, namely, through their role in the immunology of reproduction [1,8,52]. Characterization of the components of seminal vesicle secretion and understanding of its regulation are hence of utmost importance.

In the work summarized in this review, the secretory activity of seminal vesicle epithelial cells has been approached from a morphofunctional point of view, in connection with endocytosis and testosterone interference. The main trend of such work seeks to gain further insight into the regulation of secretory activity in seminal vesicle epithelial cells and to unravel the specific functional role of endocytosis in such cells.

2. Secretory Cycle

Seminal vesicle epithelial cells contribute a protein-rich secretion containing a wide variety of ions and small molecules to the seminal plasma, thus making up a substantial part of this plasma in many species, including man [6,19]. The time sequence and pathway of seminal vesicle secretory protein has been traced by electron microscope autoradiography (EMAR) in the hamster [30], rat [16], and mouse [48]. In the hamster, ^{3}H-leucine was used in vitro in pulse-labeling experiments, whereas in the rat and mouse in vivo labeling was performed using either ^{3}H-leucine or ^{3}H-threonine, respectively. Despite these differences in experimental protocols, the results obtained are substantially similar.

Incorporation of radioactive amino acids, as studied by EMAR in seminal vesicle secretory cells, shows a wave of label moving through the RER, Golgi complex, and apical secretory granules reaching the luminal content within 30 minutes. Maximum labeling in the RER is observed within 5 minutes from the onset of labeling, whereas in the Golgi complex the labeling peak occurs after 15 minutes [30,48].

The secretory pathway of exportable protein in the seminal vesicle conforms to the general pattern first described in the exocrine pancreas [24], but the secretory cycle duration is shorter than in other exocrine glands [7], including the ventral prostate [17] and coagulating gland [47,48].

3. Endocytic Kinetics and Pathways

Although the most conspicuous activity of seminal vesicle epithelial cells is manufacture of secretory protein for export, some of their ultrastructural features, as first noticed in the mouse [12], indicate that these secretory cells might also take up macromolecules from the gland lumen.

In epithelial cells of hamster seminal vesicle,

Riva A., Testa Riva, F., and Motta, P.M., (eds.), Ultrastructure of Male Urogenital Glands: Prostate, Seminal Vesicles, Urethral, and Bulbourethral Glands. © *1994 Kluwer Academic Publishers. ISBN 0-7923-2800-0.*

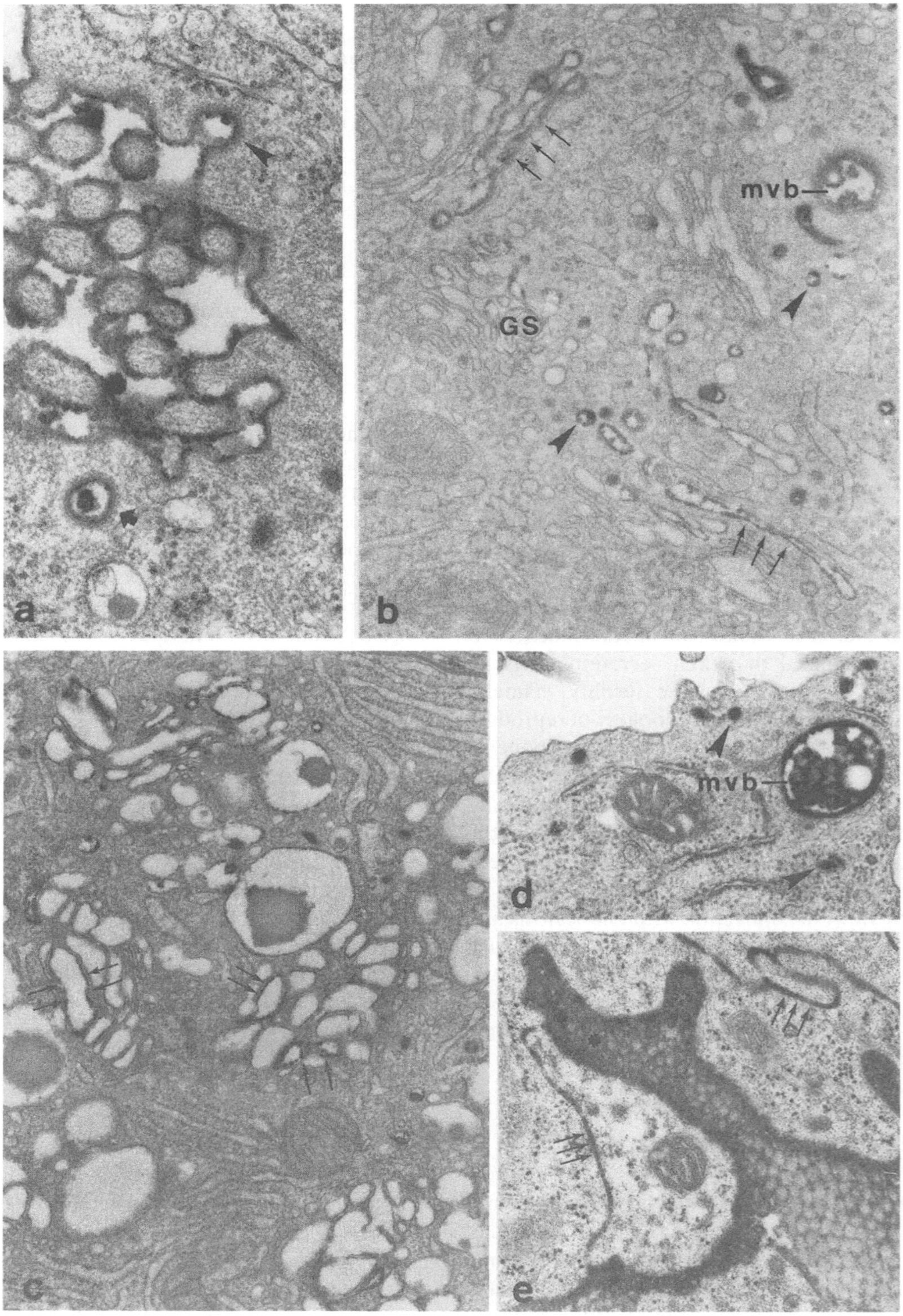

Fig. 1. Electron micrographs illustrating endocytosed HRP labeling in seminal vesicle epithelial cells of guinea pig (a,b), hamster (c), and rat (d,e). *a:* A coated pit (arrowhead) and an apical vesicle (arrow) containing HRP. *b,c:* HRP in Golgi cisterns (arrows), Golgi vesicles (arrowheads), and multivesicular bodies. *d,e:* HRP in apical vesicles (arrowheads), multivesicular bodies, intercellular spaces (arrows) and subepithelial region (asterisk) (a, ×60,000; b, ×42,000; c, ×25,000; d,e, ×30,000; GS = Golgi stack; mvb = multivesicular body).

apical coated vesicles, known to be involved in protein endocytosis, are observed in adult animals as well as during postnatal differentiation, as soon as secretory material starts to be released into the lumen [31]. This observation and the presence of complex interdigitations between cells suggest their possible involvement in the absorption and transcellular transport of substances stored in the gland lumen.

In fact, endocytosis was confirmed in the hamster seminal vesicle using either horseradish peroxidase (HRP) [29,33] or radioiodinated secretory protein [37] as tracers. HRP is taken up from the gland lumen by endocytic vesicles, which after pinching off from the apical membrane fuse with the membrane of other cell compartments, thus allowing their labeling. The endocytic pathway includes, besides the endocytic vesicles, multivesicular bodies and lysosomes, secretory vacuoles, and Golgi cisternae, from where HRP is later cleared, probably along with secretion. Endocytosis in hamster seminal vesicle epithelial cells is cyclic [29] and correlates with the secretory cycle [36]. Endocytosed secretory proteins follow the same pathway as HRP [37]. Transcellular transport of tracers through the intercellular spaces below tight junctions is also observed in these secretory cells.

The endocytic pathway shown in the hamster seminal vesicle secretory cells is not unique, as it is also observed in rat and guinea-pig seminal vesicle (Fig. 1). The endocytic activity of seminal vesicle secretory cells has been interpreted in connection with membrane recovery [29,33], which is of utmost importance in exocrine cells, and with a possible feedback mechanism for the regulation of protein secretion [37].

4. Membrane Recycling

As first pointed out by Palade [44], a mechanism must exist to remove the excess membrane added by exocytosis to the apical cell surface of exocrine cells in order to maintain a constant cell size. Whether the membrane to be removed would be degraded, dismantled into constituents to be subsequently reassembled, or reutilized as such, was for some years a matter for debate. The inclusion of secretory vacuoles and Golgi cisternae in the endocytic pathway of seminal vesicle secretory cells [33] provided the first evidence of the possible reutilization of internalized membrane in those compartments of exocrine cells. Comparable results were obtained in endocrine cells [45] and were later extended to other secretory cells [15].

Membrane reutilization and recycling were recently demonstrated in seminal vesicle secretory cells [32]. Apical glycoproteins of the seminal vesicle secretory cells were covalently labeled with ^{3}H-galactose, and their pathway during endocytosis was followed by EMAR. Quantitative analysis of autoradiograms showed that the internalized membrane is transferred to several compartments, including Golgi cisternae, secretory vacuoles, and the basolateral domain of the cell membrane, and later is recycled back to the apical surface of seminal vesicle secretory cells. This study, by using covalently labeled membrane components, provides for the first time the direct evidence required to establish membrane reutilization in the exocytic pathway and the involvement of Golgi cisternae and secretory vacuoles in the recycling pathway. The possible involvement of the basolateral domain of the cell membrane in the recycling pathway is also suggested by data obtained in this work.

5. Effect of Testosterone

It is well established that testosterone withdrawal induces a decline in the secretory activity of the seminal vesicles as well as alterations in the pattern of their secretory proteins and ultimately leads to gland involution (for a recent review see Aumuller and Seitz [5]). The morphologic equivalents of this process as shown in the rat [11] include a decrease in epithelial cell size and number, a reduction in the endoplasmic reticulum and Golgi complex, and a pronounced decrease in secretory granule size and number, leading to the disappearance of secretory material. This general pattern of involution applies to other species as well, with variations in chronology and extent of regressive events [53,55]. The hamster seminal vesicle epithelial cells keep their secretory activity up to at least 6 months after castration and are one extreme of such variation [35].

The effect of testosterone withdrawal on the

secretory activity of the hamster seminal vesicle was approached at the ultrastructural level by morphometric analysis [35] and autoradiography [34]. These studies showed a reduction in epithelial cell size and number to about 50–60% and a significant decrease in the rough endoplasmic reticulum and Golgi complex. Nevertheless, the number and size of apical secretory granules, as well as the amount of intracellular secretory material, are increased following castration. This apparent contradiction is a consequence of the fact that the synthesis of secretory proteins is not abolished, whereas their intracellular transport and exocytic rate are delayed, in epithelial cells lasting after orchidectomy [34,36]. In fact, quantitative analysis of autoradiograms showed that in castrated animals a relatively higher amount of newly synthesized secretory proteins was retained in the RER and Golgi complex, whereas a relatively smaller amount was transported to the secretory vacuoles and released to the lumen.

Castration-resistant secretion detected in the hamster seminal vesicle is useful for disclosure of testosterone interference with the transport and exocytosis of secretory proteins, which is otherwise impossible to perceive. The presence of secretion in seminal vesicle secretory cells after testosterone withdrawal has also been noted in the guinea pig [55] and, to a certain extent, the mouse [53] and has been attributed to a possible extratesticular source of androgens, most likely the adrenals. This hypothesis has been tested in guinea pig [51] and hamster seminal vesicles [46].

In castrated hamsters no further changes were observed in seminal vesicle secretory activity following either treatment with cyproterone acetate (CPA), which is an established antiandrogen, or adrenalectomy. The ultrastructure of the components involved in seminal vesicle secretion, as well as total protein synthesis and the electrophoretic pattern of secretory proteins, were similar in nontreated and CPA-treated or adrenalectomized castrated hamsters [46]. Therefore, in the hamster, apparently unlike the guinea pig [51], the secretory activity that lasts after testosterone withdrawal does not depend on nontesticular androgens. Hormonal control of this castration-resistant secretion is still an open question.

Testosterone withdrawal affects the endocytic activity of seminal vesicle epithelial cells as well. In the hamster, endocytosis is decreased in seminal vesicle secretory cells, and its kinetics is delayed following testosterone withdrawal [36]. The endocytic pathway in castrated hamsters involves the same compartments as in intact animals, but labeling of Golgi cisternae is delayed by 20 minutes following testosterone withdrawal. Labeling of Golgi cisternae coincides with a significant peak in the number of endocytic vesicles, which is also significantly smaller following castration. The slowdown of Golgi labeling kinetics and the decrease in number of endocytic vesicles are reversed by increasing exocytosis with pilocarpine treatment of castrated hamsters [36], thus showing that endocytosis is coupled with exocytosis in seminal vesicle secretory cells.

6. Cultivated Seminal Vesicle Epithelial Cells

As discussed above, epithelial cells of the seminal vesicle displaying a short secretory cycle are very active in secretion as well as in endocytosis, and these activities depend on testosterone, which allows their experimental manipulation. Because of these features, seminal vesicle epithelial cells have proven to be a successful model to study secretion, endocytosis, and membrane traffic in exocrine cells. However, further insight into the effect of hormones and other factors, namely, neurotransmitters and regulatory peptides, in secretion as well as endocytosis would rather

→

Fig 2 Secretory activity of cultivated seminal vesicle epithelial cells (SVEP) *a,b* secretory granules (arrowheads) in the apical region and Golgi zone of HSVEP, GS = Golgi stack, mvb = multivesicular body (a, ×42,000, b, ×30,000) *c* Fluorography of protein recovered from HSVEP medium after incubation with ^{35}S-Met (2 hours) in the absence (lane 1) or presence (lane 2) of monensin Notice the band in lane 1 (arrow), which is much denser than in lane 2, showing that monensin partially inhibits the release of protein to the culture medium, lane 3, molecular weight markers *d,e* Fluorographs of protein released by hamster seminal vesicle slices (d) and HSVEP (e) incubated with ^{35}S-Met (d, 90 minutes, e, overnight) Five major bands are observed in both, but whereas the molecular weight range is 28–90 kD for proteins secreted by gland slices (d), it is 43–87 kD for those released by HSVEP (e) Scales in kilodaltons

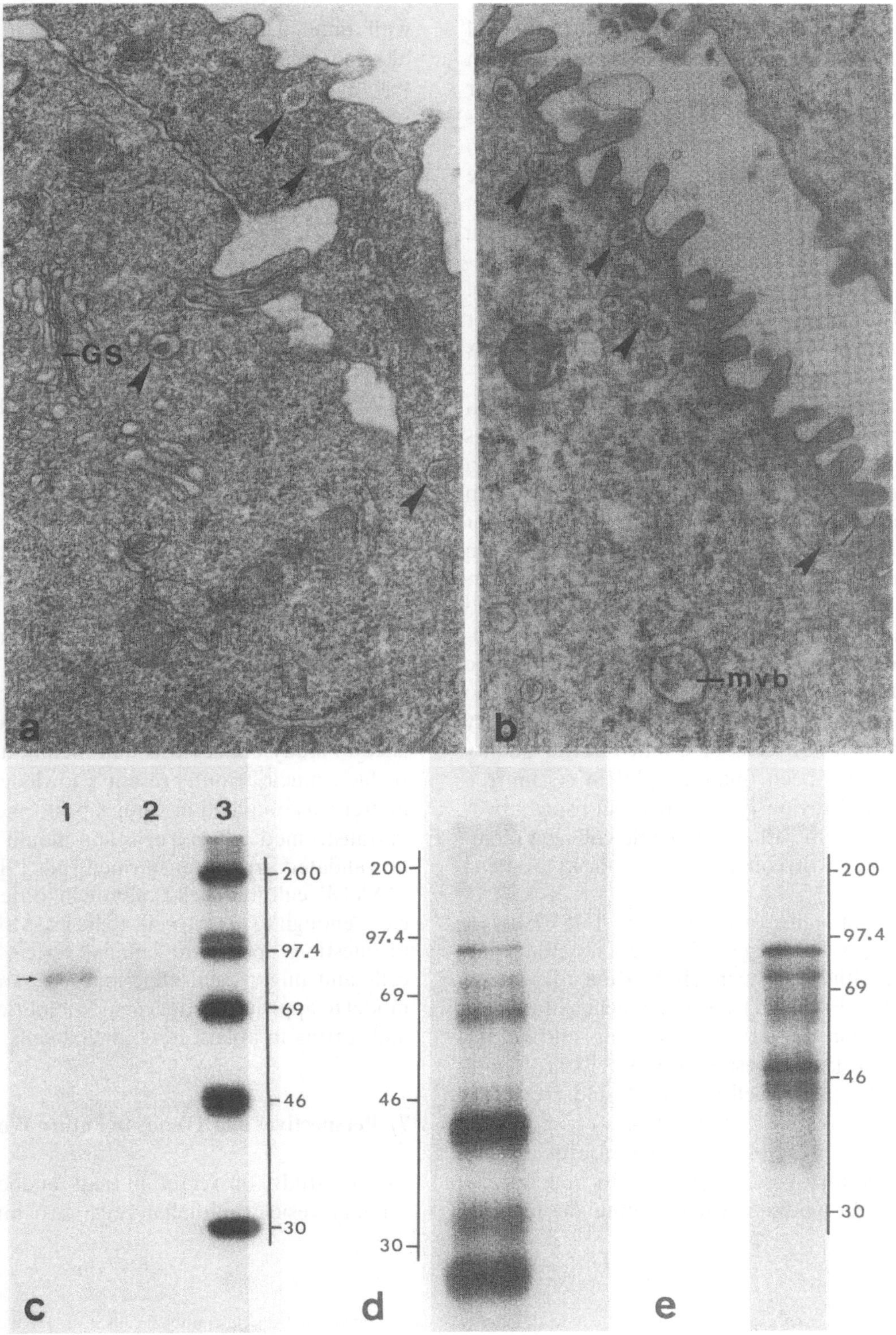

GS
a
mvb
b
1
2
3
200
97.4
69
46
30
c
200
97.4
69
46
30
d
e
200
97.4
69
46
30

require cultivation of seminal vesicle epithelial cells in a chemically defined medium, to and from which these components can be rapidly added or removed in precise concentrations.

During the 1980s, several attempts to establish seminal vesicle epithelial cells in culture were described. In most cases, 5–20% serum was required for cell growth [25,26,28,50], which is a serious drawback in hormonal studies. When cultivated in serum-free medium, the growth of seminal vesicle epithelial cells was reported either to require a three-dimensional collagen matrix [54] or to be very limited [38].

In fact, although sustained growth of guinea pig seminal vesicle epithelial cells (SVEP) was achieved for 8–10 days, allowing confluence of a few islets, full confluence was not reached in chemically defined medium and their behavior was different from in vivo [38]. SVEP cells grown in chemically defined medium were able to perform endocytosis, but the endocytic pathway did not include Golgi cisternae. They were polarized, displaying apical microvilli and desmosomelike junctions, but were rather flat in shape and no signs of secretory activity were observed. Primary cultures of SVEP cells of a much better quality have recently been obtained [39] in serum-free medium, as previously described but using a two-chamber system with a permeable collagen membrane instead of collagen-coated flasks or Petri dishes.

Epithelial cells from hamster (HSVEP) or guinea pig (GPSVEP) seminal vesicles attach and grow in either collagen (ICN Biomedicals) or transwell-col (Costar) inserts, reaching full confluence within 5–7 days after seeding, and last for at least 20 days. These cultured cells are about 10 μm tall, appear well polarized, and are active in secretion as well as endocytosis.

HSVEP cells grown in such inserts display apical secretory vesicles (Fig. 2a,b) and release protein to the medium, which accumulates linearly with time. The release of proteins is partially blocked by monensin (Fig. 2c), which is consistent with their being secretory proteins. The secretory activity of the cultured HSVEP cells is nevertheless lower than in vivo, as illustrated by (a) the size of secretory vesicles, which is about one third of the in vivo secretory vacuoles; (b) the duration of the secretory cycle, which is twice that in vivo; and (c) the amount of secreted protein, which is about 5% instead of 10% of total protein, as in vivo. The electrophoretic mobility of SVEP secreted proteins is also different from in vivo secreted proteins (Fig. 2d,e).

As for endocytic activity, HSVEP cells take up HRP and cationized ferritin (Fig. 3a–d), although displaying slower kinetics than in vivo. HRP labels the Golgi complex 60 minutes instead of 15 minutes after labeling, as in vivo. HSVEP cells grown on microporous collagen membrane (transwell-col inserts, Costar) are also able to endocytose tracers from the outer chamber medium through the basolateral domain of the cell membrane (Fig. 3e,f). Such primary cultures, where both the apical and basolateral domain of the cell membrane can be reached, might be of great importance to study endocytosis and membrane traffic. In fact, much of our present knowledge on this matter was obtained in studies performed mostly in transformed cultured cells and should therefore be validated in nontransformed cells [9].

SVEP cultured cells, although different, are close enough to in vivo cells to be used for analysis of questions specific to seminal vesicle secretory cells and might be useful, more generally, as a model to approach endocytosis, membrane traffic, and sorting in polarized epithelial cells.

7. Perspectives and Trends in Future Work

In the study of secretion and endocytosis in seminal vesicle epithelial cells, two main ques-

→

Fig. 3. Electron micrographs illustrating the endocytic activity of cultivated seminal vesicle epithelial cells. *a–c*: HRP endocytosed through the cell apex labeling tubulovesicular structures (arrowheads), multivesicular bodies, intercellular spaces (long arrows), and Golgi cisterns (small arrows). *d*: Cationized ferritin taken up through the cell apex labeling tubulovesicular structures (arrowheads) and a multivesicular body. *e,f*: HRP endocytosed through the basolateral cell membrane in tubulovesicular structures (arrowheads) and a multivesicular body and faintly labeling Golgi cisterns (arrows). mvb = multivesicular body, GS = Golgi stack (a,e,f, ×30,000; b,c,d, ×42,000)

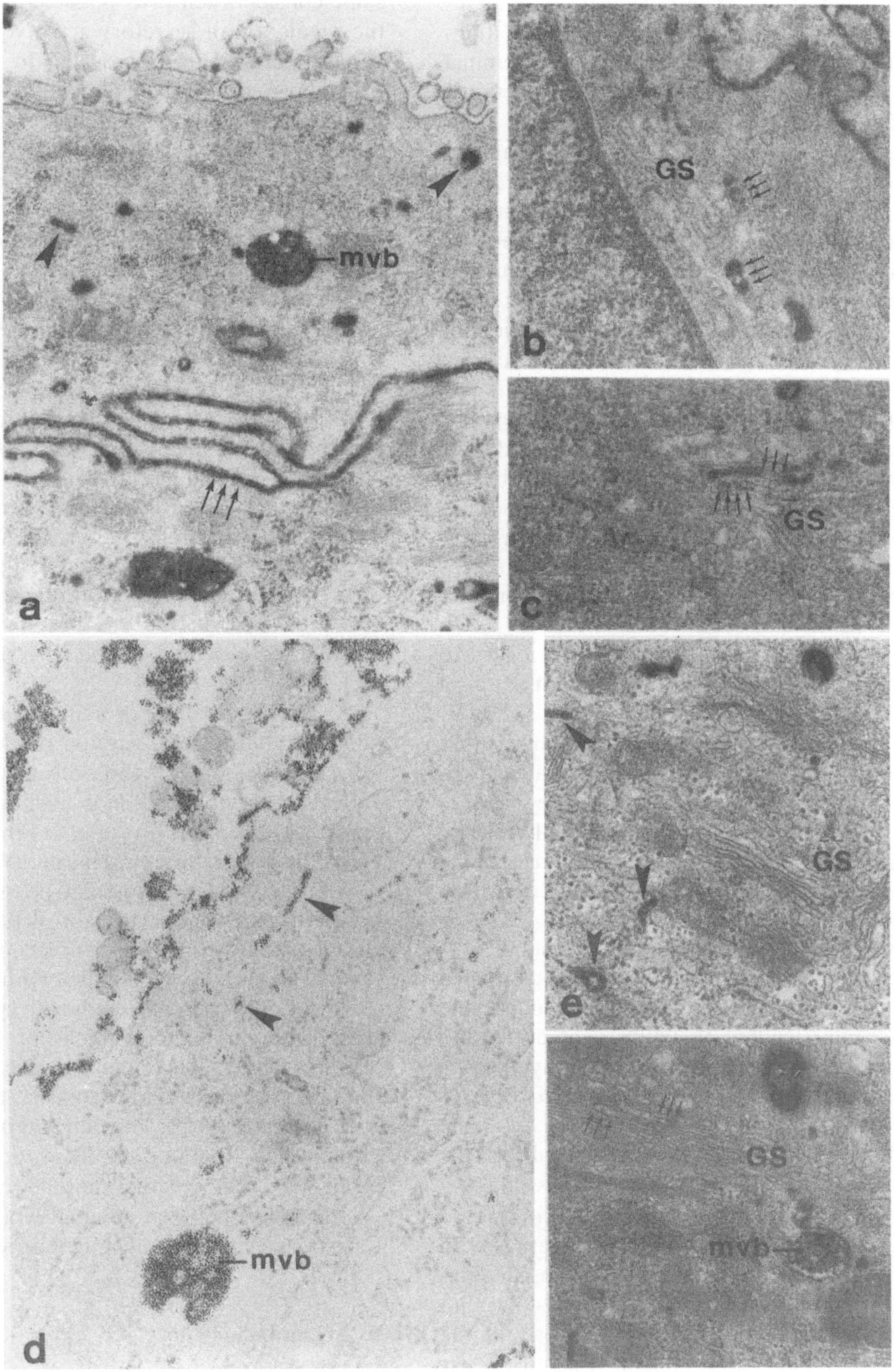
mvb
a
GS
b
GS
c
mvb
d
GS
e
GS
mvb

tions have emerged that deserve further comment. One relates to hormonal regulation of castration-resistant secretion, as detected in hamster seminal vesicle, and the other to the possible functional role of endocytosis in the entire gland.

The secretory activity observed in the hamster seminal vesicle after castration might be due either to an irreversible early action of androgens (neonatal "imprinting") or to the fact that castration-resistant secretion might be regulated through nonandrogenic hormones and/or nonhormonal factors. In fact, although the structural and functional integrity of the seminal vesicles mostly depend on testosterone, other hormones, as well as growth factors and neuropeptides, are involved in their endocrine regulation [5,10,19]. Prolactin, which seems by itself to be able to interfere with the growth and function of male accessory glands [3,41,43], is one such hormone that might be worthwhile to investigate in connection with castration-resistant secretion in the hamster seminal vesicle.

As for the role of endocytosis with regard to the entire gland, besides its involvement in apical membrane recovery in seminal vesicle secretory cells, as mentioned in this review, two other possibilities should be considered. Endocytosis might be related to the mucosal immune response and to regulation of secretion in seminal vesicles.

It is well established that epithelial cells lining the digestive, respiratory, and urogenital systems play key roles in immune defense. Antigens endocytosed from the lumen by epithelial cells are transcytosed and presented to intraepithelial lymphocytes, thus triggering the mucosal immune response and leading to delivery of antibodies into secretions [27,42]. Intraepithelial lymphocytelike cells, sometimes referred a *halo cells* or *migratory cells*, have been observed in the male reproductive tract [4,11,14,23], specifically, in the seminal vesicles [2,40], and their possible immunological significance has been considered [2,23]. The presence of such cells together with the transepithelial transport of proteins demonstrated in the seminal vesicles is consistent with the possible involvement of endocytosis in the mucosal immune response of these glands.

Another physiological role of endocytosis in the seminal vesicles that should also be given some consideration is its possible involvement in the regulation of secretory activity. The seminal vesicle secretory cells are able to take up and transcytose to the subepithelial region and to blood-vessel secretory proteins stored in the gland lumen [37]. One can speculate that transcytosed protein might bind to androgens and somehow modulate their action on secretory cells. There are suggestions in the literature that make this possibility reasonable.

Sertoli cells secrete an androgen-binding protein (ABP) into the lumen of seminiferous tubules, which they most likely take up and transcytose basally. In fact, Sertoli cells have been shown to transcytose protein from the lumen of the seminiferous tubules [49] and to secrete ABP apically (80%) and basally (20%) [20]. The secretory pathway of ABP has not been shown, but since only 20% is released basally it may be that all the protein is first secreted to the lumen and then partly transcytosed from there. ABP in the lumen of the tubules reaches the epididymis, where it is also endocytosed by principal cells [18].

Androgen binding proteins have also been demonstrated in the secretion produced by cells of the prostate [22] and salivary glands [13]. Apical endocytosis has not been shown in the epithelial cells of the prostate, but the presence of one of their secretory proteins in the subepithelial region is consistent with that possibility [6]. In salivary glands, endocytosis of secretory proteins is well established [21], and it is conceivable that it might eventually include their androgen binding protein. Sertoli cells and epididymal principal cells share with the secretory cells of the prostate, salivary glands, and seminal vesicle the fact that they are target cells for androgens. It makes sense to hypothesize that production and/or endocytosis of androgen binding proteins in such cells might be involved in modulating androgen action exerted on them. Further experimental work is required to test this hypothesis and might prove rewarding.

8. Acknowledgments

I wish to thank Dr. Erik Christensen for his comments and useful suggestions.

References

1 Adjiman M Dysfunction of the seminal vesicle and male infertility In Seminal Vesicles and Fertility Biology and Pathology C Bollack, A Clavert (eds) Basel Karger, 1985, pp 158–161

2 Allison VF, Cearley GW Jr Electron microscopic study of cells within the epithelium of the seminal vesicle of aging rats Anat Rec 172 262, 1972

3 Arunakaran J, Aruldhas MM, Govindarajulu P Effect of prolactin and androgens on the prostate of bonnet monkeys, *Macaca radiata* I Nucleic acids, phosphatases and citric acid Prostate 10 265–274, 1987

4 Aumuller G, Greenberg J Seasonal changes in the fine structure of the accessory sex gland in the mole (*Talpa europea*) Cell Tissue Res 175 403–416, 1976

5 Aumuller G, Seitz J Protein secretion and secretory processes in male accessory sex glands Int Rev Cytol 121 127–231, 1990

6 Carmo-Fonseca M, Vaz Y Immunocytochemical localization and lectin-binding properties of the 22KDa secretory protein from rat ventral prostate Biol Reprod 40 153–164, 1989

7 Case RM Synthesis, intracellular transport and discharge of exportable proteins in the pancreatic acinar cell and other cells Biol Rev 53 211–354, 1978

8 Clavert A, Gabriel-Robez O, Montagnon D Physiological role of the seminal vesicles In Seminal Vesicles and Fertility Biology and Pathology C Bollack, A Clavert (eds) Basel Karger, 1985, pp 80–94

9 Courtoy PJ In Endocytosis From Cell Biology to Health, Disease and Therapy NATO ASI Series, Series H Cell Biology, Vol 62 PJ Courtoy (ed) Heidelberg Springer-Verlag, 1992, pp XIII–XVIII

10 Dadoune JP Functional morphology of the seminal vesicle epithelium In Seminal Vesicles and Fertility Biology and Pathology C Bollack, A Clavert (eds) Basel Karger, 1985, pp 18–35

11 Dahl E, Tveter KJ The ultrastructure of the accessory sex organs of the male rat III The post-castration involution of the coagulating gland and the seminal vesicle Z Zellforsch Mikrosk Anat 144 179–189, 1973

12 Deane HW, Wurzelman S Electron microscope observations on the postnatal differentiation of the seminal vesicle epithelium of the laboratory mouse Am J Anat 117 91–134, 1965

13 Dlouhy SR, Nichols WC, Karn RC Production of an antibody to mouse salivary androgen binding protein (ABP) and its use in identifying a prostate protein produced by a gene distinct from Abp Bioch Genet 24 743–763, 1986

14 Dym M, Romrell LJ Intraepithelial lymphocytes in the male reproductive tract of rats and Rhesus monkeys J Reprod Fert 42 1–7, 1975

15 Farquhar MG Multiple pathways of exocytosis, endocytosis, and membrane recycling Validation of a Golgi route Fed Proc 42 2407–2413, 1983

16 Flickinger CJ Synthesis, intracellular transport, and release of secretory protein in the seminal vesicle of the rat, as studied by electron microscope radioautography Anat Rec 180 407–427, 1974

17 Flickinger CJ Protein secretion in the rat ventral prostate and the relation of Golgi vesicles, cisternae and vacuoles, as studied by electron microscope radioautography Anat Rec 180 427–449, 1974

18 Gerard A, Khanfri J, Gueant JL, Fremont S, Nicolas JP, Grignon G, Gerard H Electron microscope radioautographic evidence of in vivo androgen-binding protein internalization in the rat epididymis principal cells Endocrinology 122 1297–1307, 1988

19 Gonzales GF Functional structure and ultrastructure of seminal vesicles Arch Androl 22 1–13, 1989

20 Hadley MA, Djakiew D, Byers SW, Dym M Polarized secretion of androgen-binding protein and transferrin by Sertoli cells grown in a bicameral culture system Endocrinology 120 1097–1103, 1987

21 Hand AR, Coleman R, Mazariegos MR, Lustmann J, Lotti LV Endocytosis of secretory proteins by salivary gland duct cells J Dent Res 66 412–419, 1987

22 Heyns W, De Moor P Prostatic binding protein A steroid-binding protein secreted by the rat prostate Eur J Biochem 78 221–230, 1977

23 Hoffer AP, Hamilton DW, Fawcett DW The ultrastructure of the principal cells and intraepithelial leukocytes in the initial segment of the rat epididymis Anat Rec 175 169–202, 1973

24 Jamieson JD, Palade GE Intracellular transport of secretory proteins in the pancreatic exocrine cell II Transport to condensing vacuoles and zymogen granules J Cell Biol 34 597–615, 1967

25 Kierszenbaum AL, DePhilip RM, Spruill WA, Takenaka I Isolation and culture of rat seminal vesicle epithelial cells The use of the secretory protein SVSIV as a funcional probe Exp Cell Res 145 293–304, 1983

26 Kinghorn EM, Bate AS, Higgins SJ Growth of rat seminal vesicle epithelial cells in culture Neurotransmitters are required for androgen-regulated synthesis of tissue-specific secretory proteins Endocrinology 121 1678–1689, 1987

27 Kraehenbuhl JP Michetti HR, Perregaux C, Mekalanus J, Neutra M Role of transepithelial transport in triggering a mucosal immune response and in delivery of mucosal antibodies into secretions In Endocytosis From Cell Biology to Health, Disease and Therapy NATO ASI Series, Series H Cell Biology, Vol 62 PJ Courtoy (ed) Heidelberg Springer-Verlag, 1992, pp 363–366

28 Lieber MM, Barham SS, Veneziale CM In vitro propagation of seminal vesicle epithelial cells Invest Urol 17 348–355, 1980

29 Mata LR Dynamics of HRPase absorption in the epithelial cells of the hamster seminal vesicle J Microsc Biol Cell 25 127–132 1976

30 Mata LR The secretory cycle of the hamster seminal vesicle epithelial cells as studied in vitro by electron microscopic autoradiography Biol Cell 36 25–28, 1979

31 Mata LR Estudo morfo-funcional das celulas secretoras

da vesicula seminal do Criceto (summary in English) Doctoral thesis, University of Lisbon, 1981

32 Mata LR, Christensen EI Redistribution and recycling of internalized membrane in seminal vesicle secretory cells Biol Cell 68 183–193, 1990

33 Mata LR, Davi-Ferreira JF Transport of exogenous peroxidase to Golgi cisternae in the hamster seminal vesicle J Microsc 17 103–106, 1973

34 Mata LR, David-Ferreira JF Testosterone interference with the intracellular transport of secretion in hamster seminal vesicle Biol Cell 46 101–104, 1982

35 Mata LR, David-Ferreira JF Secretory cell activity in the hamster seminal vesicle following castration A morphometric ultrastructural study Biol Cell 53 165–178, 1985

36 Mata LR, David-Ferreira JF Testosterone interferes with the kinetics of endocytosis in the hamster seminal vesicle Biol Cell 68 195–203, 1990

37 Mata LR, Maunsbach AB Absorption of secretory protein by the epithelium of hamster seminal vesicle as studied by electron microscope autoradiography Biol Cell 46 65–74, 1982

38 Mata LR, Petersen OW, Van Deurs B Endocytosis in guinea-pig seminal vesicle epithelial cells cultivated in chemically defined medium Biol Cell 58 211–220, 1986

39 Mata LR, Rodrigues G, Pinho M Secretion and endocytosis in polarized seminal vesicle epithelial cells cultivated in a two-chamber system Abstracts of Coloquio Franco-Iberico de Microscopia Elctronica, Universitat de Barcelona, 1991, pp 66–67

40 Mitune H, Noda Y, Mohri S, Suzuki S, Nishinakagawa H, Otsuka J Fine structure of the seminal vesicle epithelium of the mouse and golden hamster Exp Anim 35 149–158, 1986

41 Negro-Vilar A, Saad WA, McCann SM Evidence for a role of prolactin in prostate and seminal vesicle in immature male rats Endocrinology 100 729–737, 1977

42 Neutra MR, Kraehenbuhl J-P Transepithelial transport and mucosal defense I The role of M Cells Trends Cell Biol 2 134–138, 1992

43 Nevalainen MT, Valve EM, Makela SI, Blauer M, Tuohimaa PJ Harkonen PL Estrogen and prolactin regulation of the rat dorsal and lateral prostate in organ culture Endocrinology 129 612–622, 1991

44 Palade GE Functional changes in the structure of cell components In Subcellular Particles T Hayashi (ed) New York Ronald Press, 1959, pp 64–80

45 Pelletier G Secretion and uptake of peroxidase by rat adenohypophyseal cells J Ultrastruct Res 43 445–459, 1973

46 Pinho MS, Mata LR Castration-resistant secretion in the hamster seminal vesicle does not depend on androgens Int J Androl 15 435–447, 1992

47 Samuel LH, Flickinger CJ Intracellular pathway and kinetics of protein secretion in the coagulating gland of mouse Biol Reprod 34 107–117, 1986

48 Samuel LH, Flickinger CJ The relationship between the morphology of cell organelles and kinetics of the secretory glands of mice Cell Tissue Res 247 203–213, 1987

49 Soares-Pessoa JF, David-Ferreira JF Bi-directional transport of horseradish peroxidase by the rat Sertoli cells An in vitro study Biol Cell 39 301–304, 1980

50 Tajana GF, Locuratolo P, Metafora S, Abrescia P, Guardiola J Synthesis of a testosterone-dependent secretory protein by rat seminal vesicle-dervied cell lines EMBO J 3 637–644, 1984

51 Tam CC, Wong YC, Tang F Further regression of seminal vesicles of castrated guinea pig by administration of cyproterone acetate Acta Anat 124 65–73, 1985

52 Thaler CJ, Knapp PM, McIntyre JA, Coulam CB, Critser JK, Faulk WP Congenital aplasia of seminal vesicles Absence of trophoblast-lymphocyte cross-reactive antigens from seminal plasma Fertil Steril 53 948–949, 1990

53 Toner PG, Baillie AH Biochemical, histochemical and ultrastructural changes in the mouse seminal vesicle after castration J Anat 100 173–188, 1966

54 Tomooka Y, Harris SE, Mclachlan JA Growth of seminal vesicle epithelial cells in serum-free collagen gel culture In Vitro Cell Dev Biol 21 237–244, 1985

55 Tse MKW, Wong YC Structural study of the involution of the seminal vesicles of the guinea pig following orchiectomy Acta Anat 108 68–78, 1980

CHAPTER 5

Functional Morphology of Prostate Gland

GERHARD AUMÜLLER, JÜRGEN SEITZ, & ALESSANDRO RIVA

1. Introduction

In spite of intensive research, present knowledge of the basic factors responsible for the initiation and progress of prostate cancer is nearly as limited as it was 45 years ago, at a time when Huggins inaugurated contrasexual hormonal therapy [121, 268]. Prostate cancer has become an increasingly common disease among elderly men. It is associated with a high prevalence of latent cancer, but only a small fraction of these dormant cancers will ever grow to become clinically evident [94]. Current research in this area is concentrated on identifying the biological mechanisms that hold the growing process under control, with special reference to the nature and role of growth regulatory factors present in normal, as well as neoplastic, prostate glands. These studies will advance our understanding of the mechanisms involved in the pathogenesis of prostate cancer.

The etiology and pathogenesis of benign prostatic hyperplasia (BPH) are also yet unresolved questions, although a number of hypotheses have been developed, most of which still await experimental validation. BPH was regarded as (a) a kind of adenoma, (b) a stromal disease, (c) the result of either hormonal imbalance (altered estrogen/testosterone ratio) or (d) testosterone, dihydrotestosterone, or estrogen stimulation, either perinatal or presenescent. The responsiveness of prostate gland to testicular steroid hormones has been evident for a long time. There are no reported cases of prostate cancer or benign prostatic hyperplasia in individuals who underwent castration prior to the onset of puberty, for example, soprano singers in the papal chapel in the late middle ages. Prostate cancer appears to be androgen dependent during early stages of oncogenesis, as initial stimulation of prostatic growth is mediated by androgens.

More recently, scientific interest has focused on the presence and possible function of growth factors and their receptors in the human prostate, and their autocrine or paracrine stimulatory effects in BPH development. Hypotheses on hormonal regulation as well as their interplay during epithelial-stromal interaction have been developed. The intact human prostate produces epithelial (EGF) and fibroblast (FGF) growth factors. They do not generally appear to have autocrine or paracrine effects. In androgen deficiency, as shown experimentally in castrated rats, the stromal cells express increased amounts of transforming growth factor-beta (TGFβ), its receptor, and basic fibroblast growth factor (bFGF).

With platelet-derived growth factor (PDGF), however, the respective receptor has not been demonstrated in prostate. The growth factor receptor-associated tyrosine protein kinase is present in human prostate in two different forms, but its functional significance in BPH development is not yet elucidated. A more significant role may be attributed to the recently described growth factors in cultured human stromal cells, which exert multifarious mitogenic and nonmitogenic effects on prostatic epithelium as well as neuronal and non-neuronal cells (see below). The perspective of studying hormone-regulated growth

Riva, A., Testa Riva, F., and Motta, P M, (eds), Ultrastructure of Male Urogenital Glands Prostate, Seminal Vesicles, Urethral, and Bulbourethral Glands © 1994 Kluwer Academic Publishers ISBN 0-7923-2800-0 All rights reserved

factor activities in stromal-epithelial interaction during the pathogenesis of BPH seem most promising.

The prostate and seminal vesicles are usually described in a generalized manner as *accessory sex glands*. There are, however, a number of aspects that lead one to believe this designation is inadequate. The male accessory sex glands vary considerably in mammals with respect to their topographical location, size, morphology, and function. Reflecting the diversity of species-specific requirements of these glands for reproduction, their structure may be due to differences in environment and sexual habits. Secretions from highly developed and specialized accessory sex glands, for example, in rodents, are responsible for formation of the so-called copulatory plug (*bouchon vaginal*; for review see Williams-Ashman [276]), which was thought to serve as a means to prevent superfecundation. However, carnivores such as dogs and cats possess a prostate gland but lack a seminal vesicle. In boars and stallions, the seminal vesicles reach a substantial size, providing a large amount of seminal fluid (for review, see Mann and Lutwak-Mann [163]). In the human prostate, the major anion secreted is citrate, while in the rat citrate is secreted in the seminal vesicle in addition to the ventral and dorsolateral prostate. However, the prevalent anion in canine prostate is chloride, which is present in the human prostate in much lower concentrations. Another example is the distribution of zinc, which is homogeneous in human and canine prostates but is concentrated in the lateral prostate of the rat.

In addition to species variability, embryonic origin, topographic situation, the structure of the individual gland, and the temporal sequence in release of the secretion must be taken into consideration when comparing the functions of these glands in different species. The seminal vesicle, as well as the ampulla of the deferent duct, are derivatives of the Wolffian duct, that is, their postnatal development and maturation depend completely on the presence of androgens. The prostate is derived from the epithelium of the urogenital sinus (for review, see Cunha [62]) and serves both as an accessory sex gland as well as a urethral gland. An abortive form of the prostate is present in the female [275].

Both morphologically and functionally, there are a number of distinctive differences in the general organization of the prostate and seminal vesicles, which apply to several species, although with exceptions. The seminal vesicles are paired, elongated, saclike or tubulelike structures surrounded by a thick coat of smooth muscles. Each seminal vesicle empties into the posterior urethra separately through the ejaculatory ducts, allowing momentous bulk secretion. Their proximal and ampullary portions are capable of fluid reabsorption and spermatophagy.

The prostate, however, consists of branching secretory tubules and acini, which are surrounded by a fibromuscular stroma. The muscular component condenses peripherally to form the prostatic capsule and centrally merges into the muscle layers of the prostatic urethra. During ejaculation, the prostatic acini are compressed by their surrounding fibromuscular coat, emptying their contents into the posterior urethra. The internal organization of the gland allows a wavelike release of secretion covering the internal surface of the urethra. Thus, many a time the evacuation of prostatic acini remains incomplete and residual secretion condenses, forming prostatic calculi [263]. Immunohistochemistry of organ-specific proteins shows that there is considerable reflux and redistribution of prostatic secretion into the ejaculatory ducts, and of seminal vesicle secretion into the proximal portions of prostatic ducts (unpublished observations).

There is growing evidence of functional heterogeneity within the prostatic secretory duct system. In canine prostate, a gradual increase in the expression of morphological equivalents of secretion at the expense of surface cell structures is observed in the periurethral portion of the prostatic ducts along the direction of the capsule. Many cells contain estrogen receptors [218] in the periurethral zone. In the same zone, perinatal squamous epithelial metaplasia is observed and endocrine cells [2] are common. In the view of the authors, the internal structure of the prostate reflects both its role as an accessory sex gland and its origin as a urethral gland.

In addition to its contractile function, prostatic stroma plays a major static role, as it forms the mechanical scaffold of the capillaries, lymphatics, and nerves, providing the required oxygen, hormones, ions, and transmitter signals to the epithelium, and in removing metabolites from the cells. From a morphological [24,133,275], functional [44,209], and embryological point of view [60,136,239,238,240], prostatic epithelium and stroma form a functional unit that is connected by the matrix system (cytoskeleton, extracellular matrix), representing a common superstructure [124].

The search for suitable animal models, both in prostate cancer research and reproductive biology, has stimulated the morphological examination of a number of different species with regard to secretions of individual glands, hormonal responsitivity, and the relationship to the respective human gland, using electron microscopy, stereology, histochemistry, or immunohistochemistry. The canine [29,265] and monkey prostates [107, 216] represent the most suitable models for the human gland, though considerable differences exist, particularly with regard to innervation.

The human male genital tract receives dual autonomic innervation, sympathetic from the last thoracic and lumbar roots via the hypogastric nerves and parasympathetic via the pelvic nerves from the sacral roots [78,259]. In the prostate a more or less dense network of both adrenergic and cholinergic nerves [26,190,256] innervates smooth muscle septa as well as blood vessels. Nerve fibers containing vasointestinal polypeptide (VIP), predominantly associated with the epithelium [6], and met- and leu-enkephalin have been found in the human prostate [15,69,257,258]. Regional distribution pattern of the opioidergic nerves in the human and the canine prostate, respectively, suggests their possible involvement in the control of myovascular functions and reflexes, for example, in the regulation of vascular perfusion and fluid transport from the vessels into the acinar lumen. Alm et al. [6] suggested that VIP-containing nerves could be characteristic of sphincters, as they are numerous surrounding the ducts of the prostate at their openings in the urethra.

When combined, the aspects of innervation, general construction of the glands, internal structure, and means of voiding into the urethra are responsible for the regular sequential pattern of emission in the human, starting with the wave of secretion from the prostate (and Cowper's gland) required for the conditioning of the urethral surface. This is followed by sperm release through the ejaculatory ducts, ending with bulk secretion of the gelating content of seminal vesicle, which liquifies after deposition under the influence of prostatic secretion [155].

2. Developmental Aspects

2.1. Prenatal Development

Human fetal prostatic differentiation begins with mesenchymal proliferation in the urogenital sinus [136,139]. Epithelial bud formation occurs in the 10th developmental week [137]. Acinar cells differentiate into "secretory" prostatic cells at the time of highest androgen production in the fetal testis. Kellokumpu-Lehtinen [140] studied prostatic differentiation in human embryos by measuring crown-rump lengths of 43–130 mm (corresponding to an age of 9–15 weeks). At the age of 10 weeks, when the verumontanum is developed, histological development begins close to the openings of the mesonephric ducts by outgrowth of several buds of the urethral epithelium into the surrounding mesenchyme (Figs. 1–5). The epithelium of these outgrowths resembles that of the neighboring stratified urethral epithelium. It consists of cells with a large round or oval nucleus with smooth outlines, prominent nucleoli, and heterochromatin locally detached from the nuclear envelope. With the exception of rare Golgi complexes, cytoplasmic organelles (mitochondria, polysomes, some granular endoplasmic reticulum) are well developed, and usually are more prominent in the cells close to the urethral origin. The cells rest on an undulating or folded continuous basement membrane, which separates the epithelium from the surrounding mesenchyme. The initially solid buds acquire a lumen at their terminal or central portions by the end of the 11th week. During this time, cells with neuroendocrine characteristics already appear in the basal portions of the buds.

Between the 11th and 14th weeks, when the number of epithelial outgrowths increases, the lumen-containing buds transform into tubuloacinar gland anlagen. The epithelium of the primitive glands consists of layers of three to five

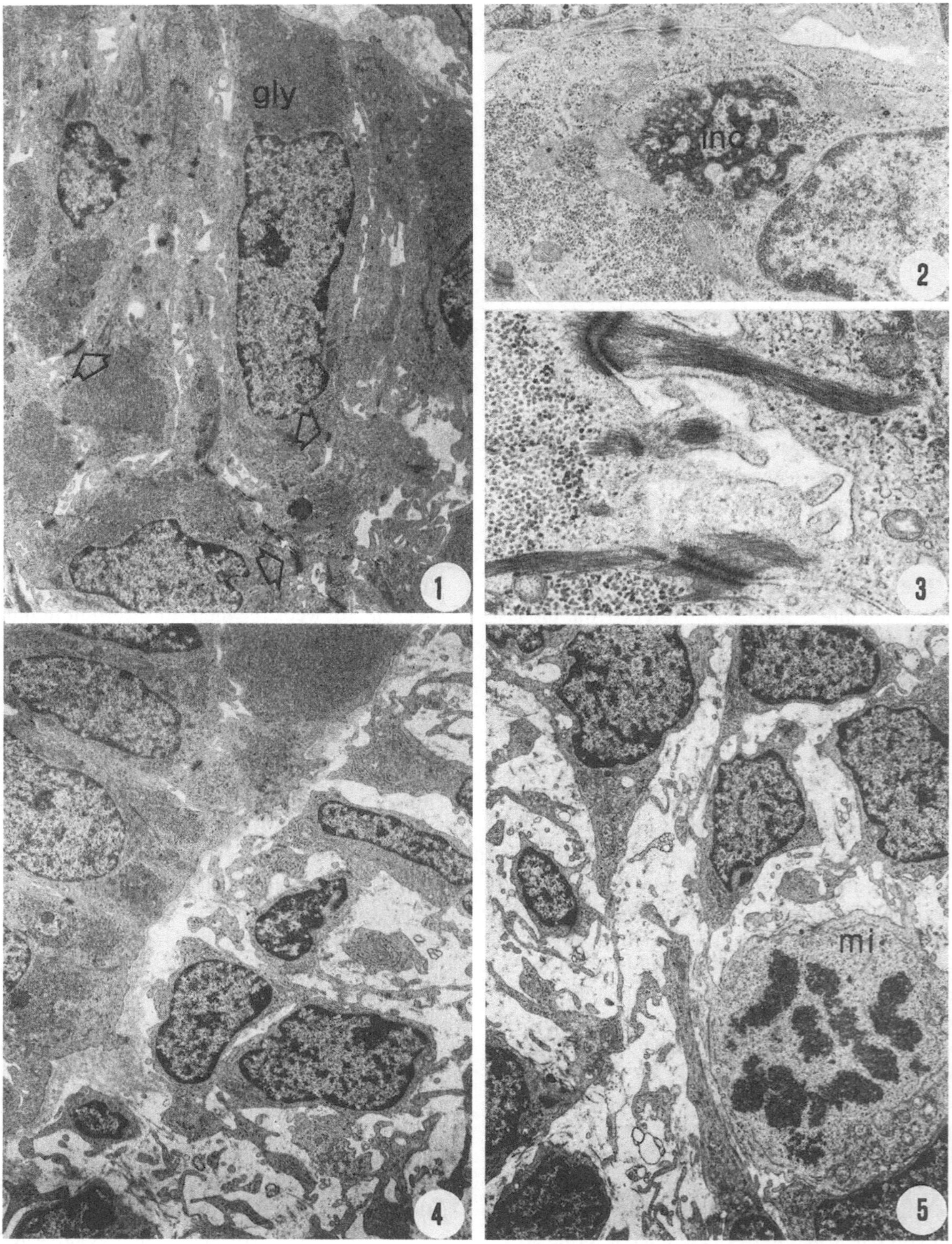
gly
1
inc
2
3
4
mi
5

cells, most of which are round and apolar. They have numerous slender cytoplasmic processes extending into wide intercellular spaces. Some apical cells have become columar and polarized apico-basally, with a large elongate to oval nucleus in the center of the cell and a supranuclear Golgi apparatus. Very few cells contain apical cytoplasmic granules, with electron-dense or flocculent material resembling incipient secretory activity of the epithelium. Even though after the 13th week some apical cells become polarized and have dense secretion granules in the apical cytoplasm, and the secretory material is seen in the acinar lumen, these cells still look rather quiescent when compared with the secretory cells of mature human prostate.

Kellokumpu-Lehtinen [139,140] found enzyme histochemically demonstrable acid phosphatase in urethral and prostatic epithelium throughout the development period from the 8th to 14th week, when fetal androgen production begins and reaches its maximum, although estrogen is also present in high amounts [284]. In early developmental stages, acid phosphatase activity was predominantly localized in lysosomes and in the Golgi complex. Later, when some of the prostatic anlagen cells became polarized and had increased amounts of rough endoplasmic reticulum and a larger Golgi apparatus, reaction products were also seen in the apical secretory complex.

In unpublished observations made using specific antibodies against different acid phosphatase isoenzymes, we found that the enzymehistochemical method demonstrates the lysosomal element (at least the nonsecretory form of acid phosphatase) in these immature glands. There is no immunoreactivity of secretory acid phosphatase (PAP) or of prostate specific antigen (PSA) in the prenatal prostatic secretory cells. Most of the secretions of immature glands stain intensely with the PAS reaction and Alcian blue at pH 3.0, indicating the presence of neutral and acidic mucopolysaccharides (proteoglycanes). These immature secreting glands are retained in the prostatic epithelium until the onset of puberty.

The perinatal increase in estrogen sensitivity of the prostatic anlagen results in a strong squamous epithelial metaplasia, preferentially in the portions of the glandular ducts close to the verumontanum. Perhaps under the influence of maternal estrogens, during the 15th and 16th weeks, the height of the cellular cords decreases, but otherwise the histological organization and ultrastructure of the epithelium remain unchanged. Triangular cells similar to the postnatally observed basal cells are seen in the basal portion of the epithelium. According to Kellokumpu-Lehtinen et al. [137, 140], the basal lamina becomes discontinuous in a few places and the outgrowing epithelium comes into contact with the underlying mesenchymal cells. Specializations of the cell membrane to maintain close cell-to-cell contact at the epithelio-mesenchymal boundaries have not been observed. The authors presume that the mesenchyme may regulate epithelial differentiation into secretory cells [137,138].

In postnatal infantile monkey specimens, we found a most prominent and thickened basement membrane, separating prostatic epithelium from the surrounding stroma; such thickened basement membranes are also seen in human prenatal and postnatal specimens (Fig. 7). The immature, prepubertal prostatic epithelium is obviously functionally separated from the surrounding stroma. This would mean that direct epithelial stromal interactions in the prostate are restricted to prenatal development.

←

Figures 1–5 show a prostate gland anlage close to the urogenital sinus of a human embryo of 60 mm CRL

Fig 1 Epithelium of the prostatic duct anlage from a human embryo (60 mm CRL) Columnar epithelial cells contain large amounts of glycogen (gly) and are connected by broad desmosomes (arrows) ×6700

Fig 2 Unidentified inclusion body (inc) in a prostatic duct anlage from the same specimen (×22,000)

Fig 3 Desmosomes from embryonic prostate epithelial cells Note the thick bundles of tonofilaments (×55,000)

Fig 4 Epithelial-mesenchymal interface of a human prostate duct anlage Basement membrane is thin and contains protrusions of adjacent mesenchymal cells (×6700)

Fig 5 Mesenchymal cells from the prostatic anlage of a 60 mm CRL human embryo One cell is in mitotic division (mi) (×6700)

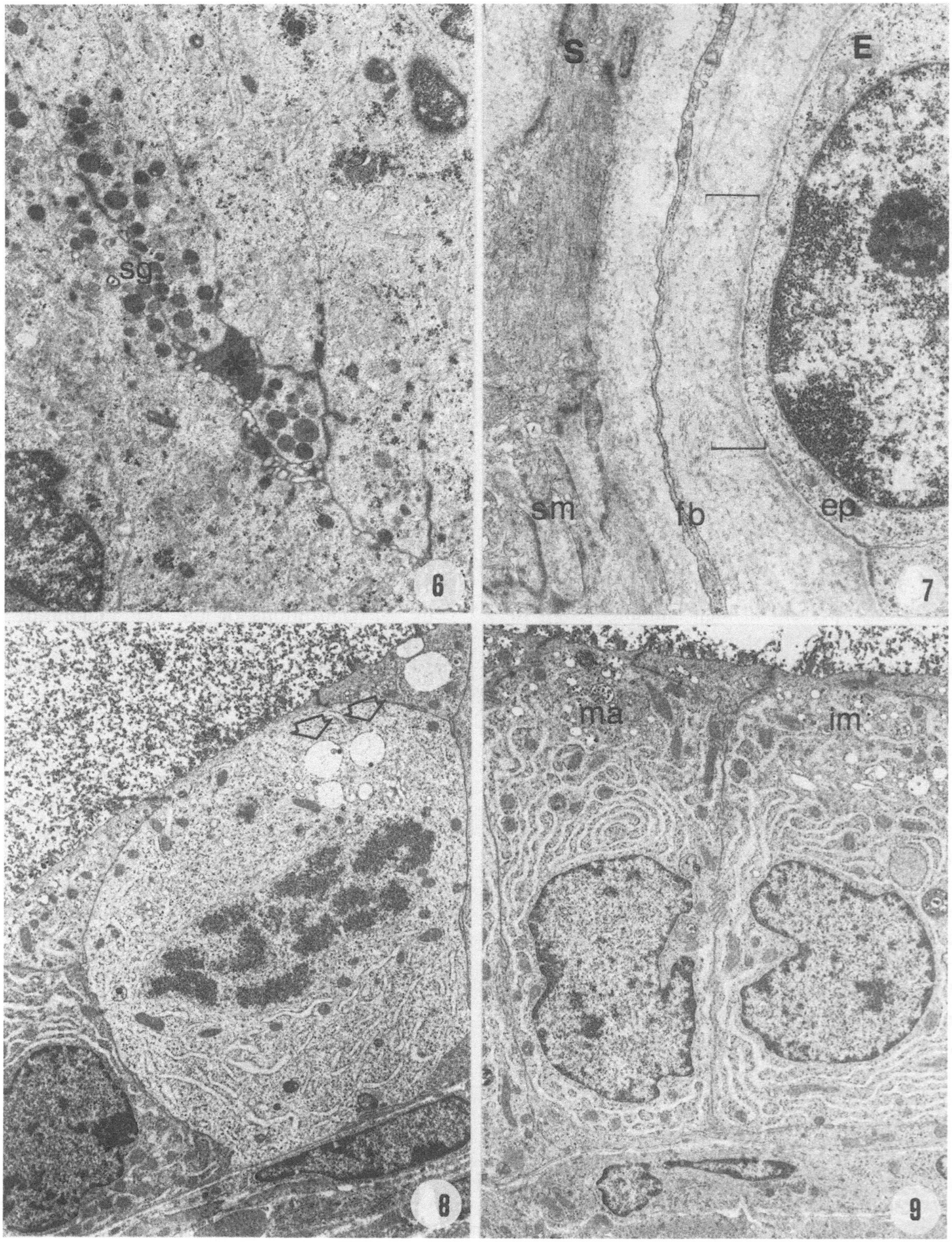
sg
6
S
E
sm
fb
ep
7
ma
im
8
9

2.2. *Postnatal Development*

Postnatal development of the human prostate proceeds in three phases: (a) a regression period after birth; (b) a quiescent period up to 12–14 years and (c) a maturation period at 14–18 years [17,23]. At birth, the collicular portion of the urethral wall contains prostatic gland ducts that display strongly metaplastic stratified squamous epithelium elicited by maternal estrogens. A few weeks later, usually at 6–8 weeks, metaplastic epithelium is replaced by cuboidal pseudostratified epithelium. In the periphery of the developing prostate, the epithelial anlagen form solid cords with numerous buds surrounded by a thick basement membrane. During infancy these cords acquire a lumen that is also invested by pseudostratified cuboidal epithelium (Figs. 6 and 7).

The cytology of the infantile prostate is almost identical with that of the adult gland. A nearly continuous layer of basal cells is immunoreactive after cytokeratin staining, while the adluminal cells are not. Forms intermediate between basal and adluminal cells are never seen. Most of these developing glands contain small, solid outpocketings consisting of only basal type cells. These appear to represent the pacemakers during morphogenesis of the acini. The outgrowth of developing acini occurs in close contact with the stroma.

This can be seen, for example, in the prostate of a 5-year-old boy immunostained for smooth muscle specific actin, where a close relationship between smooth muscle cells and developing gland ducts is easily recognized. In the central portion of the gland, the number of smooth muscle cells surrounding the epithelium is clearly less, but there is barely one acinus without making contact with a few muscle cells separated only by interposed fibrocytes. In the seminal vesicle, the situation is completely different: The smooth muscle cells of the glandular wall are always separated from the epithelium by a thick layer of connective tissue. The close association of epithelium and smooth muscle cells in the developing prostate is certainly of functional significance [241].

Functional maturation of the epithelium in the prostate can easily be traced by immunohistochemical studies of prostatic secretory proteins [17,18]. In the rat postnatal development and functional maturation of the prostate proceed rather rapidly, starting from the 12th postnatal day onwards and reaching the glandular periphery at about 30 days. On survey light micrographs of ventral prostate from 12-day-old rats immunostained for prostatic binding protein, the major secretory component of this gland, the portion intermediate between the urethral opening and the subcapsular termination of the gland ducts, displays a positive immunoreaction. On the 16th day, the diameter of the glandular lumen is considerably increased and so is the amount of immunoreactive cells and secretion. In 16- and 18-day-old animals treated with vincristin and sacrificed 6 hours later, the cells containing secretory granules are in mitosis. The number of mitoses is far less in basal cells and is prevalent only in the periphery of the glandular tips. Once the epithelium has differentiated into secretory and basal cells, replication of secretory cells is the normal means of cell renewal in the prostate.

At the ultrastructural level, the concomitant differential steps of both the epithelium and stroma of rat prostate are more evident. On the first day of postnatal life, the prostate consists

←

Figures 6–9 display postnatal changes in primate and rat prostate during puberty

Fig 6 Prostatic epithelium of a pubertal rhesus monkey Formation of acinar lumen (asterisk) and secretory granules (sg) has already started Cells contain sparse cytoplasmic organelles and clusters of glycogen (×8600)

Fig 7 Interface between prostatic epithelium (E) and stroma (S) of a pubertal rhesus monkey prostate Note the thickness of the basal lamina (brackets) Interspersed between epithelial (ep) and smooth muscle cells (sm) is seen a thin process of a periacinar fibroblast (fb) (×17,000)

Fig 8 Epithelium of rat ventral prostate from an 18-day-old animal Dividing secretory cell contains immature secretory granules (arrowheads) (×6700)

Fig 9 Maturating secretory cells of rat ventral prostate from an 18-day-old animal Rough endoplasmic reticulum and Golgi apparatus are well developed Part of the secretory granules is immature (im), containing a single granule, whereas the mature vacuoles (ma) contain flocculent material (×6700)

of solid cords of cuboidal epithelial cells, which protrude as paired buds from the urethral epithelium into the surrounding stroma. The ensuing division into ventral, lateral, and dorsal parts is already evident. Dorsal portions originate both from a sulcus lateral to the colliculus seminalis and from an area slightly cranial to it. From here they grow dorsally into an area of dense connective tissue (lateral to the future site of the seminal vesicle) where the rudiments of the coagulating glands are found. Paired epithelial buds that are ventral to the urethra will form the ventral portions of the prostate. No regional differences in fine structure are evident between prostatic cells from various locations at this time. A round to oval nucleus with a distinct nucleolus occupies most of the cytoplasm of the cuboidal epithelial cells. Mitochondria with lamelliform cristae, some RER cisternae, and many free ribosomes are scattered throughout the cytoplasm. The Golgi apparatus is small and consists of a few stacks of cisternae and associated smooth vesicles. Adjacent cells are connected by distinct junctional complexes in the center of the buds. The lumen of the prostatic acinus is not yet open, but is occupied by microvilli, which arise from the apical surface of the epithelial cells [89]. Several layers of flattened, undifferentiated mesenchymal cells surround the epithelial buds and merge with the remainder of the interstitium. The mesenchymal cells that are located next to the basal lamina later differentiate into fibroblasts, whereas more peripherally situated cells develop into smooth muscle cells. During the first week, cells of the prostatic buds increase somewhat in size, but their fine structure remains essentially the same.

Cells of the prostatic epithelium begin to acquire characteristics of the adult prostate during the second and third postnatal week (Figs. 8 and 9). Distinct differences can be seen between epithelial cells in the different regions of the prostate complex for the first time, and these occur somewhat earlier in the ventral portions of the prostate than in other regions. The epithelial cells become polarized, that is, organelles of the low columnar cells are partially stratified. The nuclei move to the basal part of the cells. Basal, supranuclear, and apical regions with microvilli can be distinguished. The amount of RER and the size of the supranuclear Golgi apparatus increase greatly 2–3 weeks after birth. A patent lumen is formed in the acini of the ventral, lateral, and dorsal prostate between postnatal days 7 and 14 [39,119]. The lumen of the coagulating gland appears several days later (day 10–17). Secretory granules are first seen during the second and third week of postnatal development (ventral prostate: day 10; dorsal prostate: day 12; lateral prostate: day 15; coagulating gland: day 17). The granules are discharged into the lumen of the acini in increasing amounts from day 10 to 21 and form a moderately dense, flocculent material. Basal cells can be clearly differentiated from those of the secretory epithelium in all regions of the prostate. The former are small triangular cells with heterochromatic nuclei. Their cytoplasm contains only a few organelles, glycogen, and an increased number of microfilaments [248]. Secretory cells have more organelles and fewer microfilaments. Pronounced changes also occur in the stroma of the glands during the second week of development. Differentiation of smooth muscle cells first appears to be completed in the ventral prostate (day 10), followed some days later by other glands (coagulating gland, day 12; dorsal prostate, day 14; lateral prostate, day 19). The capillaries of the stroma migrate closer to the acini and are eventually situated very close to their basal lamina.

2.2.1. Later postnatal development: 4th week to maturity. The prostatic cells gradually take on the appearance of those of mature prostate during this period. Developmental changes are characterized by a further increase in the amount and complexity of the RER and the size of the Golgi apparatus [92]. An adult appearance is seen as early as 28 days postnatum, but is not complete in all cells until about 35 days postnatum [90–92, 119,248]. In the human prostate, functional maturation of the epithelium generally follows the same pattern as in other mammals. In a prostate section of a 14-year-old boy, most glands have a more or less ductlike appearance, but already display some immunoreactivity for acid phosphatase [17,23] or prostate specific antigen (PSA). In the prostate of a 15-year-old boy, some of the prostatic acini have developed papillary projections, which are still rather thick, although only part of the cells are immunoreactive. In simple histological stains, secretory activity seems to be present in some of these nonimmunoreactive epithelia. Histochemical staining shows these nonimmunoreactive secretory cells to represent mucus-producing cells, as can be easily shown in PAS-stained sections processed for acid phosphatase immunoreactivity. The PAS-positive cells are numerous during infancy and gradually decrease in number during glandular maturation. In the normal adult gland, these cells have disappeared. In benign prostatic hyperplasia, and especially in prostate cancer, these cells reappear. The prostate has achieved its fully mature state if the following criteria are fulfilled:

1. Differentiation of the epithelium into secretory, basal, and neuroendocrine cells is finished.
2. PAS-positive mucus cells are lacking in prostatic epithelium.
3. All glandular cells, including those of the subcapsular periphery and the urethral contact zone, display a positive immunoreaction for acid phosphatase, prostate specific antigen, and β-microseminoprotein.

2.3. Experimental Studies of Epithelio-Mesenchymal Interactions

The prune-belly syndrome (PBS) is a congenital defect with prostatic aplasia, especially the primary absence of prostatic smooth muscle, that, on the one hand, causes weakness of the prostatic wall with resultant sacculation of the prostatic urethra, bladder distension, and eventual hydronephrosis [176] and, on the other hand, points to the decisive role of the mesenchyme in inducing prostatic epithelium. The fundamental work of Cunha and collaborators on mesenchymal epithelial interactions during prostatic development [59] resulted in the following salient sentences (cited by Cunha et al. [61], Table 1, p. 69):

1. Interactions between epithelium and mesenchyme are required for development of accessory sexual structures.
2. Mesenchyme induces and specifies patterns of epithelial morphogenesis, cytodifferentiation, and functional activity.
3. Urogenital mesenchyme can reprogram the differentiated statement of adult epithelium (e.g., bladder, vagina).
4. Androgen-sensitive wild-type urogenital mesenchyme is the actual target and mediator of morphogenetic effects of androgens upon developing male accessory sex glands.
5. Mesenchyme determines the expression of hormonal sensitivity of epithelial derivatives of the urogenital sinus.
6. Epithelial-stromal interactions play important roles during embryonic, neonatal, and adult periods.
7. During urogenital development morphogenetic mechanisms are similar and are highly conserved in different mammalian species.

The methodology of homotypic or heterotypic recombination of epithelial and mesenchymal portions of organs and characterization of the resultant structures has also been applied to prostate tumors, as embryonic induction was suggested to be operative both in normal and neoplastic development of the prostate gland. It is assumed that the mesenchymal and epithelial components of the prostate gland interact with each other in vivo through short-range signals that determine the developing structure resulting from the interacting tissues. Chung et al. [54–56] employed the concept of embryonic induction and defined the directive roles of fetal urogenital sinus mesenchyme (UGM) in prostatic epithelial growth and hormonal responsiveness. Improved tissue culture methods and growth conditions have allowed the establishment of human prostate cell lines or stains that can be used for analysis of this inductive or target potency.

Rowley [213] derived mesenchymal cell lines from fetal rat urogenital sinus organ cultures. Continuous passaging of one of these lines resulted in cells that in monolayer cultures constitutively express negative growth activity that is different from transforming growth factors, interleukin and rat fibroblast-derived interferons α and β. Additional aspects of extracellular matrix and growth factors are discussed in Chapter 3.

3. Functional Properties of Stromal Cells

3.1. General Structure of the Stroma

The stroma of adult human prostate consists mainly of smooth muscle cells, fibrocytes, and connective tissue, with numerous free cells, predominantly macrophages and mast cells, and ramifications of blood and lymph vessels, as well as nerve bundles and axons. More or less thick bundles of smooth muscle cells extend radially from the composite musculature of the urethra and merge peripherally into the prostatic capsule, which is made up of an outer vascular, intermediate fibrous, and inner muscular layer. Secondary bundles form a sometimes circular and sometimes oblique or tangential interlobular or periductal layer, which is continuous with thin tertiary bundles that are arranged in a basketlike manner around the acini.

3.2. Ultrastructure of Smooth Muscle Cells

The ultrastructure of prostatic smooth muscle cells is rather similar in various species and locations within the gland. The cytoplasm of these cells is occupied primarily by fine filaments (6 nm in diameter) that are mainly oriented parallel to the long axis of the cell. Spindle-shaped dense bodies are scattered through the course of the filaments. The latter extend into dense plaques subjacent to the plasma membrane. The arrangement and distribution of cell organelles is nearly identical with that in smooth muscle of the seminal vesicles. Surface vesicles (caveolae) have been found arranged in clusters separated from each other by a smooth cell surface on freeze-etch replicas. Each cell is surrounded by a basal lamina about 50 nm in thickness. At some locations on the surface of a cell, projection of one smooth muscle cell protrudes into a cup depression in an adjacent cell. At these locations, the external laminae surrounding the cells are absent, and the extracellular space between the two apposed plasma membranes is narrowed to 15–20 nm, forming intermediate-type junctions. These are more frequent in rat than in human prostate. Intermediate junctions are particularly frequent between smooth muscle cells close to or within the muscle layer of the prostatic urethra. Muscle cells are often intermingled with a dense network of elastic fibers.

Bundles of unmyelinated nerve processes are numerous in rat prostatic stroma, and the distance of accompanying muscle cells ranges between 50- and 500 nm. At certain points, axon varicosities that contain aggregations of numerous small clear vesicles 30–60 nm in diameter, some dense-core vesicles 15–20 nm in diameter, and rare large vesicle 100 nm in diameter make closer contact with smooth muscle cells. In some instances, the axons lie on the unindented surface of the muscle cell and sometimes in a shallow groove on its surface (Fig. 10). In other cases, deep indentations are found in smooth muscle cells surrounding an axon. The plasma membrane of the axon is separated from the muscle cell by a space 15–20 nm wide. No membrane specialization at these points of contact have been observed, although myofilaments are usually absent from the underlying cytoplasm. Experimental studies in rat and dog have demonstrated that the ultrastructure of prostatic smooth muscle cells is strongly hormone dependent, which is important with respect to the pathogenesis of benign prostatic hyperplasia.

3.3. Experimental Studies

In a recent study on ultrastructural changes in smooth muscle cells of the rat ventral prostate

→

Figures 10–13 show ultrastructural changes in prostatic smooth muscle cells after hormonal challenge

Fig 10 Smooth muscle cells from an intact mature rat ventral prostate One nerve terminal (t) is seen apposed to a muscle cell (×8600)

Fig 11 Prostatic smooth muscle cells from an animal castrated 6 week previously Cells are thin and elongate, with an increased amount of interstitial connective tissue (×6700)

Fig 12 Smooth muscle cell from rat ventral prostate after 6 weeks estradiol treatment The cell is slightly hypertrophied and contains glycogen flakes Surface vesicles (caveolae) and dense plaques are reduced in number (×27,000)

Fig 13 Prostatic smooth muscle cells 6 weeks after castration and estradiol treatment Cells have an irregular outline and are reduced in size (×17,000)

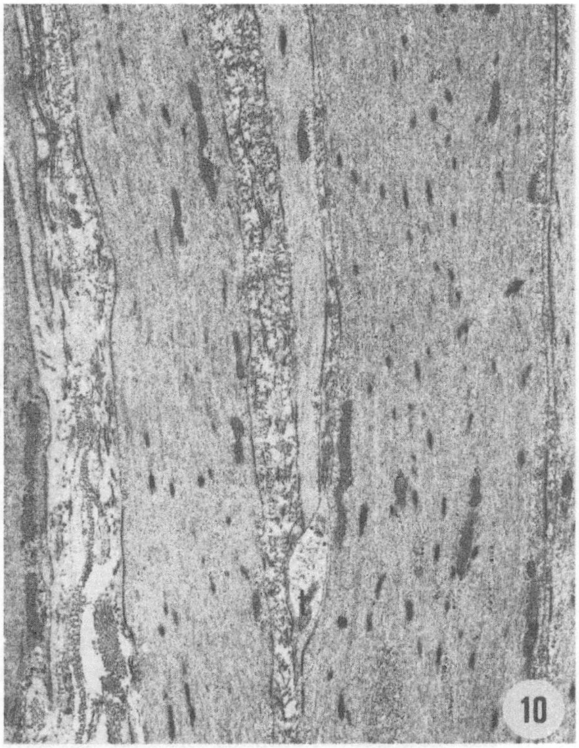
10

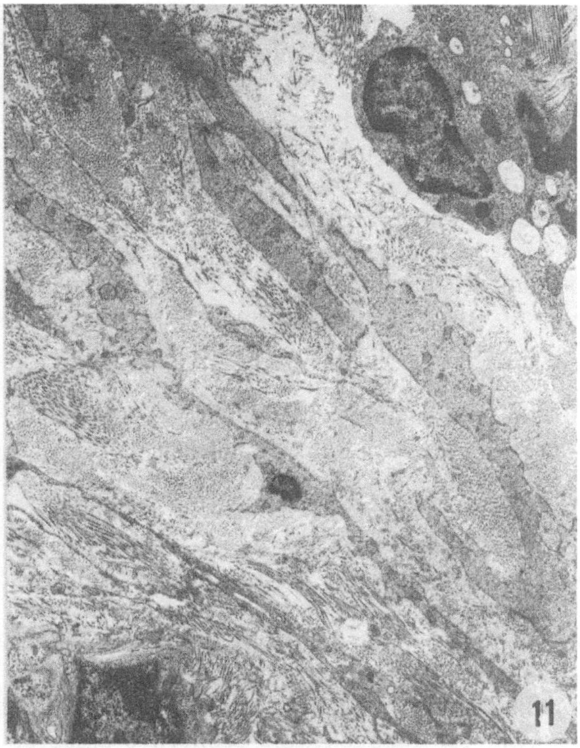
11

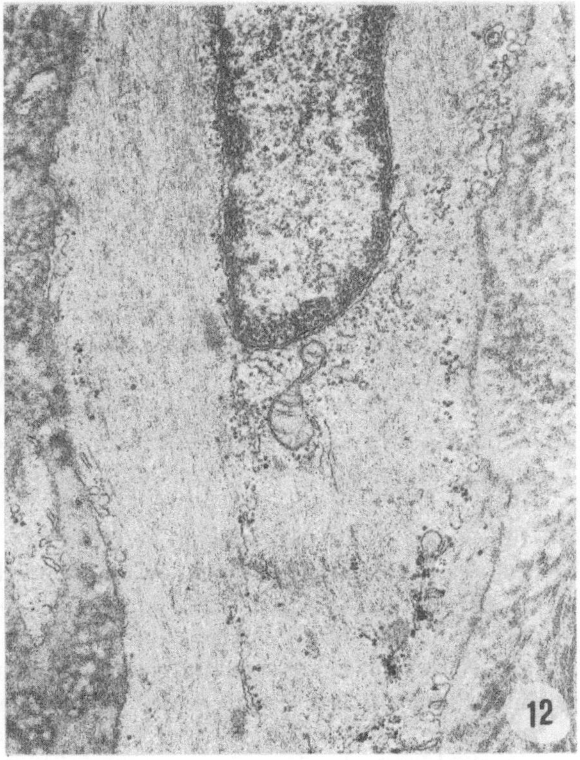
12

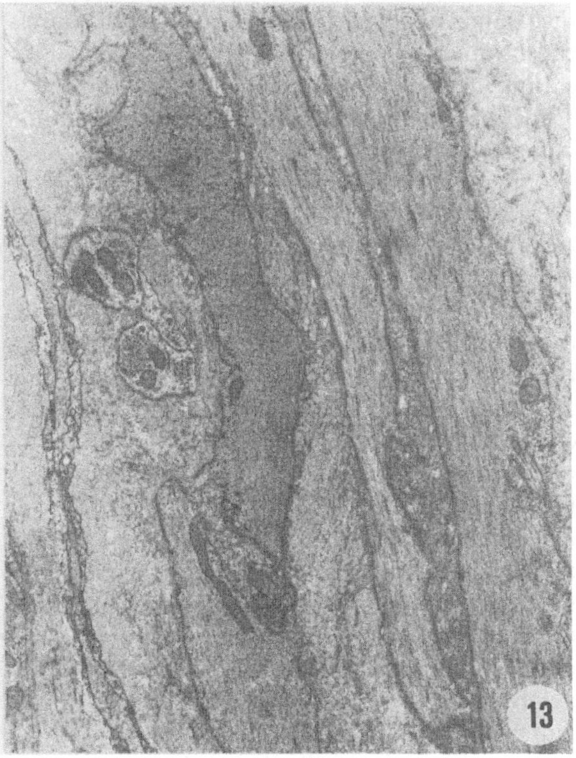
13

after castration, estrogen treatment, or combined treatment (Figs. 10–13), we found characteristic changes in structure, arrangement, and quantity of smooth muscle cells [282]. In control specimens, actin- and desmin-immunoreactive smooth muscle cells formed narrow sheaths surrounding the acini and were separated by thin layers of loose connective tissue, which formed more prominent bundles only in interlobular spaces. Smooth muscle cells consisted of three to four layers with few slender fibroblasts interspersed in connective tissue between extended muscle cells and the epithelium. Smooth muscle cells contained regularly arranged intermediate filaments and myofilaments, and scarce cytoplasmic organelles close to the nuclear region.

In estrogen-treated animals, the layer of smooth muscle cells was more prominent due to the reduced glandular diameter. An increase in connective tissue resulted in larger distances between smooth muscle cells, which showed a positive immunoreaction for both actin and desmin. After 12 weeks of treatment, the connective tissue of the animals had partly replaced smooth muscle cells, which often incompletely surrounded the shrunken acini. Smooth muscle cells showed a reduction in actin immunoreactivity, while desmin immunoreactivity appeared unchanged. Ultrastructurally, the cells displayed a wrinkled outline and were indistinguishable from those seen in castrated animals. Between the cells, however, less fibrous connective tissue was seen, and more ground substance was noticeable. By 1 week after castration, and more pronounced after 12 weeks, the periacinar smooth muscle cells had formed an irregularly arranged and thickened layer of clumsy elongate cells that displayed immunoreactivities of actin and desmin. Connective tissue fibers were interspersed in the muscle cell layer and separated the cells from each other as well as from the epithelial acinar lining. Connective tissue fibers within the stromal septa had increased considerably. At the end of the experiment, some of the smooth muscle cells were replaced by connective tissue. At the ultrastructural level, smooth muscle cells had gained a very irregular outline, with numerous spinelike extensions containing densely packed caveolae (surface vesicles) and areae densae. The density of contractile filaments appeared unchanged or was slightly reduced, while cytoplasmic organelles were scattered in groups throughout the cytoplasm.

In estrogen-treated, castrated animals, the increase in periacinar and interstitial connective tissue at the expense of smooth muscle cells was less obvious. The layer of smooth muscle cells was thickened and less densely packed, and the interstitial connective tissue also had increased, but these features were clearly less pronounced than in castrated animals. After 12 weeks of treatment, irregularly arranged desmin- and actin-immunoreactive cells surrounded the acini, but their number appeared as reduced as in castrated animals. The cells contained condensed polymorphic nuclei surrounded by a narrow rim of cytoplasm with few cytoplasmic organelles. Caveolae and areae densae were numerous in slender and irregularly formed projections from the cells.

In a quantitative analysis the most striking changes were observed in the relative amount of stroma, which increased by a factor of about three in estrogen-treated animals and four in castrated animals. The increase in stroma proceeded slowly in estrogen-treated animals and rapidly in castrated animals. The relative proportion of smooth muscle cells, as deduced from actin and desmin immunoreactivity, was nearly doubled in estrogen-treated animals (with or without castration) and in castrated animals reached 2.5 times the normal value. To get a more detailed view of the changes within prostatic smooth muscle cells, a stereological analysis of the cytoplasmic organelles was performed. The relative volume density in intact smooth muscle cells was 63 vol % for the cytoplasm, 19 vol % for the nucleus, 9 vol % for rough endoplasmic reticulum, 0.4 vol % for the Golgi apparatus, 5 vol % for mitochondria, 2.4 vol % for areae densae, and less than 0.3 vol % for lysosomes. There was a slight reduction of the cytoplasm in castrated animals, while the nuclear proportion was doubled by the end of the experiment. No significant changes were observed for rough endoplasmic reticulum, Golgi apparatus, mitochondria, and areae densae. The number of lysosomes was initially increased, but soon reached control values. In estrogen-treated and estrogen-treated castrated animals, there was initially a slight, but insignificant increase in volume density of the cytoplasm. At the end of the experiment, values dropped slightly below control values. After 12 weeks, nuclear volume increased from 19 vol % to about 30 vol %. The proportion of the rough endoplasmic reticulum was initially reduced but finally exceeded the control values. The relative volume of the areae densae was in the upper normal range, while those of the Golgi apparatus and mitochondria were largely unaltered. The relative volume of the lysosomes increased by the second and third week, and then reached control values.

Although the relative volume density of smooth muscle cells increased by a factor of 2.5 times in castrated animals, the cells were atrophic, and their outline characteristically changed in each group. The alterations of myofilaments and intermediate filaments were inconspicuous, with a slight reduction of actin filaments, both in castrated and estrogen-treated animals. There were no signs of functional "activation" of smooth muscle cells, that is, transition from a contractile to a metabolic state. While no dramatic reduction of actin filaments was observed in smooth muscle cells, rearrangement (formation of clusters or bundles of intermediate filaments) of the shape of cells varied characteristically. Generally speaking, there was atrophy in smooth muscle cells from all experimental groups after 12 weeks treatment, which resulted in a relative decrease in cytoplasm and a concomitant increase in the relative volume of the nucleus. An only slight and insignificant increase was observed in the volume density of rough endoplasmic reticulum in castrated animals. Bartsch and Rohr (see Zhao et al. [282] for references) were the first to devote a detailed morphometric, ultrastructural, and endocrinological study to smooth muscle cells in human BPH. They reported on activated smooth muscle cells with increased endoplasmic reticulum and Golgi vesicles. Their ultrastructural figures are not conclusive in all respects, as cross-sectioned cells were compared with longitudinally oriented cells. In our analysis we only used longitudinally sectioned cells for evaluation.

3.4. *Paracrine Effects of Prostatic Stromal Cells*

Different isolation procedures for prostatic stromal cells have been reported [197,242] that allow the collection and subsequent cultivation in vitro of isolated prostate stromal cells [52,242, 243]. These cells were identified as either smooth muscle cells [243] or fibroblasts [20,75]. In our own experiments we found no morphological differences between isolated stromal cells and fibroblasts grown out from BPH explants (Figs. 14–17). The cells have a flat, nearly rectangular, form with very few pseudopodia and surface differentiations. At their contact sites, lamellar interdigitations are observed, although no membrane differentiations occur. Immunohistochemically the cells express vimentin, actin-stress fibers (cross-reactive with smooth muscle-specific actin antibodies), androgen and estrogen receptor, tissue-type transglutaminase, tenascin, and fibronectin. Their growth is stimulated by androgens and moderately inhibited by estrogens, and at the ultrastructural level the stromal cells contain dense arrays and strands of microfilaments extending parallel to the underlying surface of the culture dish. In the perinuclear area these filaments intermingle with the loosely arranged network of intermediate filaments. The number of cell organelles is relatively sparse. A few rodlike mitochondria with dense matrix are interspersed between short profiles of communicating and interlacing cisternae of rough endoplasmic reticulum and clusters of polyribosomes. The Golgi apparatus is small and consists of a few stacks and a small number of vesicles. At the cell surface, several micropinocytotic vesicles occur as well as rather few coated vesicles. The nucleus holds a central position in the cells and bulges above the average level of the cytoplasm. Its chromatin is loosely arranged; coarse clumps of chromatin are found adjacent to the unusually large nucleolus and are often indistinguishable from the nucleolus. After androgen stimulation, and still more pronounced after sodium butyrate treatment, the cells loose their rectangular shape and produce elongated tender extensions with knoblike terminations that contain several stress fibers and deposit tenascin spots at the underlying surface.

Prostatic stromal cells, either cocultured with testicular Sertoli cells [243], prostate cancer cells [73,75], prostate epithelium [52], neural tissue [20,73], or by means of conditional media, exert positive paracrine effects on their respective targets that result in enhanced or selective secretion of certain proteins [75], mitogenic or pro-

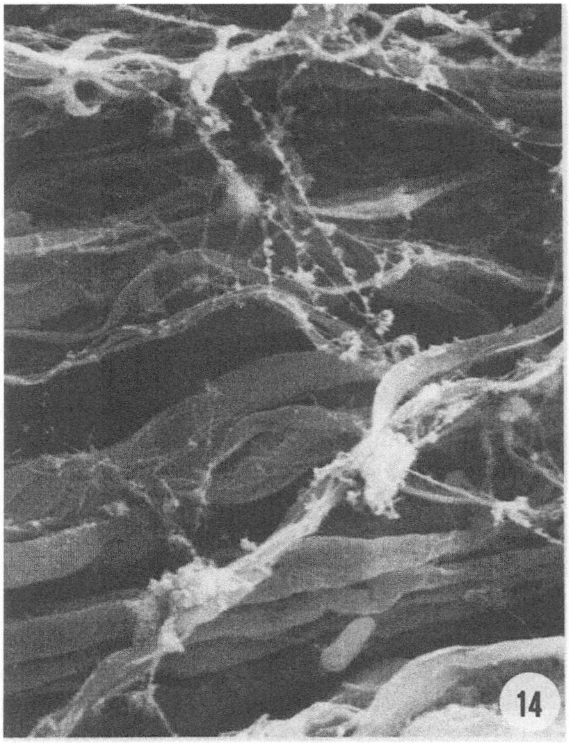
14

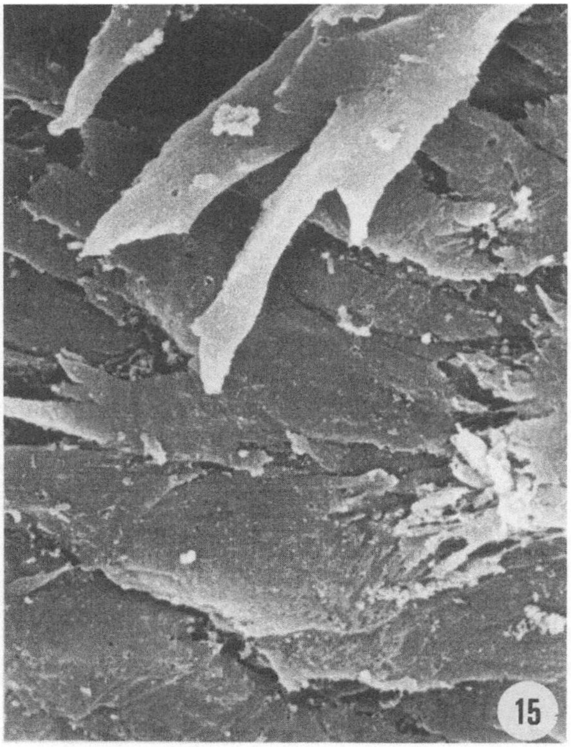
15

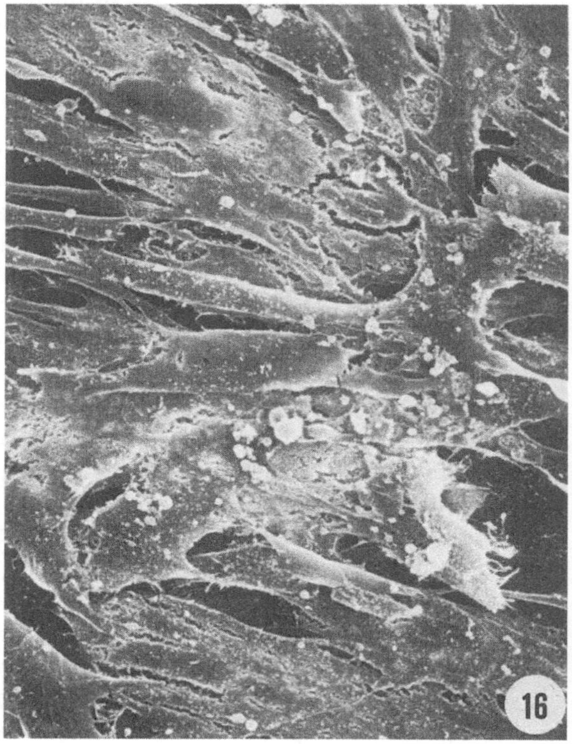
16

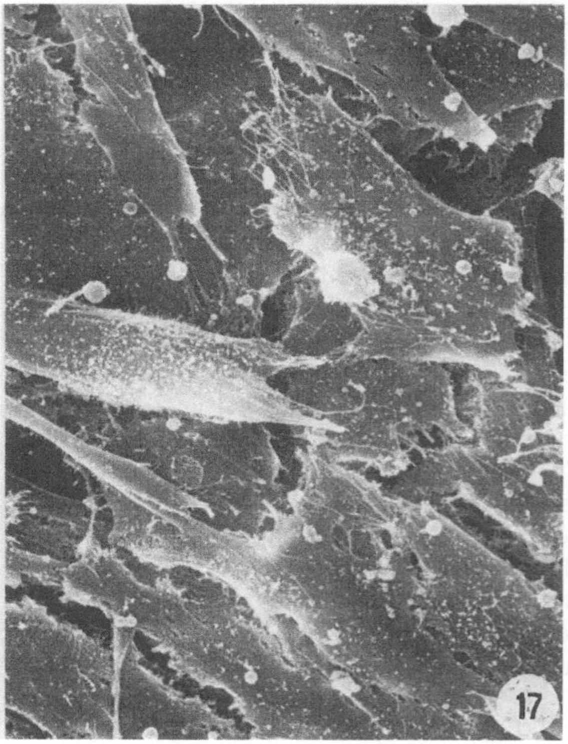
17

liferative activity [20,52], or neurotrophic activity [20]. These effects are species dependent in that rat, but not human, prostate stromal cells exert mitogenic effects on PC-21 pheochromocytoma and C6-glioma cells, while their neurotrophic effects (survival of chicken sensory, sympathetic, and parasympathetic neurons) are nearly identical [20].

Graham et al. [103], extending the work of Djakiew et al. [75], localized nerve growth factor (NGF)-like immunoreactivity predominantly in the stromal component of BPH, adenocarcinoma, and normal human prostatic tissue. However, the NGF receptor (NGF-R) was localized predominantly in the epithelial cells of these tissues. Renal tissues provided a negative control and testes provided a positive control for both NGF-like protein and the NGF receptor. These results indicate the production of an NGFβ-like protein by human prostatic stromal cells that interact with an NGF-R on the adjacent epithelial cells, thereby mediating paracrine interactive growth regulation of the human prostate.

Several growth factors have been identified that may function as putative paracrine regulators of prostatic growth. In this context epidermal growth factor (EGF)-like [127] and bFGF-like [235] proteins account for a considerable amount of growth factor activity in the prostate. The EGF receptor is present in the basal cell layer [166] of prostatic epithelium, and its expression is obviously under hormonal control [64,160,161, 182]. In addition, aFGF [164] and transforming growth factor β [179] have been identified in the prostate or prostatic tumor cells. Chang and Chung [52] proposed a model of epithelio-stromal interaction in growth regulation of the adult prostate exerted through a DHT and growth factor pathway. Close metabolic cooperation between prostatic fibroblast and epithelial cells, with DHT produced by the epithelial cells and growth factors, serves as an important molecular signal. The interaction of these factors may determine the responsiveness of prostate gland to androgenic steroids.

3.5. Immunoregulatory Cells

Contrary to the marginally studied macrophages that constitute a major compartment of migratory elements of prostatic stromal cells [96,97] lymphocytes and mast cells in the prostate have recently attracted some interest [96]. Like most mucosal surfaces of the male genital system, the prostatic epithelium contains intraepithelial lymphocytes, which are mainly T suppressor/cytotoxic CD 8+ cells. Cells of the inducer/helper phenotype are mainly localized within the interstitium of the prostate, while very few B lymphocytes have been identified.

IgA is present in relatively high amounts of prostatic fluid, especially in prostatitis. As the migration pattern of IgA blasts is accepted as an essential characteristic of a common mucosa-associated lymphoid tissue (MALT), the question is whether mucosa of the male genital tract could also be included in the MALT due to a preferential entry of IgA lymphoid blasts into the prostate. Fritz et al. [97], therefore, labeled in vitro proliferating lymphoid cells from peripheral and mesenteric lymph nodes in male rats and studied their migration pattern. A low, but significant, migration towards the male genital organs was found, but with no difference between blasts from peripheral and mesenteric lymph nodes. There is thus no evidence to include the male genital tract in the common mucosal secretory immune system.

The mast cells form a heterogeneous population differing in number and localization in organ compartments. Due to different functions, "mucosal mast cells" have been distinguished

←

Figures 14–17 represent scanning electron micrographs of prostatic stromal cells in situ and in vitro

Fig 14 Scanning eletron micrograph of interstitial stroma of rat ventral prostate Thick bundles of connective tissue fibers obscure the periacinar smooth muscle cells (×2500)

Fig 15 After chemical dissection with hydrochloric acid, prostatic smooth muscle cells from an animal castrated and estradiol-treated 6 weeks previously display the characteristic elongate fusiform or multipolar outlines (×2300)

Fig 16 Survey scanning electron micrograph of human prostatic stromal cells grown in vitro (×1250)

Fig 17 At higher magnification the stromal cells grown in vitro display the structural characteristics of fibroblasts (×2500)

from "connective tissue mast cells." Gupta [105] described an increase in mast cells in the prostate from birth to young adulthood with clearly greater numbers in BPH. Fritz et al. [97] found nearly twice the number of mast cells after lead citrate fixation compared to formalin fixation. It is not clear whether or not the number of mucosal mast cells exceeds that of connective tissue mast cells in the prostate and if they were hormonally regulated such as those in the testis [99].

4. Growth Patterns of Epithelium

4.1. Concepts of Internal Prostate Gland Organization

The conventional description of prostatic "lobes" (middle, lateral, anterior, posterior) was based on embryological observations [157]. Several different definitions of the lobes have subsequently been suggested [32,250]. In a series of papers, McNeal [168–170] criticized the older concepts and developed a model based on special dissection techniques, taking into account comparative, embryological, as well as pathological considerations. According to McNeal, the gland consists of four subdivisions: (a) the central zone, (b) the peripheral zone, (c) the transition zone, and (d) the anterior nonmuscular stroma. He describes the central zone as a histologically distinct organ within the prostate capsule, contributing as much as 40% of the epithelium of the prostate. Its acini are much larger and more elaborate than the remainder of the gland. Its more crowded, darker staining epithelium was described as the exclusive site of production of pepsinogen II [205] and plasminogen activator [206]. The remainder of the prostate has been divided into a large peripheral zone (approximately 70% of the glandular prostate) and a tiny transition zone, which is medially in contact with an outer border of the preprostatic sphincter. Anteriorly, the transition zone forms the anterior glandular border of the prostate in its midportion just below the bladder neck. According to McNeal [168] the boundary between the transition zone and the more posteriorly situated peripherally zone extends laterally from the urethral wall and then curves anteriorly to meet the anterior aspect of the prostate.

Neglecting the topographic position of the individual prostatic tubuloalveolar system in relation to the ejaculatory ducts and the urethra [16], the prostate may be regarded as consisting of branching secretory tubules and acini, which are surrounded by a fibromuscular stroma. The muscular component condenses peripherally to form the prostatic capsule and centrally merges into the muscle layers of the prostatic urethra.

4.2. Regional Differentiation of the Prostatic Ductal System

As early as 1939, Rabl [204] demonstrated regional differences in the tubuloalveolar glands of the human prostate, which consist of a relatively straight main duct with numerous ramifications and diverticula. The diverticula adjacent to the main duct are connected by short connecting pieces that form sharp angles with the main duct, whereas in the periphery the diverticula join the connecting pieces in a rectangular manner.

We have pointed to the collicular region, where the various cell types of the prostatic gland duct allow the discrimination of four different zones (see Aumüller [24] pp. 75–77, Figs. 41 and 61). To the contrary, in the subcapsular peripheral portion of the gland ducts were described as immature, nonsecretory acini prior to full maturation of the gland. A similar gradient of differentiation of prostatic glandular cells is found in the canine prostate [19]. A recent confirmation of our hypothesis on the differentiation gradient within the proximal portions of the prostatic gland ducts was made by Frazier et al. [95], who observed PSA-immunoreactive cells within the urethral epithelium and periurethral gland ducts.

Based on the studies of morphogenesis of the ductal networks in mouse prostate by Sugimura et al. [238,239], Lee et al. [149] systematically studied the regional variation in morphological and functional activities in prostatic ductal systems in rats. They found that in rat prostate, the ducts form a complex system with branches and subbranches extending from one end to another. The entire length of the ductal system can be arbitrarily divided into three segments — the proximal, intermediate, and distal segments — the epithelial lining of which has a regional variation in cellular activities. Epithelial cells lining the distal segments were tall-columnar type and were engaged in mitotic activity. Cells in intermediate segments were also tall-columnar type; however, they were mitotically quiescent but actively secreting proteins. No sign of programmed cell death was evident in these cells. Cells in proximal segments, however, were low-columnar or cuboidal in shape, and were heavily stained for cathepsin D, a marker associated with late manifestation of cell death. Following castration, a reversal in the site of cell death occurred in the epithelium lining the ductal system. By the fourth day of postcastration, distal segments contained many epithelial cells with intense cytoplasmic staining for cathepsin D, while proximal segments showed a reduction in the number of positively stained cells. Three days later, cells in proximal segments were atrophied and devoid of staining for cathepsin D. Movement in the location of cell death from proximal toward distal segments was attributed to regional variations in responsiveness of epithelial cells to androgen stimulation and androgen depletion along the prostatic ductal system.

From a cell kinetic point of view, observation of an extensive number of cells undergoing programmed cell death offers a mechanism for maintaining epithelial population homeostasis. This would be achieved by having cell proliferation in distal segments and cell degeneration in proximal segments, implying that a migration of epithelial cells along the basement membrane, from the distal end toward the proximal end, is required to satisfy this epithelial population homeostasis in the prostatic ductal system.

To verify this hypothesis, Bettuzzi et al. [30] studied the regional and cellular distribution within the rat prostate of two mRNA species undergoing opposite regulation by androgens. Sulphated glycoprotein-2 (SGP-2) is identical with the testosterone-repressed message-2 (TRPM-2 [45]), which is reported to be induced in castrated rat ventral prostate during programmed cell death [177]. A number of other systems have been described in which SGP-2 is involved in the apoptotic process. An increase in ornithine decarboxylase (ODC) activity accompanies normal or pathological cell growth in rat prostate, and mammalian tissue, where it was first recovered [192]. It belongs to the group of androgen-induced prostate proteins in that its activity drops dramatically upon castration and is restored by androgen replenishment. Using ^{35}S-labelled RNA probes derived from SGP-2 and ODC-cDNAs, respectively, for in situ hybridization, Bettuzzi et al. [30] found in whole prostate sections from intact rats that the SGP-2 transcript was only detectable in restricted areas and not evenly distributed over the whole gland. The ODC transcript, however, was not detectable in areas where the SGP-2 transcript was located, but instead in the complementary residual of the gland. Furthermore, each of the two mRNAs preferentially accumulated in a cell population of cuboidal cells that was morphologically different from the columnar epithelial cells, where ODC-mRNA was localized. Castration caused a dramatic accumulation of SGP-2 and a decrease in ODC-mRNAs in the cells of the columnar epithelium 4 days later. The authors infer that in the intermediate and distal parts of the ductal system of the rat ventral prostate, the ODC gene would be expressed at a high rate, while being turned off in the proximal ducts. Castration resulting in apoptosis of the epithelial cells of the intermediate and distal ducts caused SGP-2 to be actively expressed and ODC to be repressed in the latter segments. They argue that SGP-2 participates at the onset of programmed cell death in those cells that become insensitive to androgens when migrating to the proximal ducts (as hypothesized by Lee et al. [149]), while ODC may have a role in cell multiplication and secretory protein biosynthesis of epithelial cells that exhibit androgen sensitivity.

Such a presumed difference in androgen sensitivity along the proximo-distal gradient of the prostatic ducts, however, is difficult to reconcile with the homogeneous distribution of the androgen receptor in the prostate reported by Lubahn et al. [158], Tan et al. [245], Chang et al. [51], Sar et al. [217], and Prins et al. [198]. To determine possible differences in androgen sensitivity within the prostate, Prins [199] examined the androgen receptor (AR) levels and 5α-reductase activity along the proximal-distal axis of microdissected ventral prostatic ducts of 15-, 30-, and 100-day-old rats. The results revealed no discernible differences in AR levels, or binding activity in any cell type along the ductal length in prepubertal,

pubertal, or adult rats. In addition, 5α-activity was the same in the distal and proximal ductal regions. The authors therefore concluded that regional heterogeneity in prostatic growth and function is not the result of differences in levels of AR and 5α-reductase, but that perhaps other region-specific structural or intracellular, or perhaps paracrine, factors may be responsible for the differences in androgen responsiveness along the duct.

These differences may be due to the pattern of steroid hormone receptors [42] or differences in steroid hormone metabolism. Pylkkänen et al. [201] studied the immunohistochemical and biochemical distribution of estradiol-17β hydroxysteroid oxidoreductase in the urogenital tract of control and neonatally estrogenized male mice. They found the highest ratios of NADPH-dependent ^{3}H-estrogen reduction to oxidation ratio in cell-free homogenates from coagulating gland and seminal vesicle, as well as from the prostatic and lower intrapelvic urethra, which are considered the most estrogen-sensitive parts of the male urogenital system. The epithelium of the lower and prostatic urethra as well as the periurethral collecting ducts were stained with an antibody prepared against (human placental) 17β-hydroxysteroid oxidoreductase. Both biochemical activities and immunohistochemical staining patterns were not significantly altered after neonatal estrogenization. According to Pylkkänen et al. [201], it is possible that there are specific sites, preferentially in the prostatic urethra and collecting ducts, in which the changes in 17β-oxidoreduction of estrogen does play a role in the regulation of androgen action. This interpretation is well in line with the reported localization of estrogen receptors in the stroma underlying urethral epithelium and surrounding periurethral collecting ducts in monkey and mouse prostates [38,202], and in the basal cells of the acinar and ductal epithelium in human and canine prostates as well [218,274].

Prins [199] observed in neonatally estrogenized rats permanently altered prostatic growth and lobe-specific changes in androgen receptor expression in the adult gland. Immunohistochemistry revealed a marked reduction or absence of epithelial AR in the ventral and dorsal prostate of estrogenized rats, whereas the epithelial cells of the lateral prostate expressed AR similar to controls. The incidence of AR-positive fibroblastic stromal cells increased in lateral prostates from 5% in controls to ~25% in estrogenized rats. These alterations in AR distribution may partially explain the aberrant growth responses observed in these tissues.

In summary, the heterogeneity in estrogen sensitivity within the prostatic duct system along with the homogeneous androgen sensitivity of epithelium in the proximal-distal axis of prostatic ducts may be regarded as essential prerequisites in the different functional behavior of prostatic cells, which in addition may be under the influence of local paracrine modulators in stroma (fibroblasts) or epithelium (neurendocrine cells).

4.3. Pathological Considerations

Franks [93] established the concept of the "outer prostate" that was uniformly susceptible to carcinoma and encompassed all Lowsley's lobes. He also described a tiny "inner prostate" composed of mucosal and submucosal glands oriented around the urethra. This region was identified as the site of origin of benign nodular hyperplasia (BPH), but was reported to be immune to carcinoma. McNeal [168] reinvestigated the site of origin of adenocarcinoma in a series of over 200 radical prostatectomy specimens. In the central zone, contributing as much as 40% of the epithelium of the prostate, only between 5% and 10% of cancer origins were found, whereas the remainder larger proportion originated both in the peripheral zone and the anteromedial transition zone, where BPH also develops. Carcinomas originating in both zones were nearly equivalent to clinical stage A and B, respectively. Transition zone cancers showed much less capsule penetration due to the boundary function of the stroma in the transitional zone. In carcinomas from the peripheral zone, capsule penetration depended largely on facilitated spread along the perineural spaces, and its distribution was determined by the location of the superior and inferior nerve pedicles. Prognosis of tumor progression is obviously related to tumor volume. Both in autopsy cancers as well as in clinical and incidental surgical tumors according to McNeal [168], poor differentiation was most infrequent at small cancer volumes. Areas of high grade (malignancy) became more common among about one third of autopsy carcinomas that were larger than 1.0 cc. Autopsy cases with distant metastases were consistently larger than 5 cc and had a large proportion of high grade tumor. He therefore infers prostate cancer to be a single biologic species with "latency" being simply a function of small volume. Clinically manifest disease would only be found among this small subset of carcinomas that are larger than 1 cc and also show large areas of poor differentiation. Such a volume-related sequence of changing biologic malignancy would be conceivable by spontaneously evolving tumor cells heterogeneity and the accumulation of successive mutational events with time, resulting in development of hormone and drug resistance, and metastatic capacity. This latter view is opposed by the opinion of Gleason [100], who suggests that prostate cancers have more or less fixed degrees of malignancy and growth rates, indicating a kind of "biologic determinism" rather than a steady increase in malignancy with time. Such a "biologic determinism" would favor the idea that larger tumors were more malignant from the beginning and grew more rapidly to larger size than the slow-growing, low-grade tumors.

The aforementioned concept of a proximodistal gradient in the prostatic duct system (with proximal portions engaged in programmed cell death, intermediate portions of active secretion, and a terminal portion of reserve or proliferative function) would explain the possibility of development of biologically differently determined carcinomas of the prostate: (a) those with relatively low growth rate, (b) those with a higher degree of glandular organization, but considerable growth rate, and (c) those with low degree of glandular organization and high proliferative potency, and would reflect the biological determination of their respective site of origin.

5. Epithelio-Stromal Interface and Nonsecretory Cells

5.1. General Structure

The strict histological separation of prostatic epithelium and prostatic stroma into two distinctive functional entities is an oversimplification. In functional terms, both compartments must be viewed as mutually interdependent, acting as a "prostatic functional unit" (Fig. 18). The prostatic functional unit consists of the secretory cells and their auxiliary structures, namely, basal cells, the basal lamina, capillaries, fibrocytes, smooth muscle cells, free connective tissue cells, nerve axons, and lymphatics, which are all destined to provide the secretory cells with the required oxygen, hormones, ions, transmitter, and growth factor signals, and to remove the metabolites from the cells [22] (see Fig. 2). The element connecting all these structures is the so-called biomatrix system, consisting of the cytoskeleton of the respective cells, the nuclear envelope and nuclear matrix, and the extracellular matrix [124].

5.2. Epithelio-Stromal Interface

The epithelio-stromal interface of the prostate is made up of periacinar fibroblasts, intercalated between stromal smooth muscle cells and epithelium. Capillaries and nerve axons, the basal lamina of the epithelium, and the bases of the epithelial cells, mostly basal cells, small portions of the secretory cells, and a few neuroendocrine cells are engaged in this extended contact area. During prenatal and postnatal development, aging, and hormone-induced regression, the epithelio-stromal interface undergoes characteristic changes.

The basal plasma membrane of prostatic basal and secretory cells is fixed to the basal lamina mainly by a number of hemidesmosomes. The basal lamina is usually smooth, measuring 70–100 nm, and consists of a typical lamina rara and lamina densa. It adheres firmly to the epithelium, to which it remains attached during mechanical separation of epithelium and stroma. The outline of the basal lamina is undulating in some specimens, serrating or developing footletlike protrusions. In some instances a reticulate network of the basal lamina is seen partially in connection with the basal plasma membrane of the epithelial cells.

Characteristic changes are observed in the basement membrane of rat prostate (dorsal, ventral, coagulating gland) after androgen deprivation or estrogen treatment [118,233]. In the coagulating

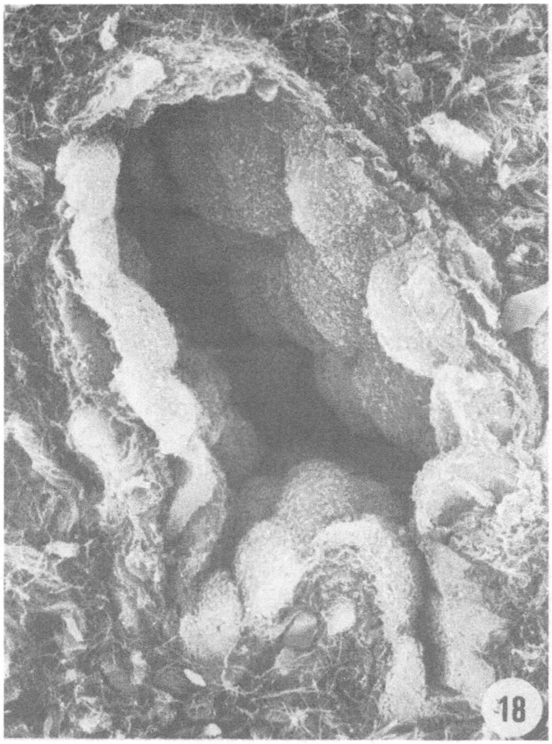

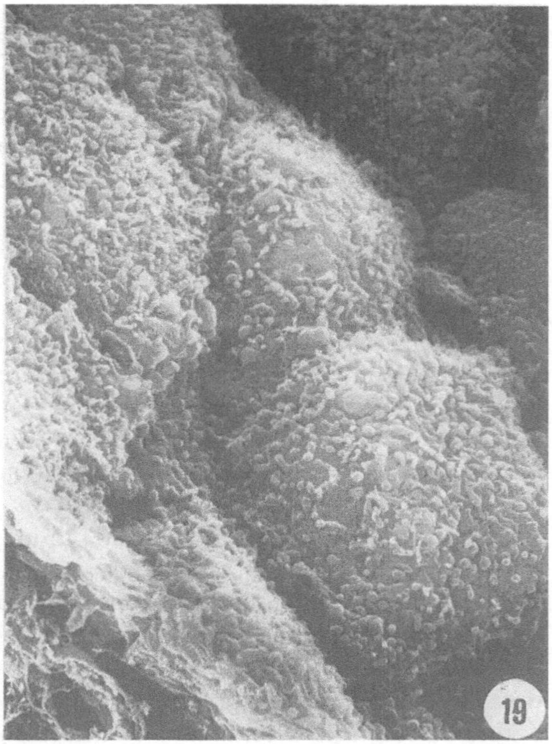

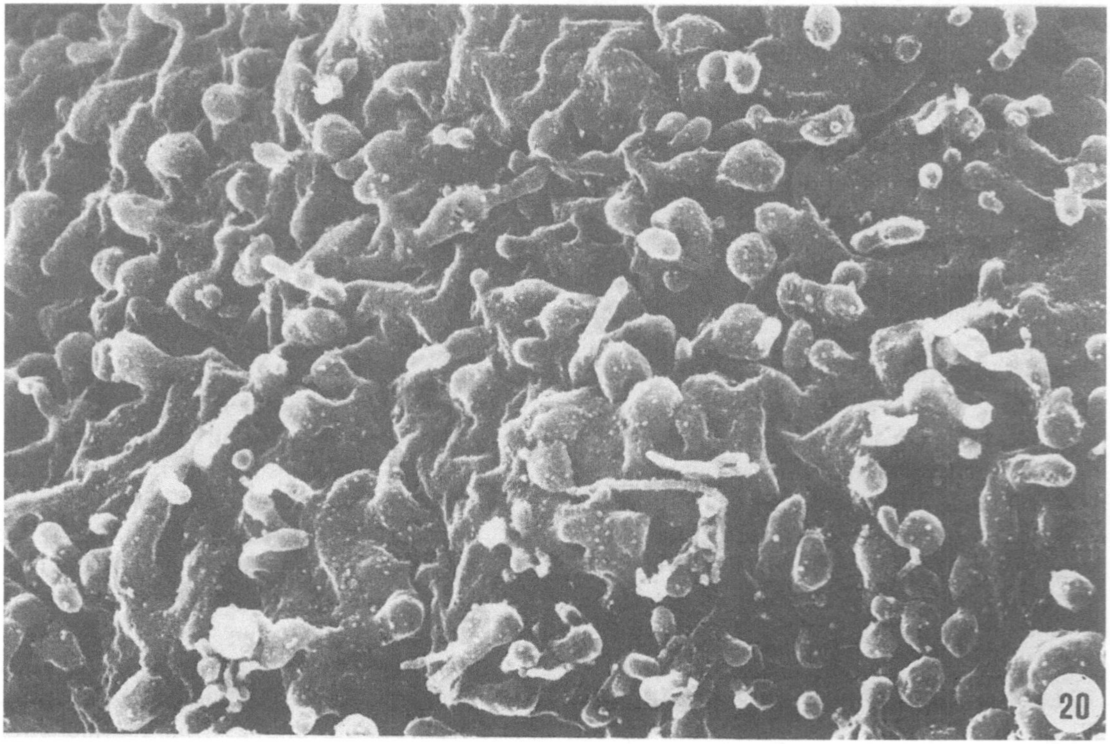

Figures 18–20 show the surface structure of human prostatic epithelium

Fig 18 Human prostatic acinus from a case of benign prostatic hyperplasia Epithelial cells are rather low (atrophic) (×1500)

Fig 19 Apical portions of human prostatic secretory cells bulging slightly into the lumen (×4500)

Fig 20 Irregular clublike protrusions of the apical plasma membrane of a human prostatic secretory cells (×15 000)

gland for instance, the relative volume percentage of subepithelial basement membrane increases by a factor of 4.5 at 6–12 weeks after castration. In the dorsal prostate, castration also induces proliferation of the subepithelial fibroblasts with massive deposition of basement membrane components, rendering the epithelio-stromal interface highly irregular. This resulted in a typical deformation of the basal outline of the epithelial cells. Just as altering cell morphology alters DNA synthesis and gene expression, the hormone induced changes in epithelial cell basal surface may play a significant role.

Murphy et al. [185] studied the effects of the individual matrix components collagen I and IV, laminin, and the complete basement membrane (Matrigel) on the morphology, motility, growth rate, and secretion of a human prostate cancer cell line (LNCaP) in the absence or presence of dihydrotestosterone (DHT). Dynamic cell structure as measured by cell motility was very sensitive to the extracellular matrix (ECM) components and the presence of DHT. Interdependence of growth, secretion, and ECM mediated effects was less clear in this transformed prostatic cell line. Fixation of cells to the extracellular matrix is one of the prerequisites for polarized secretion. In an elegant experimental study using a bicameral culture system, Djakiew et al. [74] studied the density dependent polarized secretion of the PA III rat prostate cancer cell line grown in a serum-free defined medium. The cells form morphologically polarized, hydrodynamically impermeable layers, whereas culture in 5% calf serum results in formation of squamous cell layers that are hydrodynamically permeable. These cells are comparable to the anaplastic phenotype and exhibit an inversion of polarized total protein secretion with an increased protein proportion (especially of proteases) secreted in a basal direction (at lower cell densities). Analysis of protease secretion under these conditions showed that metalloproteinases, tissue-type plasminogen activator, and a 72 kD gelatinase were secreted in a predominantly basal direction, as well as urokinase and a gelatinase of 26 kD that were secreted more or less equally into the apical and basal compartments of the chambers. The consequences of such a loss or inversion of polarized secretion would be to increase the localized concentrations of proteases along the basal domain of cells, thereby facilitating degradation of the basement membrane and interstitial tissue in vivo [74].

In addition to the characteristic basement membrane proteins (collagen IV, laminin, fibronectin), tenascin is expressed in a hormone-dependent manner [20]. Human prostatic stromal cells grown in vitro produced only little tenascin under control conditions, reflecting the adult state in situ, where rather little tenascin was detected immunohistochemically in the basement membrane. Stimulation with DHT, however, clearly induced tenascin expression. This effect was exceeded by the strong induction of tenascin production with sodium butyrate.

Glycosaminoglycanes (GAGs) of the epithelio-stromal interface are not well characterized. Chan and Wong [49] studied glycoconjugates in the lateral prostate of the guinea pig using gold-labeled lectins. In general, the stromal extracellular matrix as well as the epithelial basement membranes demonstrated a weak lectin binding. Mannosyl, N-acetylglucosamine, galactose/N-acetylgalactosamine residues, and complex glycoconjugates, such as chondroitin sulphate, were noted in the stromal tissues of the guinea pig lateral prostate, including the extracellular matrix, capillaries, and smooth muscle.

5.3. Basal Cells

Morphologically, the basal cells of the prostate in different species resemble each other very closely (see Fig. 23). They are flat, trigonal, ovoid, or lense-shaped cells, measuring 4–6 μm in height and 9–11 μm in width, which are located between the glandular cells and basement membrane. Their shape varies considerably. Columnar basal cells, with their long axis in the same plane as that of the columnar glandular cells, are not infrequent. Occasionally, cells resembling basal cells are seen interposed between the glandular cells. Their apex appears to extend toward the acinar lumen, making their true identity uncertain. The plasma membranes of the basal cells display a strong activity of ATPase and 5′-nucleotidase; the latter may therefore be used as a marker enzyme for these cells. The basal cells are fixed with hemidesmosomes on the basal lamina and exhibit

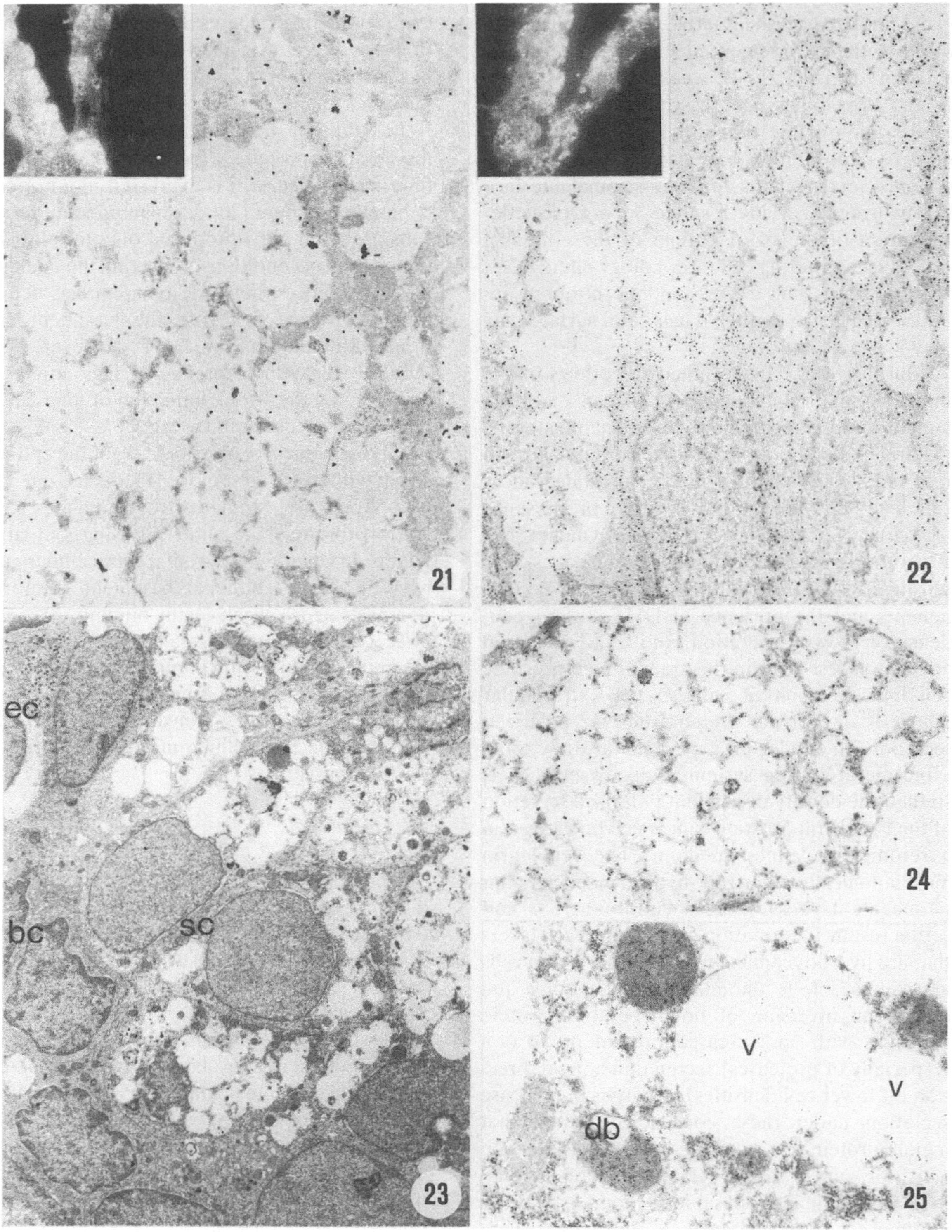
21
22
ec
bc
sc
23
24
v
v
db
25

a linear attachment to the columnar cells, but desmosomes are also found [24,35], and in some instances an intricate system of microplicae is seen to interdigitate with adjacent plasma membranes.

The cytoplasmic matrix is more electron dense than that of the columnar secretory cells and in some instances it seems remarkably condensed. Cytoplasmic organelles are scanty, as in poorly differentiated cells. The cytoplasmic/nuclear ratio is clearly in favor of the latter. The nucleus is oval, with its long axis parallel to the basement membrane and often indented or even markedly lobulated. The chromatin is more dense than that of secretory cell nuclei and is concentrated on the nuclear membrane. Nucleoli are often conspicuous and present in most of the basal cell nuclei. The cytoplasmic matrix contains rough endoplasmic reticulum, free ribosomes, mitochondria, a Golgi apparatus, lysosomes, microfilaments, microtubules, lipid droplets, and glycogen. No polar arrangement of the cytoplasmic organelles is recognizable.

The rough endoplasmic reticulum is sparse. Only a few short narrow membrane profiles are seen, irregularly studded with ribosomes. Most of the latter are encountered in the cytoplasmic matrix, where they form the majority of cytoplasmic structures. A few polyribosomes are also seen. Mitochondria of usual size and configuration with matrix granules are present and are frequently clustered in foci of the cytoplasm. They are usually round, oval or rod shaped, and often smaller than those of the glandular cells. The intimate contact of rough endoplasmic reticulum and mitochondria common in the glandular cells is never seen in the basal cells.

The Golgi apparatus is present, but often appears poorly developed. It is composed of a few stacks of flat cisternae and vesicles. Vacuoles are usually absent and secretory vacuoles have not been observed. Multivesicular bodies, dense bodies, and lysosomes are occasionally present in the Golgi region. They display lysosomal acid phosphatase activity. Occasional acid phosphatase-positive lipid droplets may be observed. Secretory acid phosphatase activity has never been noted in the basal cells. The lack of such enzymic activity, absence of attachment plates and surface vesicles, and a perinuclear distribution of organelles help distinguish its cytoplasm from that of smooth muscle cells.

The plasma membrane of the basal cell adjacent to the basement membrane is occasionally undulating, but is usually straight and lacking hemidesmosomes or attachment devices. Pinocytotic vesicles are rare, but coated vesicles are relatively frequent. The lateral and apical aspects of the plasma membrane are often thrown into complex folds and interdigitations with adjacent basal or glandular cells. Microvilli or microplicae are present in the intercellular space. Desmosomes are present between basal and glandular cells. In inadequately fixed specimens, the intercellular space between the basal cells exhibits lacunar distensions, which contain fine granular material of low electron density.

Immunohistochemically, strong immunoreactivity of epidermal growth factor receptor has been described in basal cells of human prostatic

←

Figures 21–25 represent examples of immunocytochemical reactions of human prostatic epithelium

Fig 21 Secretory cells from a hyperplastic human prostate gland Immunogold staining of secretory vacuoles using an antibody against secretory prostatic acid phosphatase (PAP) The size of the gold particles is 20 nm (×13,000) *Inset* PAP immunofluorescence of the same specimen (×1500)

Fig 22 Secretory cell from human hyperplastic prostate gland Immunogold staining using an antibody directed against prostate specific antigen (PSA) is confined to the cytoplasmic matrix Secretory vacuoles are only slightly labeled The size of the gold particles is 20 nm (×6700) *Inset* PSA immunofluorescence Serial section adjacent to that shown in inset of Figure 21 (×1500)

Fig 23 Survey electron micrograph of human prostatic glandular epithelium consisting of basal (bc), enterochromaffin (ec), and secretory cells (sc) Note the structural diversity of the secretory vacuoles (×11,000)

Fig 24 High power electron micrograph showing the subcellular distribution of PSA immunoreactive material in the cytoplasmic matrix of a human prostatic secretory cells (×11,000)

Fig 25 High power electron micrograph showing the PAP immunoreactive vacuoles (v) and dense bodies (db) in a human prostatic secretory cells (×27,000)

epithelium by Maygarden et al. [166]. In all cases of intact prostate or benign prostatic hyperplasia, the authors found strong immunostaining in a continuous or nearly continuous pattern, with staining restricted to the basal layer of the glands. This distribution pattern closely resembles that described for prolactin binding [279] or the localization of stratum corneum keratin described by Wernert et al. [275] in the adult prostate. In the fetal and prepubertal prostate, the multilayered epithelium of the prostatic ducts is positive for all keratin antibodies. Only after puberty, the immature multilayered epithelium becomes double layered, consisting of the peripheral, flattened to cuboidal basal cells (immunoreactive for stratum corneum keratins) and an inner cylindric epithelium positive for keratins 8 and 19 [275].

Wilson et al. [278] studied the distribution of cathepsin D, an apoptosis-related enzyme in both the normal and castrated ventral prostate of the rat. In regressing ventral prostate, they described the appearance of cells parallel to the basement membrane that are laden with immunoreactive cathepsin D and resemble macrophagelike cells. The origin of these basally positioned cathepsin D-positive cells in the epithelium was not fully established, but the authors hypothesize that these cells differentiate from a cell originating in the epithelium, that is, the basal cells, as they had not observed an invasion of the epithelium by macrophages. The possibility of the basal cell differentiating into a phagocytic cell is a new concept for the yet unresolved functions of this cell type and is difficult to accept from a mere morphological point of view.

Because of its relatively indifferentiated appearance, basal cells have been thought of as stem or progenitor cells [27,57,70,220,234] whose progeny would eventually differentiate into secretory cells [50,172,260]. This concept is not supported by studies that show both secretory and basal cells of castrated mice incorporate ^{3}H-thymidine and divide following testosterone replacement [81,83].

Early ultrastructural studies [212] suggested prostatic basal cells to be myoepithelial cells because of structural similarities with the salivary myoepithelial cells. Although the term *myoepithelial* has been applied to basal cells of the prostate by a number of authors, this point of view was rejected by others [18,22,24] for a number of reasons:

1. Immunohistochemistry using cytokeratin isotype specific antibodies [13,36,150,172,187, 200,260] demonstrated cytokeratins 5, 13, 14, and 16 to be expressed in human prostatic basal cells by Feitz et al. [85] and Srigley et al. [230].
2. Unlike the prostatic basal cells, Srigley et al. [230] found myoepithelial cells of salivary glands strongly positive for smooth-muscle specific actin (antibody HHF35) and negative for cytokeratins 7, 8, 13, 16, 17, and 18 (antibodies 8.12 and PKK1).
3. Myoepithelial cells are usually found in ectodermally and entodermally derived glands, such as the sweat, mammary, tracheobronchial, salivary [230] and bulbourethral glands [208]. They have a hybrid phenotype intermediate between epithelial and mesenchymal cells in that they contain muscle-specific myofilament proteins together with keratin-type intermediate filaments. They can therefore be discriminated immunohistochemically from smooth muscle cells, which usually contain desmin as an intermediate filament protein, and from myofibroblasts, which contain the intermediate filament protein vimentin along with myofilament proteins.
4. An additional constant feature of myoepithelial cells present in the mammary gland is their interposition between luminal cells and the basement membrane (as can be visualized by laminin staining). Glands containing myoepithelial cells are usually devoid of smooth muscle cells in the stroma and vice versa.

Srigley et al. [230], in a very meticulous immunohistochemical and ultrastructural study on basal cells in human prostate, found the cells negative with the rhodamine-tagged phalloidin, a chemical that binds specifically to actin microfilaments. At the ultrastructural level they also report on the absence of thin microfilament bundles, dense bodies, and micropinocytotic vesicles in prostatic basal cells. This varies with earlier reports. In our own specimens, microfilaments were seen in basal cells, and these reacted with smooth-muscle specific actin. Microfilaments of a variable amount are present in basal cells. They are approximately

5 nm in width, of indeterminate length, and are scattered throughout the cytoplasm. Their orientation appears at random and follows no definite axis. They occasionally form bundles similar to those seen in the basal region of the secretory cells. The number of these filaments appear to be inversely proportional to the amount of cytoplasmic free ribosomes.

Basal cells exhibiting a great abundance of microfilaments in the cytoplasm are common in the human genital tract and occur in the epididymis [108] and the deferent duct [115]. Hoffer [115] discusses the possibility that the dense network of filaments in basal cells may serve as a cytoskeleton and that this feature, in turn, stabilizes the epithelium at a time of maximum distension or compression. Under certain conditions, the basal cells of the human prostate apparently undergo a kind of metaplastic transformation and develop a myoepithelial phenotype. Grignon et al. [104] studied cases of sclerosing adenosis of the human prostate, a rare lesion characterized by the proliferation of variably sized glands in a cellular stroma. In addition to typical PSA-positive secretory cells, the glands contained a distinct population of cells reacting to muscle specific actin and the S-100 protein antibodies. Ultrastructural studies localized these cells between the basement membrane and the secretory cells, a position typical for myoepithelial cells. They were also different from cells observed in basal cell hyperplasia [57].

Basal cells are also suggested to play a role in the transportation of substrates or fluids between the periacinar stroma and the secretory cells of the acini. Adenosine triphosphatase activity was described on the basal cell plasma membrane, and micropinocytotic and coated vesicles are found on their basal surfaces [249]. In addition, complex plasma membrane infoldings and interdigitations between basal and secretory cells were found. These ultrastructural features and the frequent close proximity of blood capillaries in the stroma to basal cells [249] support the concept of their transport role.

5.4. *Neuroendocrine Cells*

In addition to the basal cells underlying the secretory cells, the prostate is peculiar in having basally located (neuro-) endocrine cells (see Fig. 23) [2,24]. Endocrine cells in the human prostate were regarded by Feyrter [88] as "paracrine." They have been identified both by different silver staining procedures [2,87] as well as by electron microscopy [3,24,71,87]; review [2]. In addition to the human prostate and urethra [264], they have also been found in different animals. The paracrine/neuroendocrine cells of the human prostate are represented by at least two types of cells [2]:

1. Serotonin-producing cells, immunoreactive also for neurone-specific enolase (NSE), chromogranin A (Chr A), and a TSH-like polypeptide (32 kD). In some of these cells, calcitonin has been demonstrated immunohistochemically.
2. Much less frequent neuroendocrine cells are immunoreactive for somatostatin.
3. In addition, Fetissof et al. [86] found calcitonin secreting cells in prostatic carcinomas and numerous other hormones have also been described [72]. The cell types appear in the open (lumen reaching), closed, and dendritic forms [71]. Abrahamsson and Lilja [1] have shown the TSH-immunoreactive cells to contain a peptide (32 kD) that has certain structural homologies with the pituitary β-subunit of TSH and is secreted into the seminal fluid [194,271].

The endocrine cells of the human prostate have recently attracted the interest of a number of authors [33,66,71,271]. A detailed discussion is presented by de Mesy Jensen and di Sant' Agnese in this volume.

6. Secretory Cell Maturation and Function

6.1. *Significance of Prostatic Secretion*

The secretions from male accessory sex glands interact with each other and with spermatozoa, their predominant functions being semen gelation, coagulation and liquefaction, coating and decoating of spermatozoa, ionic and metabolic exchange reactions between seminal plasma and spermatozoa, and interaction with cervical mucus [18, 163]. While the method of split-ejaculates yielded only rough estimates of the nature of various

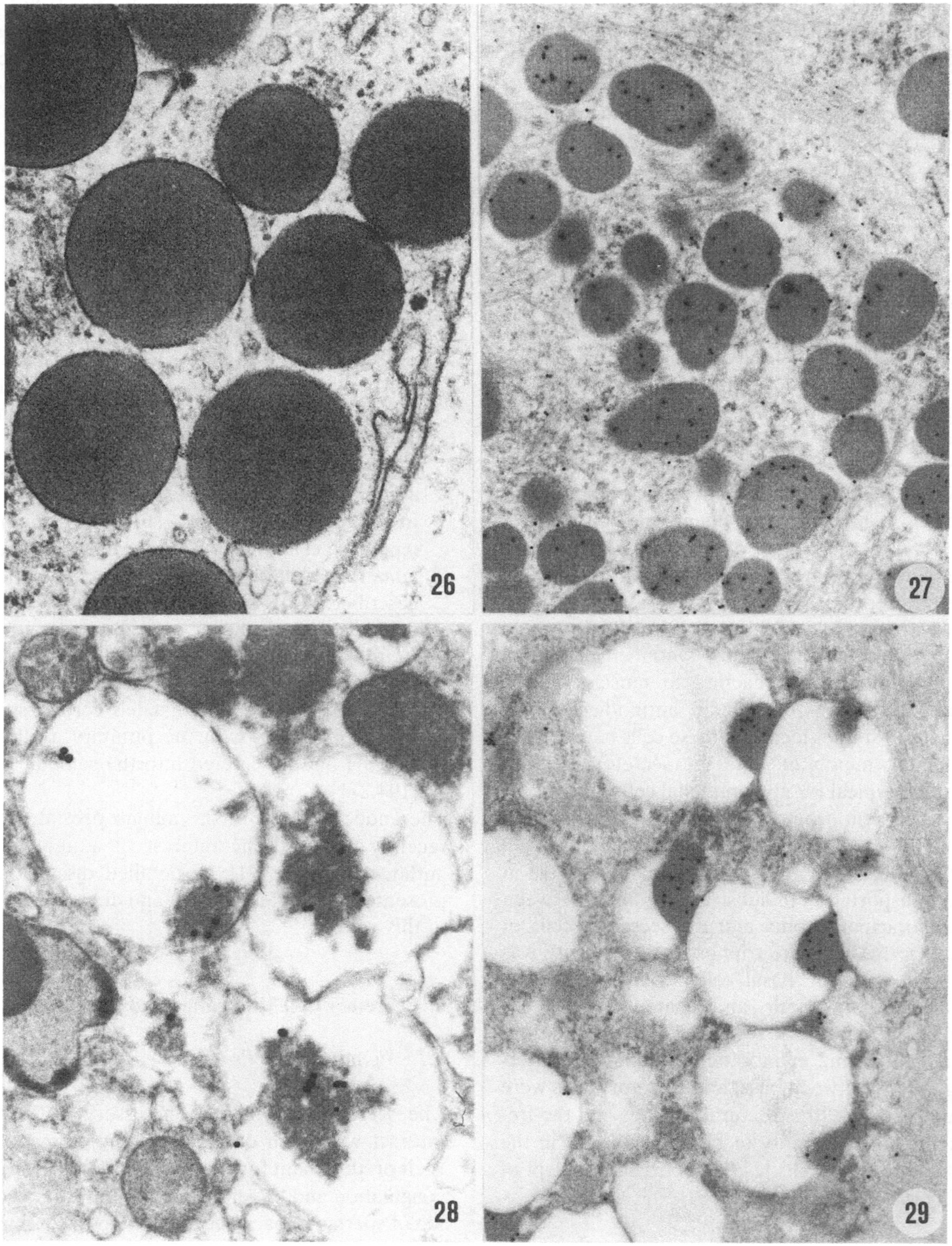
26
27
28
29

compounds and their respective source, two-dimensional gel electrophoresis (2D-PAGE) of semen or isolated glandular secretion [153], or of organ homogenates [150], led to the identification and molecular and functional characterization of several proteins, both in human and experimental animals. In addition to immunosuppressive material [128], sperm-motility blocking agents, an antifertility compound, and a sperm-binding protein have recently been described in human semen [16]. The search in forensic medicine for specific markers of human semen following sexual assault has revealed a variety of different proteins, one of which turned out to be the essential gel-forming substance delivered from seminal vesicles into semen, semenogelin [154], and MHS-5 [111]. The differences in clotting and liquefaction observed in human semen can now be determined quantitatively, since both the clotting and the liquefying system, prostate specific antigen (PSA) [267], have been isolated and characterized. Although quite a number of secretory proteins are known in the human prostate, only three [153] have gained major importance as diagnostic tools, namely, acid phosphatase (PSA) [267,270] and β-microseminoprotein. The nature of the latter is controversial [77,272], as it shows partial sequence homology with β-inhibin [28,76,98]. In view of pathogenetic mechanisms in the human prostate, additional secretory proteins, such as prostatic growth factors [113,127,236] and hormones [1, 193,194,273], have aroused the interest of both biochemists and pathologists, as they were thought to be of particular significance in the regulation of prostatic growth [246].

6.2. *Morphology of Prostatic Secretory Cells*

The secretory cells of the prostate and seminal vesicles share a basic ultrastructural organization [34] in that they may be divided into five different functional zones, that is, basal, nuclear, supranuclear, Golgi, and apical zones, arranged in a polarized manner (Figs. 18–25). The dimensions of a secretory cell from the human prostate are about 12–13 μm (range 8–25 μm) in height and 8–10 μm in width. The diameter of the nucleus is about 5–7 μm and the supranuclear zone varies in height (2–8 μm). The round or ovoid nucleus is situated in the lower third of the cell. In the lower third, numerous mitochondria, short profiles of rough endoplasmic reticulum, free ribosomes, lysosomes, and dense bodies, along with round lipid droplets and clusters of glycogen, are found. This region is stabilized by a dense meshwork of intermediate filaments and microfilaments that are fixed to basal hemidesmosomes and lateral desmosomes. This compartment is continuous with the perinuclear region, where endoplasmic reticulum, mitochondria, few Golgi vesicles, dense bodies, and secretory vacuoles may be present. The bulk of the extremely pleomorphic secretory vacuoles interspersed with dictyosomes of the Golgi apparatus, mitochondria, dense bodies, lipofuscins, multivesicular bodies, short profiles of rough endoplasmic reticulum, free ribosomes, glycogen, and cytoskeletal elements is found in the supranuclear region. The apical region comprises the apical plasma membrane, with a varying number of short stubby microvilli, a few vesicles, and several secretory vacuoles, often bulging out at the apical pole into the lumen. Microfilaments as well as intermediate filaments in this area concentrate at the junctional complex.

The ultrastructure of the monkey prostate is rather similar to that of the human prostate. The secretory vacuoles differ only slightly in structure. In the monkey prostate, the secretory vacuoles (2.5–4.0 μm in diameter) are either empty or contain flocculent, or condensed granules (0.4–

←

Figures 26–29 illustrate the polymorphism of the secretory granules of the prostate in different species and their hormone dependence

Fig 26 High power electron micrograph of secretory granules from a canine prostatic granular cell Secretory material homogeneously distributed and granular structure is very regular (×83,000)

Fig 27 Slightly irregular-shaped secretory granules from a canine prostatic glandular cell after 6 weeks of estradiol treatment Immunogold staining with a PAP antibody is confined to the secretory granules Size of gold particles 5 nm (×27,000)

Fig 28 High power electron micrograph of secretory vacuoles in prostatic glandular cells of a cynomolgus monkey PSA immunoreactivity is confined to electron-dense material (×65,000)

Fig 29 Immunogold staining with anti-SVS II of the dense core of secretory vacuoles in the epithelium of the rat lateral prostate Gold particle size 10 nm (×41,000)

1 0 μm in diameter) These granules contain a protein crossreactive with human PSA antibody (Fig 28)

In the canine prostate, the secretory cells vary in height from cuboidal to tall columnar Nuclei occupy a basal position and are round to slightly elongated in shape, sometimes indented, and contain a prominent nucleolus surrounded by coarse clumps of chromatin The endoplasmic reticulum is moderately developed, mostly concentrated in the basal and perinuclear region, and is interspersed with short round, oval, or elongated mitochondria, dense bodies, lysosomes, and numerous free ribosomes The supranuclear cytoplasm contains numerous round secretory granules (Figs 26 and 27) and a well-developed Golgi complex The apical plasma membrane is studded with numerous elongated microvilli, except where it bulges into the lumen The lateral plasma membranes have numerous plications and interdigitations, as well as a few desmosomes The basal plasma membrane is smooth The size of the Golgi apparatus, the number of condensing vacuoles, and the structure of the secretory granules in different species is clearly hormone dependent When castrated dogs are treated with 5α-androstanediol, a significant increase in the number of secretory granules is observed, often reaching the extent found in glandular hyperplasia Bulging of the apical plasma membrane into the lumen is frequently observed

Abnormal growth of the prostate (benign prostatic hyperplasia, BPH) occurs frequently in dogs and humans, in both cases associated with increasing age Brendler et al [37] demonstrated that prostatic weight increased steadily in beagles between 2 and 6 years of age, paralleled by a progressive increase in the incidence of BPH This was primarily due to proliferation of the epithelial cells lining the acini of the prostate, with some proliferation of stromal tissue In a quantitative analysis of epithelial and stromal tissue and cellular compartments in immature, normal, and hyperplastic canine prostates, Zirkin and Strandberg [283] found significant differences in the volume densities of glandular and stromal tissue but not in glandular epithelial cells The volume density of glandular tissue was significantly lower, and stromal tissue significantly higher, in the immature prostate than that in prostates characterized as normal or hyperplastic The volume densities of these tissues were not significantly different in normal and hyperplastic prostates In contrast, the absolute volumes of each of the glandular, epithelial, are stromal compartments were significantly greater in prostates of dogs with BPH than in normal prostates, and greater in normal than in immature prostates The numbers of epithelial cells per prostate and the volume of an average epithelial cell were also different in the three groups, being greater in prostates of dogs with BPH than in normal prostates and greater in normal than in immature prostates The results of stereological analyses of the volume density of cytoplasmic organelles in prostatic epithelial cells of immature, normal, and hyperplastic prostates showed significant differences in rough endoplasmic reticulum, free ribosomes, and secretion granules Organelle volume density did not differ significantly in epithelial cells of the normal and BPH groups, but free ribosome volume density was higher, and RER and secretion granules were lower in cells of the immature prostate than in the normal and BPH groups

In summary, in the immature canine prostate,

→

Figures 30–33 display characteristic features of rat dorsal prostate and coagulating gland

Fig 30 Survey electron micrograph of secretory cells from rat coagulating gland Note polymorphic apical blebs (asterisks) (×11 000)

Fig 31 Survey electron micrograph of secretory cells from rat dorsal prostate Numerous intraluminal secretory blebs (asterisks) (×6600)

Fig 32 Membrane apposed endoplasmic cisternae in rat dorsal prostatic secretory cell neighboring a Golgi apparatus (×51 000)

Fig 33 Polymorphic deformed and partly demembranated (arrows) apical blebs released from secretory cells of rat dorsal prostate 15 minutes after carbamylcholine stimulation of secretion (×21 000)

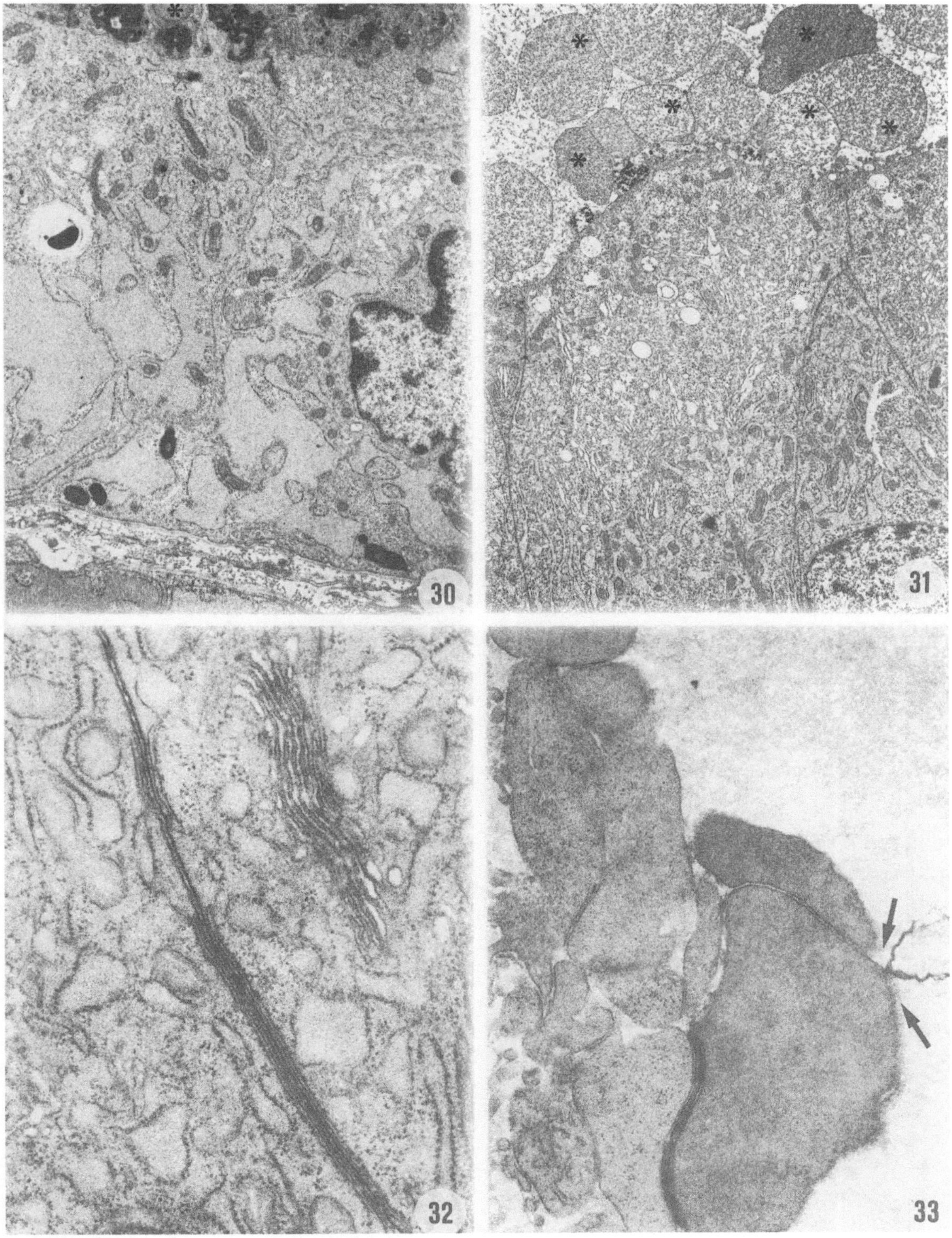
30
31
32
33

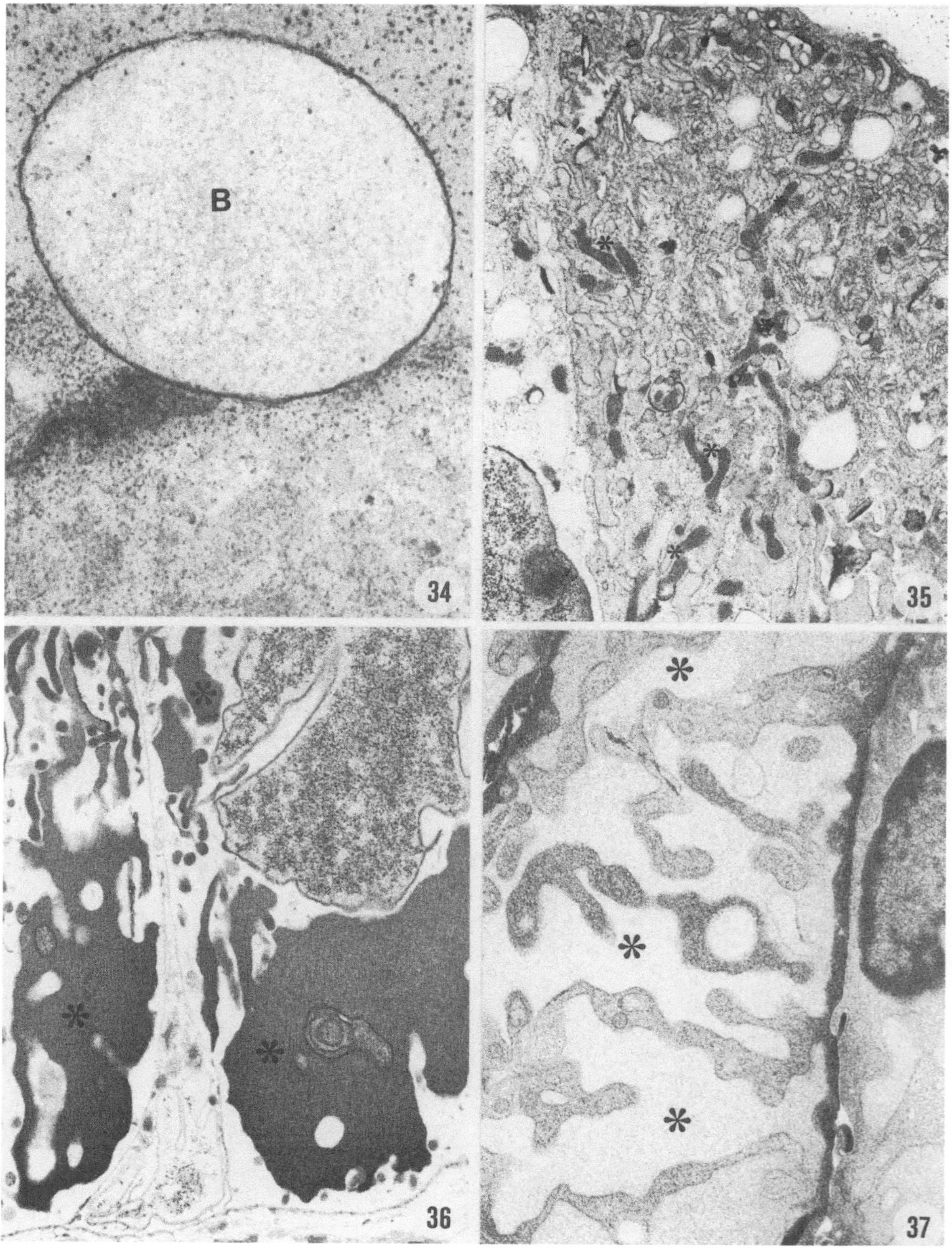
B
34
35
36
37

the absolute volumes of glandular tissue, epithelial cells, and stromal tissue were significantly lower than in the normal and hyperplastic gland, as were epithelial cell number and average volume. Ultrastructural differences in prostatic epithelial cells were obvious from the significantly diminished volume density of secretion granules in epithelial cell cytoplasm, reflecting the very low secretory activity in these dogs. The lacking difference in the volume density of cytoplasmic organelles in secretory cells from normal and hyperplastic canine prostates resembles the same situation in the human gland.

In rodents, the prostate is a complex organ, made up of the ventral, lateral, and dorsal lobes [24,34]. The lateral prostate (Fig. 29) shares several functional features with the seminal vesicles [11,18], as does the dorsal lobe with the coagulating gland (Figs. 30–41) [277]. The different lobes of the prostate have several histological features in common, being built up of acini of various sizes, composed of columnar epithelium resting on a thin basement membrane. A systematic study of the fine structural difference of the rat prostatic complex has been performed by Dahl et al. [63]. The ventral prostate is easily identified immunohistochemically by its prostatic binding protein (PBP) content [14,112]. The epithelium of the coagulating gland forms branching papillary projections and shows clear vacuoles in the basal cytoplasm, as well as apical blebs projecting into the lumen. The same applies for the dorsal prostate. The lateral prostate is peculiar in that in older animals the acinar lumen is filled with condensed secretion, which has a tendency to cause a sterile inflammation [183]. There are considerable ultrastructural differences between the prostatic lobes in a given species as well as between different species. Since the rat prostatic complex is one of the best studied, a brief survey of the ultrastructure based on earlier reviews [24,34] and recent findings [122,123,214,215] is given.

The epithelial cells of the ventral prostate vary in height depending on the sexual activity of the animal [11]. In sexually inactive animals, the cells are low columnar, lining the lumen filled with condensed secretion. The cytoplasm contains microtubules distributed longitudinally from the apical region to the basal region, but no microtubules are found in the nuclear region. Most of the microfilaments are localized beneath the apical plasma membrane [145]. The apical and supranuclear portions of the cells contain many densely packed, round secretory granules. In ventral prostate of sexually active animals, the cells increase in height, the rough endoplasmic develops, and its turnover appears enhanced, as deduced from the numerous lysosomal structures. The Golgi apparatus, condensing vacuoles, and the rather polymorphic secretory granules increase significantly in extent and amount. Intraluminal secretion achieves a flocculent to granular character, which may be due to enhanced fluid transport through the epithelium. Stimulation of the rat prostate with either pilocarpine or testosterone [142] results in protrusion of the apical compartment of the secretory cells. In freeze fracture replicas, Kachar and Pinto da Silva [131] were able to distinguish between condensing vacuoles of the Golgi zone, apical condensing vacuoles, and secretory granules, showing a low density of membrane particles, the lowest found among all cytoplasmic structures.

In the lateral prostate of sexually inactive rats, the secretory granules are still more condensed, consisting of a central granule in a large vacuole. In sexually active animals, this type of secretion granule is rare in the lateral prostate, but the secretory vacuole is instead replete with dispersed

←

Figures 34–37 illustrate different compartments found in secretory cells of rat dorsal prostate

Fig 34 Rat dorsal prostate, 1300 nm thick section, impregnated copper ion Impregnation precipitate is excluded from the contents of the bleb (B) (×12,600)

Fig 35 Same specimen as in Figure 34 Preferential impregnation of the mitochondria (asterisks) in the supranuclear compartment (×6000)

Fig 36 Same specimen as in Figure 34 Cisternae of rough endoplasmic reticulum (asterisks) are impregnated (×6000)

Fig 37 Same specimen as in Figure 34 Preferential impregnation of the cytoplasmic matrix and exclusion from cisternae of rough endoplasmic reticulum (asterisks) (×12,000)

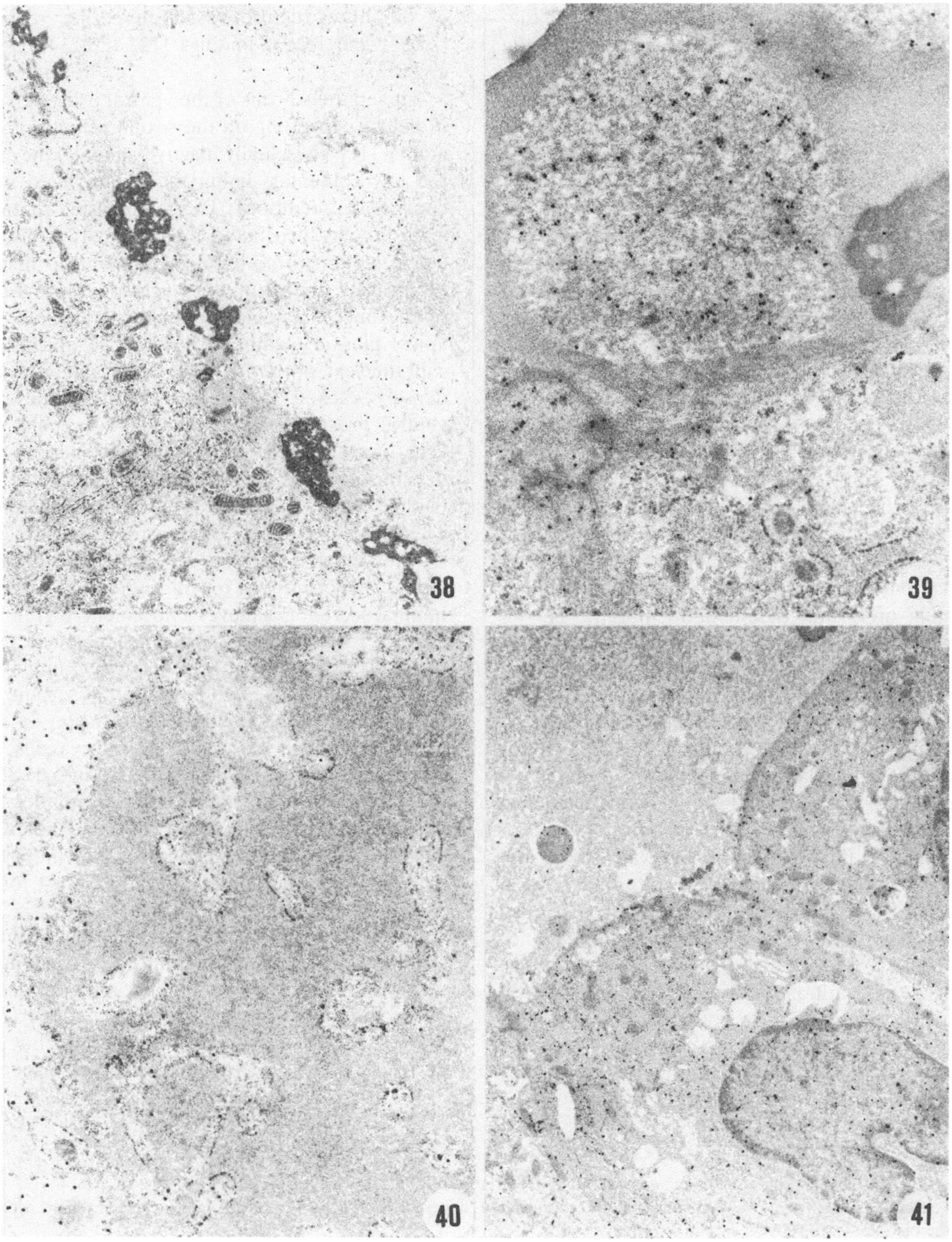
38
39
40
41

flocculent material. The Golgi apparatus is not very prominent. The endoplasmic reticulum surrounding the basally located nucleus consists of elongated and narrow cisternae, where dense bodies of different sizes occur. The microvilli of the apical plasma membrane are slender and contain a central actin bundle and peripherally located α-actinin [134].

The coagulating gland and the dorsal prostate of the rat are unique in that they are devoid of characteristic secretory granules [9]. The secretory cells contain a basally located large nucleus. A well-developed Golgi apparatus surrounded by numerous vesicles and vacuoles is located in the supranuclear region. The rough endoplasmic reticulum consists of widely dilated cisternae (Fig. 30). In the apical third of the lateral plasma membranes of adjacent cells, collapsed cisternae of rough endoplasmic reticulum are arranged in parallel with the slightly curved plasma membranes (Fig. 32). A salient feature of secretory cells is the presence of apical blebs or protrusions, which are mostly round but may also be irregular in shape. In cases where the connection of the blebs with the cells is visible, it has the appearance of microvilli. As will be discussed later, these blebs are the equivalent of apocrine secretion.

6.3. *Ultrastructural Immunolocalization of Prostatic Secretory Proteins*

The recent development in immunohistochemical methods using a potent signal enhancement systems have allowed the identification of quite a number of secretory (and cytoskeletal) proteins in the accessory sex glands, both at the light microscopic and electron microscopic levels. The importance of prostatic secretory proteins as markers of prostatic cancer has prompted a number of studies on the ultrastructural localization of these proteins as well as on their release from normal and malignant cells (acid phosphatase [10,180, 228,269]; PSA [226,269], β-microseminoprotein [10]). Lilja and Abrahamsson [153] studied consecutive paraffin sections of the human prostate using antibodies against acid phosphatase (PAP), prostate specific antigen (PSA), and β-microseminoprotein (β-MSP). The immunoreactivity against all three proteins varied only slightly in staining intensity from specimen to specimen or from cell to cell within each section. All three proteins were present in the same cell. Although a number of different proteins have been described in human prostate (e.g., metalloendopeptidase [82], acid proteinases [205,206,207]), the three most important are secretory prostatic acid phosphatase (PAP), prostate specific antigen (PSA), and β-microseminoprotein (βMSP), which will be briefly described.

6.3.1. Acid Phosphatases (EC 3.1.3.2.). The term *acid phosphatases* describes a group of enzymes catalyzing the hydrolysis of several physiological and artificial monophosphate esters into the respective hydroxyl compounds and inorganic phosphate (P_i) at slightly acidic pH values. Neither the natural substrates nor the physiological function of the enzyme are precisely known as yet. Monophosphate esters are formed during a variety of metabolic processes, indicating multiple catalytic activity of the enzyme. At the cellular level, secretory and membrane-bound forms are known, the most important of which are lysosomal and may be used as marker enzymes [181]. Secretory acid phosphatases occur in salivary and accessory sex glands, preferentially in the prostate [18].

←

Figures 38–41 show the nonclassical intracellular pathway of transglutaminase biosynthesis

Fig 38 Apical portion of a secretory cell of rat coagulating gland. Positive immunoreaction (antibody against secretory transglutaminase) is found in apical blebs (×8000)

Fig 39 High power electron micrograph showing a strongly immunolabeled apical bleb (antibody against secretory transglutaminase, gold particle size 20 nm) (×25,000)

Fig 40 Strong immunolabeling (same antibody as in Fig 39) of the cytoplasmic matrix of a secretory cell from rat dorsal prostate No labeling of the cisternae of rough endoplasmic reticulum is seen (×20,000)

Fig 41 Fourteen days after castration only few, weakly labeled apical blebs are left Enhanced labeling of the cytoplasmic and nuclear matrix (×10,000)

Kutscher and Wolbergs [146] showed that acid phosphatase activity present in urine of adult men was due to admixture of prostatic fluid. Gutman and Gutman [106] introduced acid phosphatase as a marker for metastasizing prostatic cancer. To differentiate prostatic acid phosphatase (PAP) from other phosphatases, L (+)-tartrate was used as a "specific" inhibitor of PAP. Recent studies, however, showed that neither the enzyme test nor the immunological determination is specific, but rather false-negative and false-positive results are observed.

Acid phosphatase is present not only in the human prostate, but also in the caudal portion of prostate in the rhesus monkey, somewhat less in the canine prostate, and at low concentrations in the prostatic secretion of guinea pig, cat, rat, and rabbit, while high activities are present in bovine and cynomolgus prostate. Biosynthesis of the secretory enzyme is strictly androgen dependent.

Biochemical studies indicate that acid phosphatases are a heterogeneous class of polypeptides, differing with respect to pH optimum, substrate, and inhibitor specificity. A number of quantification assays have been developed using mostly artificial substrates. Most widely used is the hydrolysis of nitrophenylphosphate, but in addition phenylphosphate, phenolphthaleinphosphate, and 1-naphthylphosphate are used. Additional test systems measure the quantity of liberated phosphate.

ACID PHOSPHATASE FROM HUMAN PROSTATE. Both human prostatic and leucocytic acid phosphatases are well characterized. The native purified enzyme has a molecular weight of 90–109 kD and consists of two subunits, the molecular weight being 46–50 kD after SDS-PAGE. The protein is glycosylated. Amino acid analyses performed by Vihko et al. [261,262] and McTigue and van Etten [171] demonstrated a relatively high number (15–18) of cysteine residues, which seem to have only limited influence on enzymic activity. There are conflicting data on the N-terminal amino acids. Using isoelectric focusing and subsequent histochemical staining of human prostatic extracts, we were able to demonstrate 20 isoforms [221]. After comparison with isoenzymes from other human tissues, we distinguished three different groups. Group I consists of 13 isoenzymes focusing between pH 3.8 and 4.8, nine of these being secretory. Cofocusing isoforms are present in extracts from seminal vesicles, epididymis, female and male liver, kidney, and leucocytes. They are perhaps identical with leucocytic isoforms 2a and 4, as described by Yam et al. [281] and Lam et al. [147]. Four isoenzymes in group II focus between pH 5.0 and 5.5, and are also present in spleen and other tissues. Group III comprises five different bands, focusing between pH 5.6 and 5.9. They are present in nearly all organs extracts and presumably represent the lysosomal forms. The band pattern described is very stable. Addition of protease inhibitors or aging of the extracts for several days at 4–8°C did not change the band pattern. Addition of 1% serum albumin or citrate buffer (0.05 M, pH 4.8) had a stabilizing effect on enzyme activity. Interestingly, the IgG fraction of an antibody directed against acid phosphatase likewise stimulates enzyme activity [224]. In the presence of albumin, the formation of the 46 kD subunit from the 50 kD form is prevented. As has been shown by electrophoretic titration [221], acid phosphatases of group I are stable in the pH range between 2.9 and 9.5. Below pH 2.4, equaling the pK value of N-acetyl neuraminic acid, the 9–12 titration curves merge into a single line. Smith and Whitby [227] were already able to relate the microheterogeneity of prostatic acid phosphatase to glycosylation differences (variation of sialic acid residues) rather than to the differences in the polypeptide chain. Ostrowski et al. [189] and McTigue and van Etten [171] analyzed the carbohydrate moiety of the molecule. They found 2–3 fucosyl, 11–14 mannosyl, 4–7 galactosyl, 10–15 glucosamine, and 7–10 N-acetyl neuraminic acid residues.

Tyrosine phosphate represents one of several amino acid phosphates that is more readily hydrolyzed by prostatic acid phosphatase than serine and/or threonine phosphate. Li et al. [152] stated that normal acid phosphatase activity is always associated with a protein tyrosyl phosphatase. In competition experiments, we have shown that both tyrosyl phosphate and 1-naphthylphosphate mutually inhibit the histochemical reaction on IEF gels. Lin et al. [156] provided evidence of phosphotyrosyl-phosphatase activity of prostatic acid phosphatase, which is inversely related to a tyrosyl kinase activity. The nature and localization of the physiological substrate, however, are completely unknown as yet. The most likely candidate is a tyrosine-phosphorylated protein on epididymal sperm, where a protein kinase activity has been found.

6.3.2. PSA or Kallikreinlike Protease (EC 3.4.21.). Prostate specific antigen (PSA) is a protein highly specific for the human prostate, where it has been detected by Wang et al. [266]. Under native conditions and after SDS-PAGE, PSA has a molecular weight of 33–34 kD, a pI value of 6.9, and is glycosylated (2.7% w/w hexose, 2.8% w/w hexosamines, and 1.1% sialic acid). Comparing the N-terminal sequence of the protein to other proteases, Ban et al. [25] classified the protein into the kallikrein family. Lilja et al. [154] demonstrated that PSA hydrolyses semenogelin, the major coagulating product from human seminal vesicles.

Isolation of a PSA-coding mRNA from prostatic mRNA [159], in situ hybridization of PSA-mRNA in human prostate [203], and the lack of immunoreactivity with antisera to PSA in the other male sex glands [186] provides conclusive evidence of the prostate being the secretory origin of PSA in the male genital tract. Recently, Frazier et al. [95] detected immunoreactive PSA and PAP in male periurethral glands. Along with its previous immunolocalization in female Skenes ducts (prostate homologue [196]), certain forms of cystitis [188], urachal remnants [101], and cloacogenic remnants [132], this finding disproves the prostate specificity of this protein. Complete antigenic identity between PSA and γ-seminoprotein (γ-SM) [5] was shown in double immunodiffusion systems and by the establishment of the primary structure of PSA [159] and that of γ-SM.

6.3.3. β-Microseminoprotein (β-MSP). Lilja [154,155] isolated a low-molecular mass protein from seminal plasma as a byproduct during the purification of PSA from pooled seminal plasma. The protein had a molecular mass of about 15 kD on SDS-PAGE (after reduction). The amino acid composition of the purified protein largely resembled that of β-inhibin, β-MSP, and the secreted form of PSP 94 [77]. The immunohistochemical localization in human prostatic epithelium of β-inhibin [98] and of β-MSP [153] are identical and support the prostatic origin of β-MSP. Conclusive evidence of the prostatic origin of β-MSP was provided by detection of its mRNA in the prostate and by its subsequent molecular cloning and cDNA sequencing. The biological effect of β-MSP in human semen is as yet unknown. A proposed inhibitory effect of β-MSP (or β-inhibin) on the secretion of pituitary FSH secretion is at least doubtful and has been challenged by Gordon et al. [102]. Weiber et al. [272] have shown that β-microseminoprotein is not a prostate-specific protein. Immunohistochemically, they localized it in goblet cells of tracheobronchial epithelium and submucosal glands, in mucosal cells of the stomach, duodenal Brunners glands, colon, and the ciliated epithelium of the Fallopian tube and the Gartner ducts adjacent to the uterine cervix.

All three proteins (PAP, PSA, β-MSP) colocalize in prostatic epithelial cells, indicating their biosynthesis in the same cell (Figs. 21, 22, 24, and 25). However, a number of different proteins [158,192] show deviant localizations and have, therefore, been used to distinguish between the acini of the central zone and peripheral zone of the prostate. Lactoferrin was prevalent in epithelium of the central zone, periurethral glands, and lining epithelium of the prostatic urethra. Whether it is synthesized in these cells or whether its presence is due to trans-sudation from the dense capillary network of this area has not been solved.

At the electron microscopic level, some divergent results have been obtained by the different groups that have studied the ultrastructural localization of prostatic secretory proteins (acid phosphatase [10,180,228,269], PSA [226,269], β-MSP [2,153]. While Aumüller and Seitz [10] found acid phosphatase immunoreactivity restricted to the electron-translucent vacuoles and their electron-dense cores of the glandular cells and labeling of other cytoplasmic organelles in the background range, Song et al. [228] reported labeling of the Golgi apparatus. Warhol and Longtine [269] localized both PAP and PSA throughout the endoplasmic reticulum and the cytoplasmic vesicles as well as the intraluminal secretion of the prostate. Abrahamsson [2] found PSA and β-MSP immunoreactivity distributed throughout the endoplasmic reticulum and secretory vesicles, whereas acid phosphatase immunoreactivity was confined to lysosomal granules. He infers from this localization pattern that PSA and β-MSP, on one hand, and PAP, on the other hand, were separated into different storage compartments within the secretory cells. Divergent results obtained by different groups may be due to the fact that immunoelectron microscopic localization of secretory proteins is very much dependent on handling and fixation of the tissue, the quality of the antiserum used, and the detection method. Mori and Wakasugi [180], for example, used the unlabeled antibody-enzyme method and found that acid phosphatase was distributed at microvilli of the apical plasma membrane and the secretory granules of the supranuclear portion of the glandular cells. They assume that acid phosphatase may be a metabolite, converted from primary lysosomal acid phosphatase in the Golgi complex. It would then be translocated to the apical plasma membrane. The positively staining vesicles and the positively stained plasma membrane were extruded into the lumen according to an apocrine secretion mechanism.

The clearly limited structural preservation of prostatic tissue in all the studies mentioned forbids any definitive deductions on the intracellular transport and release mechanisms different from the classical pathway. In our specimens presented here (Figs. 21 and 22), we found a divergent localization of PSA (present in cytoplasm and mostly absent from secretory vacuoles) and of acid phosphatase (confined to secretory vacuoles and dense bodies). It is not clear, however, whether there is a functional compartmentalization in the secretory vacuoles, for example, in those of the rat seminal vesicles. The low degree of structural preservation does neither allow one to develop definite ideas on the morphogenesis of the highly complex prostatic secretory vacuoles.

7. Release Mechanisms

7.1. Merocrine Exocytosis

In the prostate secretory cell of different species, three different modes of secretion have been described (a) merocrine [18,24,34,110], (b) apocrine [34,130,131,135], and (c) diacytosis of prostasomes [41] (for review see [210]). Kachar and Pinto da Silva [130] described the coexistence of the apocrine and merocrine modes of secretion in epithelial cells of rat ventral prostate. They do not, however, rule out the possibility that these observations may be due to artifacts appearing during specimen preparation. As stated above, the secretory cells of the prostate are particularly sensitive to alterations in osmolarity, reduced oxygen tension, and mechanical compression. Differences in the resulting alteration (swelling of mitochondria, apical blebbing) may be due to differences in membrane thickness and stability [195]. Kawai and Aumüller [134] observed that the characteristic ultrastructure of apical microvilli in prostatic secretory cells is not sufficiently preserved after perfusion fixation with mild fixatives. Mild fixation results in changes of internal organization and actin distribution of the apical cell pole [145]. Certain experimental conditions, such as androgen deprivation or muscarinergic stimulation, result in a changed pressure within the tissue and may lead to apical blebbing in prostatic epithelial cells [135]. This should not be confused with apocrine secretion. In the canine prostate, light microscopic studies often report this phenomenon, but electron microscopy failed to support such findings [116,175]. Hohbach and Ueberberg [117] only found merocrine secretion in the prostate of the normal dog. Exocytosis that persisted after stimulation with pilocarpine was quantitatively increased to a great extent. Apocrine or holocrine types of secretion were neither found under resting conditions nor under extreme stimulation of the gland with pilocarpine.

In human prostate, and similarly in monkey prostate, the supranuclear portion of the secretory cells contains a highly complex system of vacuolar, vesicular, or granular structures (Fig. 24). The most prominent organelles of the supranuclear region are the secretory vacuoles. They are abundant in number and of extreme polymorphism, measuring between 0.8 and 2.2 μm. In current literature, the various forms of secretory vacuoles have been described insufficiently and no classification of morphogenesis has been attempted. A diagrammatic representation of the secretory granules together with their probable morphogenesis has previously been proposed [24].

Of course, the true morphogenesis of secretory granules remains uncertain until immunoelectron microscopic studies using several antibodies are performed. The morphological classification was based on mere morphological analysis, taking into account progressive development of vacuoles from those adjacent to the Golgi complex to the most apically situated ones. This assumption seems probable, as several authors describe an enlargement of the vacuoles from the Golgi region to the plasma membrane. At least six different forms can be seen [24]:

1. Clear empty membrane bound vacuoles
2. a) Membrane bound vacuoles with little floccular content
   b) Membrane bound vacuoles densely filled with floccular content
3. Clear membrane bound vacuoles containing small granules
   a) Without
   b) With central electron dense core
4. Membrane bound vacuoles with floccular content and a single granule
   a) Without
   b) With electron dense central core
5. Membrane bound vacuoles with dense floccular content and several
   a) Empty
   b) Dense core granules
6. Membrane bound vacuoles with an electron dense matrix and several
   a) Empty
   b) Dense core granules

The different secretory vacuole forms seem to have their common origin in the clear empty membrane bound vacuoles found around the Golgi apparatus. It is not clear whether lysosomes seen in this area fuse with the growing vacuoles or whether these vacuoles independently concentrate a floccular matrix resembling that of the lysosomes. The degree of condensation of this floccular matrix varies, but seems to depend on the presence of the small intravacuolar granules. These granules develop from invaginations of the vacuole membrane. The origin of the central core of the granules remains uncertain [34]. Different forms of secretory vacuoles are simultaneously seen in the supranuclear and apical regions of the cells. Brandes [34] described the fusion of cytoplasmic organelles, preferentially mitochondria and rough endoplasmic reticulum, with these vacuoles and discussed a probable autophagic mechanism. Indeed, these fusions are frequently seen, but no lysosomal membrane is apparent. Therefore, these fusions of secretory vacuoles and mitochondria seem more likely to be artifacts than autophagic processes.

The apical plasma membrane is smooth in rare cases and in most instances is bordered by a varying number of short stubby microvilli, containing a core of microfilaments. In some instances micropinocytotic vesicles, as well as dense bodies, seem to arise from invaginations of the apical cytoplasmic membrane.

Extension of the apical region is quite different in the individual acini and even in neighboring cells. The differences in height of the epithelial cells are due to the varying extension of the apical zone. In high columnar cells the apical zone protrudes bleblike into the lumen. The length of the bleb, extending from the plane between the apical tight junctions of the lateral plasma membrane to the plane of the bleb tip, measures about 3–4 μm in high columnar cells and about 0.5–1 μm in low columnar or cuboidal cells. The cytoplasmic matrix of the apical region is of very low electron density and contains a network of microfilaments, which is predominantly orientated parallel to the apical surface of the cell.

7.2. *Prostasomes and Diacytosis*

In a series of papers, Ronquist, Brody, and collaborators described the ultrastructure of secretory granules and vesicles from human prostatic fluid of healthy men, infertile patients [4,40,41, 109,211,231], and even in bulls [4]. These structures ranged in size from 20 to 150 nm and were surrounded by tri-, penta-, or multilamellar membranes. They were termed *prostasomes*, having been identified in prostatic secretory cells [41]. Prostasomes isolated by preparative ultracentrifugation and Sephadex G 200 chromatography displayed characteristic enzyme activities associated with their surrounding membranes [211]. These enzymes were (a) Mg^{2+}- and Ca^{2+}-dependent adenosine triphosphatase (ATPase), (b) protein kinase, and (c) Zn^{2+}-dependent peptidase. While ATPase has been suggested to represent the molecular basis for vectorial transport of Ca^{2+} into prostasomes [211], Zn^{2+}-dependent peptidase was thought to play a key role in the liquefaction of semen. Protein kinase activity was described to be effective during ATP-induced autophosphorylation, which in turn resulted in a significant increase in thickness of prostasome membrane [231]. Alteration in the properties of organelle membranes may promote fusion or facilitate other steps during interaction between spermatozoa and prostasomes. This may be essential during the prostasome induced increase in sperm forward motility. Ronquist and Brody [210] described the export of intact prostasomes from the interior to the exterior of the cell into the prostatic fluid.

The secretory vacuoles in human prostate have been named *storage vesicles* by Brody et al. [41], and the granules found within these storage vesicles were given the name *prostasomes*. Two different modes of release of secretory cells are described as follows [41]: (a) Prostasomes are delivered into the lumen by exocytosis, which is preceded by fusion of adjacent membranes belonging to the storage vesicle and the secretory cell; (b) alternatively, the whole intact storage vesicle is translocated from the interior of the cell into the acinar lumen through the plasma membrane — a mode of secretion named *diacytosis*. Human prostate specimens used for electron microscopy are always immersion fixed, and their removal from the patient by needle biopsy or by other surgical procedures is usually associated with more or less severe tissue damage. The observation of storage vesicles surrounded by an intact outer membrane and containing prostasomes is not compulsory, because any type of membrane rearrangement subsequent to release is conceivable in such a highly organized complex of different proteins. The concept of prostasomes has proven to be fruitful with respect to the functional properties of prostatic secretory particles.

7.3. Apocrine Secretion

The term *apocrine secretion* was coined by a german histologist, P. Schiefferdecker in 1922 [18] to define the release of secretory material from cells by apical bulging and pinching of the vesicle. A number of studies from the light microscopic era describe apocrine type of secretion in the human and canine prostate, and in the rat ventral prostate [24]. As indicated earlier, apical blebbing is observed in rat ventral prostate epithelium only after castration [123]. True apocrine secretion, that is, the release of secretory material through apical protrusions or blebs in the absence of secretory granules, is convincingly shown, although only in the dorsal prostate and the coagulating gland (Figs. 30, 31, 33, and 34) [9,53, 109,251,280]. As shown by Aumuller and Adler [9] in an experimental study, radioactively labeled secretion accumulates in the apical blebs of cells from the dorsal prostate. The apical blebs arise mostly from microvilli and their structure is hormone dependent. In human prostate in rare cases the apical plasma membrane is smooth and forms bleblike protrusions in contact with the rest of the cells, often only by a narrow stalk. Comparable appearing cytoplasmic fragments, may be recognized within the acinar lumen, and these two morphologic features are interpreted as evidence for an apocrine type secretory activity [34,133]. The contents of these apical blebs, however, vary greatly and in several cases are quite a homo-

→

Figures 42–45 illustrate the hormone-dependent changes in the ultrastructure of the rat coagulating gland

Fig 42 Rat coagulating gland 12 weeks after castration Acini are shrunken and invested by cuboidal cells containing only few cytoplasmic organelles No signs of a secretion are left (×6700)

Fig 43 Coagulating gland from a rat 12 weeks treated with estradiol Epithelium is shrunken, but some equivalents of secretory activity are left (endoplasmic reticulum, Golgi apparatus) (×8000)

Fig 44 Same specimen as in Figure 43 at slightly higher magnification Atypical apical blebs are found on several cells (×11,000)

Fig 45 Higher magnification of the portion marked on Figure 44 Incomplete demarcation of the apical bleb and supranuclear portion of a secretory cell Remnants of the apical plasma membrane (am) are seen Contents of the blebs consists of ribosomes and matrix substance (×51,000)

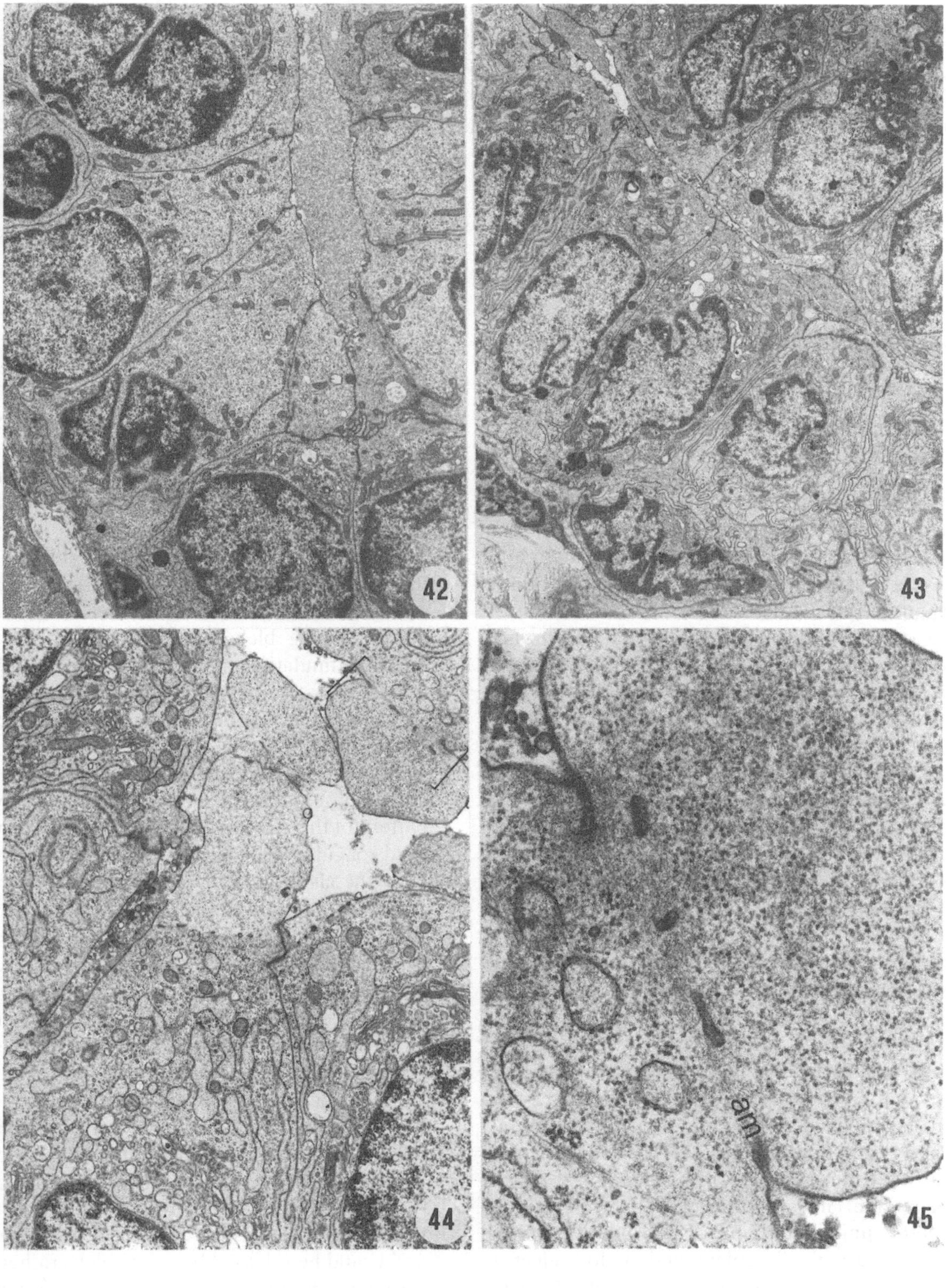
42
43
44
am
45

geneous mass. Moreover, true apocrine secretion is not well documented at the ultrastructural level, and it is doubtful to assume this type of secretory activity in the human prostatic epithelium. We have recently proven that in rat dorsal prostate and in the coagulating gland these blebs are required for the release of a specific compound, as was anticipated in a previous paper [223]. This compound seems to be secretory type transglutaminase (TGase) released both from the dorsal prostate as well as the coagulating gland (Figs. 38–41).

We purified transglutaminase from rat coagulating gland secretion [222]. The purified protein was homogeneous and had a molecular weight of 65 kD after SDS-PAGE. Under native conditions (pH 7.4), it aggregates into larger oligomers that elute in the void volume during FPLC on a Superose 12-column. During the purification procedure the pI changes from 7.6 to 8.3–8.5 (isomers). Mild hydrolysis and subsequent separation of acylated carbohydrates by gas chromatography revealed a prevalence of mannosyl residues. Mannose-specific lectins such as concanavalin A are only weakly bound by the native enzyme. Nonsaturated fatty acids (not yet specified) can be extracted by use of chloroform/methanol from the hydrolysate. Using detergents such as CHAPS or octylglucoside and enzymes such as phosphoinositol-specific phospholipase C (PI-PLC), the enzyme can be solubilized from homogenates of rat coagulating gland. There is circumstantial evidence that this protein has a lipid anchor that is lost during secretion. Recently, TGase present in keratinocytes was identified to represent an anchor protein. Perhaps, other tissue-type or membrane-bound transglutaminases may be suggested to be acylated by a phosphoinositol anchor. Ho et al. [114] recently cloned the cDNA of rat dorsal prostate transglutaminase. Using an antibody against the highly purified native antigen, we were able to show its release from dorsal prostate and coagulating gland secretory cells in a clearly apocrine fashion [223]. Blebs originate (mostly from the microvilli) at the apical plasma membrane and are surrounded by a typical bilayered unit membrane. The content of these blebs is usually flocculent and of low electron density. The outer leaflet gets readily detached from the bleb membrane and the residual leaflet forms vesicular structures that dissolve completely in the luminal content. Frequently, only a clear large vacuolar structure sharply demarcated against the residual secretion indicated the site where a bleb had formed. Less frequently, the contents of the blebs condense during the process of membrane dissolution and thereafter dissolves in intraluminal secretion.

Number, size, and morphology of the blebs are clearly dependent from hormonal or nerval stimuli (Figs. 42–45). Shortly after castration, their number greatly decreases, and 5–7 days after castration nearly no bleb is left on the luminal surface of the cell. After prolonged estrogen treatment, bleb formation is also impeded; instead, the complete apical cell pole or at least broad areas of the apical plasma membrane bulge into the lumen, rendering the apical cell pole a crescentlike or clublike shape. Remnants of the terminal web and portions of microfilament crossovers expand at the level of the junctional complex and separate the interior of the cell from the apical bulges. After enhanced sexual activity of the animals, the number of recently formed and detaching blebs is clearly increased. Cholinergic stimulation enhances the number of blebs dramatically, which then loose their characteristic shape and form polymorphic figures that reach far into the lumen of the acini.

Immunoelectron microscopy using our transglutaminase antibody showed a peculiar labeling pattern of the secretory cells of the dorsal prostate (and coagulating gland) that diverges significantly from the classical infracellular pathway of merocrine secretion. Contrary to the conventional staining pattern (e.g., in pancreas), the cisternae of the rough endoplasmatic reticulum were unlabeled, although the cytoplasmic portion of the cells displayed dense labeling. Neither the Golgi apparatus nor the surrounding vesicles and vacuoles showed any immunolabeling. The cytoplasmic matrix underlying the terminal web, however, was labeled. This pattern indicates an intracellular pathway that is difficult to reconcile with current concepts of intracellular transport. It suggests that the protein synthesized in the cytoplasm would not pass through the Golgi apparatus and would be released by apical blebs rather than through secretory granules. There are a number of structural peculiarities of the protein that are in favor, and others, that are against, such a presumed nonclassical pathway: Glycosylation of the protein, for example, must necessarily occur at a site different from the Golgi apparatus; N-terminal blockage by an acyl residue, on the other hand, would explain its not entering endoplasmic cisternae. Studies are underway to shed some light on this enigma.

8. Cellular Plasticity

Several morphological and biochemical studies have shown that in experimental animals androgen deprivation (affected either by orchidectomy, hypophysectomy, antiandrogen treatment, or LH-RH agonist treatment) results in a dramatic decrease of prostatic size, weight, and function, both in terms of proliferative and secretory activities [24,79]. Morphological studies focus on regressive changes that are observed after androgen withdrawal [225]. Biochemical studies showed several genes to be depressed after castration. It is not clear as yet whether the increased activity of some prostatic enzymes measured after castration is due to cell degradation, programmed cell death [125], or the development of androgen insensitivity [178].

Because of the rather complex situation in the human accessory sex glands, and especially as an attempt to understand the pathogenesis of benign prostatic hyperplasia, different experimental models using rats [7], monkeys [67], and dogs [116,216,265] have been developed, based on an unbalanced estrogen-androgen ratio as a challenge for prostatic growth [29]. The canine prostate has proved particularly suitable, as it shows a clear cut androgen-dependence in function [283]. Hyperplasia in canine prostate develops either spontaneously [29] or under the influence of different androgenic compounds in the presence of elevated estrogen levels [253,265]. Depending on the experimental protocol (use of different androgens in castrated and estrogenized dogs in the presence of antihormones), a rather heterogeneous structural alteration develops, seemingly dependent on the location within the gland [12,13]. The differences both in structure and secretion determine the limits of this model, which nevertheless has contributed much to our understanding of the phenotypic plasticity of the canine secretory cells. In a series of very thorough studies Merk et al. [148,173–175] analyzed the multiple phenotypes of prostatic glandular cells in castrated dogs after individual or combined treatment with androgen and estrogen. Characteristic alterations are found in secretory granules of the dog prostate using immunoelectron microscopy [12]. Castration-induced atrophy in canine prostatic epithelium results in an increase in the amount of scattered intermediate filaments. Secretory granules are sequestered into autophagic vacuoles and the previously peanut-agglutinin-positive luminal membrane becomes negative [175]. Treatment with estrogen causes a basal cell proliferation, which yields squamous cell progeny. The atrophied glandular epithelium hypertrophies and presents the so-called estrogen-modified glandular cell (EMG-phenotype) [173], which includes small secretory granules, bundles of filaments, and lectin-positive luminal granules. Combined androgen and estrogen treatment results in androgen-dominated, estrogen-modified glandular cells ("A-EMG" phenotype) [175], which display granules of the size found in androgen-dominated cells, but tonofilament bundles and peanut agglutinin-positive luminal membranes resemble their counterparts in EMG cells. Studies of estrogenic challenge of the prostate in rat [282] and monkey (baboon [48]) show that metaplastic changes occur far less impressively compared to dogs. In the human prostate, estrogenization results only in slight metaplasia of the epithelium and a largely unaltered prostatic volume [68].

9. Selection of Proliferative Cells

9.1. Prostate Growth

Different models have been designed to explain the homeostatic constraint mechanism [43,255] controlling prostatic growth (collagen synthesis [165], collagenase activity [184], secretion [21], growth factors and inhibitors [170]), but no definite understanding is achieved. Comparing the extremely low incidence of seminal vesicle cancers to that of the prostate, several prostate-specific peculiarities, such as embryological development [59,61], neuroendocrine effects in aging and on vessels [111], stromal/epithelial interaction, receptor multiplicity, and environmental factors (diet, sexual activity, etc.) have to be considered. In addition, factors such as oncogenes [247], tumor repressor genes [191], and alterations of the intracellular signal transduction pathway [8] are to be taken into account.

Another aspect with respect to the role of secretion in prostate cancer is the autocrine growth factor hypothesis [141,229], which is widely accepted in prostate research. In addition to the presence of receptors of epidermal growth factor in the human and canine prostate [219,252], the isolation of growth factors from prostates of different species has been recently described, [58, 143,144,162,244]. Growth factors have been found to act synergistically on certain prostatic growth factors and provided evidence that it was structurally related to basic fibroblast growth factors (bFGF [31,167,237], TGFβ [232]). An excellent review of regulation of prostate growth has been presented by Davies and Eaton [65].

9.2. *Functional Aspects of Cell Renewal*

Regarding cell renewal in the male accessory sex glands, three different conditions have to be discriminated:

1. Postnatal growth and organ differentiation
2. Normal glandular function (during adolescence, adulthood, and involution, where different sets of receptors and regulatory mechanisms of the glands are conceivable)
3. Androgen withdrawal and replacement (physiologically occurring in animals with seasonal sexual activity, or experimentally induced)

The last-named condition has been widely used to study the control mechanisms of prostatic cell proliferation [254]. Stiens and Helpap [234] performed a cell kinetic study in accessory sex glands in 1-day- to 15-month-old rats. The most intensive cell proliferation was observed within the first 2 weeks after birth. Thereafter, proliferation decreased continuously and differentiation of prostatic epithelium occurred. In newborn animals the highest labeling index was found in the coagulating gland (14.9%), followed by the dorsal prostate (11.4%) and ventral prostate (8%). In the latter lobe, the mitotic index increased, reaching a maximum value of 11.7% by day 14. A second but much smaller peak of epithelial proliferation occured with the onset of sexual maturation (week 5–6 after birth). Subsequently, the labeling index dropped to values below 0.5 and remained constant.

The different lobes of the adult prostate have a comparable proliferation pattern. As the normal prostate has only a small cell turnover rate, mitotic figures are extremely rare. Only after androgen withdrawal and replacement do dramatic changes in programmed cell death and cell renewal occur [80,81,84]. While the basal cells were previously regarded as the stem cells of prostatic epithelium, Evans and Chandler [84] found no clear evidence that basal cells alone, represented the proliferative compartment. It was shown that basal and secretory cells are self-replicating cell types with discrete functions. Evan and Chandler [84] found substantial numbers of basal, as well as glandular, cells of prostatic epithelium proliferating in the intact animal. The basal cell labeling index (LI) was 3.75%, representing 1.85 ($\pm$ 0.4) $\times$ 10^5 labelled cells per prostate. For the glandular cells, the comparable figures were 0.38% and 3.32 ($\pm$ 1.5) $\times$ 10^5. Seven days after castration, the glandular cells were decreased in number by 66%. After androgen substitution each cell type followed a very similar temporal pattern of proliferative activity. A greater portion of basal than glandular cells responded, but in terms of total numbers of cells labeled during the peak of proliferative activity, the value for the glandular cells was larger. The basal cells are clearly not the sole population of proliferating cells in prostatic epithelium, both under normal conditions as well as during testosterone stimulation. This observation does not exclude the possibility that the prostatic epithelium is maintained by a single cell lineage system, in which the stem cells would comprise a subpopulation of the basal cells.

Isaacs [126] advanced a stem-cell model for the prostate gland intended to explain normal cell renewal activity, as well as the kinetic pertubation occurring in benign prostatic hyperplasia and prostatic cancer. Three hierarchic orders of cells were distinguished by the author: (a) stem cells (b) amplifying cells and (c) transit cells. Stem cells were suggested to be capable of extensive self-renewal, to exist as a small fraction of the prostatic epithelial cell population, and to be androgen-independent. The amplifying cells are believed to arise from stem cells as an extensively expanding population capable of only a limited number of cell divisions. While they were thought not to require androgen for survival, they are androgen responsive. The amplifying cells would then differentiate into transit cells significantly increasing the cell number. The transit cells, in turn, were capable of proliferating a limited number of times, the number being determined by the prevailing androgen level and, unlike the stem cells or amplifying cells, they are considered to be dependent on the presence of androgen for survival.

As yet, none of these hypothetical cell forms have been morphologically identified. Verhagen et al. [260] used antibodies to various keratins as markers for different prostatic epithelial cell types and followed staining patterns during androgen withdrawal and subsequent replacement. A heterogeneous population of luminal cells was observed in association with androgen replacement. These had keratin expression patterns intermediate between basal and luminal cells. The results of this study support the theory that basal and luminal cells are members of the same cell lineage.

Under experimental conditions that lead to sloughing of secretory cells, basal cells proliferate, and in explants of BPH tissue form a monolayer replacing the functional acini. These cells express stratifying keratin and EGF receptor, but are negative for secretory acid phosphatase and PSA [129]. Proliferation of basal cells under conditions has been classified as an emergency reaction rather than physiological cell renewal [21].

10. Outlook — Prostate Pathology: Revenge of a Transitory Organ?

Benign prostatic hyperplasia and prostate cancer are the most frequent neoplasms in men [46,120]. The age-related increase in benign or malignant growth of the prostate gland has been related to several risk factors and permissive or inductive stimuli such as diet, environmental pollution, sexual habits or activities, as well as aging and changing hormonal situations. In prostate cancer oncological factors such as oncogenes, tumor suppressor genes, programmed cell death, impaired defense mechanisms, growth factors and inhibitors, epithelio-mesenchymal interactions, as well as endocrine stimuli and genetic effects are discussed [47,65].

The apparently nearly inevitable increase in proliferative disorders of the prostate in elderly men sharply contrasts with that of the adjacent sex gland, the seminal vesicle, on one hand, and the urethral Cowper's gland, on the other hand, where carcinomas are rare. Prostate and seminal vesicle are androgen target organs and are more (seminal vesicle) or less (prostate) intimately related to male reproduction. There are obvious differences in the organ biology of both. The seminal vesicle is a derivative of the Wolffian duct, requiring exclusively androgens for its embryological realization [16]. However, the prostate derives from a composite area of the urogenital sinus, requiring both estrogens and androgens during organogenesis. It undergoes different phases of estrogen and androgen responsivity (perinatally and during puberty). During these imprinting steps cell populations develop that have lost the characteristics of their simple-structured progenitor cells and that differ in their biological determination along the prostatic ducts (resorption, surface protection, apoptosis, secretion, regeneration/reserve function) but lack a function-related characteristic structure. This means, although morphologically homogeneous, these cells are functionally heterogeneous and in this respect resemble the mammary glandular cells in the female.

To summarize, in terms of biological determination [100], the prostate has a kind of an ambiguous commitment, being a urethral gland, on one hand, and an accessory sex gland, on the other. This ambiguous degree of functional commitment is reflected by its relatively short period of intact morphological organization. It reaches its mature morphological and functional structure usually only by the age of 18–20 years, retains it for about 10 years (when at the age of 30 initial signs of structural and functional disintegration occur), and gradually looses its functionally organized structure. An additional 15–20 years later, proliferative activity is resumed due to a changed hormonal situation, but under limited regulatory conditions (changes in the biomatrix, changed receptor expression, change in efficiency of intracellular signal pathways) Presuming that the number of highly regulated replications of the functionally essential compound (secretory cells) of an organ (prostate) is limited (very low mitotic index), an extended lifespan with continued proliferative stimuli would eventually result in unregulated growth

Whereas the benign proliferative lesions of the prostate show at least a certain correlation with exogenous and endogeneous risk factors (diet, race) that can be influenced by medical care, the ambiguous functional commitment and biological determination of the prostate in our personal view will inevitably continue to produce malignant growth unless the organ has been removed from the body in time

Acknowledgments

We gratefully acknowledge the expert technical help of Mrs I Dammshauser and G Hoffbauer, who made most of the scanning and transmission electron microscope preparations, Mr G Jennemann for his excellent photographic work, Mrs C Lochmann, who mounted the photographs, and Mrs G Nicholls, who patiently typed the text and made many linguistic corrections Thanks are due to the Deutsche Forschungsgemeinschaft for continued financial support Part of the work originates from our DFG grant Au-48/7-10

References

1 Abrahamsson PA, Lilja H Partial characterization of a thyroid-stimulating hormone-like peptide in neuroendocrine cells of the human prostate gland Prostate 14 71–81, 1989

2 Abrahamsson PA Neuroendocrine differentiation and secretory proteins in the parenchyma in hyperplasia and in carcinoma of the prostate An immunohistochemical, biochemical, ultrastructural and clinical study Studentlitteratur, Lund, 1988

3 Abrahamsson PA, Wadstrom LB, Alumets J, Falkmer S, Grimelius L Peptide-, hormone- and serotonin-immunoreactive cells in normal and hyperplastic prostate glands Pathol Res Pract 181 675–683, 1986

4 Agrawal Y, Vanha-Perttula T Effect of secretory particles in bovine seminal vesicle secretion on sperm motility and acrosome reaction J Reprod Fertil 79 409–419, 1987

5 Akiyama K, Nakamura S, Iwanaga S, Hara M A chymotrypsin-like activity of human prostate-specific antigen, τ-seminoprotein FEBS Lett 265 168–172, 1987

6 Alm P, Alumets J, Brodin E, Hakanson R, Nilsson G, Sjoberg NO Peptidergic (substance P) nerves in the genitourinary tract Neuroscience 3 419–429, 1978

7 Andersson H, Tisell LE Morphology of rat prostatic lobes and seminal vesicles after long-term estrogen treatment Acta Pathol Microbiol Immunol Scand Sect A 90 441–448, 1982

8 Andrews PE, Young CYF, Montgomery BT, Tindall DJ Tumor-promoting phorbol ester down-regulates the androgen induction of prostate-specific antigen in a human prostatic adenocarcinoma cell line Cancer Res 52 1525–1529, 1992

9 Aumuller G, Adler G Experimental studies of apocrine secretion in the dorsal prostate epithelium of the rat Cell Tissue Res 198 145–158, 1979

10 Aumuller G, Seitz J Immunoelectron microscopic studies on human prostatic and leukocytic acid phosphatases Prostate 7 161–169, 1985

11 Aumuller G, Braun BE, Seitz J, Muller T, Heyns W, Krieg M Effects of sexual rest or sexual activity on the structure and function of the ventral prostate of the rat Anat Rec 212 345–352, 1985

12 Aumuller G, Funke PJ, Hahn A, Hoffbauer G, Tunn U, Neumann F Phenotypic modulation of the canine prostate after long-term treatment with androgens and estrogens Prostate 3 361–373, 1982

13 Aumuller G, Habenicht UF, El-Etreby MF Pharmacologically induced ultrastructural and immunohistochemical changes in the prostate of the castrated dog Prostate 11 211–218, 1987

14 Aumuller G, Heyns W Immunocytochemistry of prostatic binding protein in the rat ventral prostate In The Prostatic Cell Structure and Function GP Murphy, AA Sandberg, JP Karr (eds) New York Alan R Liss, 1981, Part A, pp 409–415

15 Aumuller G, Jungblut T, Malek B, Konrad S, Weihe E Regional distribution of opioidergic nerves in human and canine prostates Prostate 14 279–288, 1989

16 Aumuller G, Riva A Morphology and functions of the human seminal vesicle Andrologia 24 183–196, 1992

17 Aumuller G, Seitz J, Bischof W Immunohistochemical study on the initiation of acid phosphatase secretion in the human prostate J Androl 4 183–191, 1983

18 Aumuller G, Seitz J Protein secretion and secretory processes in male accessory sex glands Int Rev Cytol 121 127–231 1990

19 Aumuller G, Stofft E, Tunn U Fine structure of the canine prostatic complex Anat Embryol 160 327–340, 1980

20 Aumuller G, Zhao GQ Huntemann S Westermann R, Tuohimaa P, Virtanen I Paracrine effects of human prostatic stromal cells and their hormonal regulation in vitro Ninth International Congress on Endocrinology, Nice, p 452, abstr no P-13 03 060, 1992

21 Aumuller G Morphologic and endocrine aspects of prostatic function Prostate 4 195–214, 1983
22 Aumuller G Morphologic and regulatory aspects of prostatic function Anat Embryol 179 519–531, 1989
23 Aumuller G Postnatal development of the prostate Bull Assoc Anat 75 229 39–42, 1991
24 Aumuller G Prostate gland and seminal vesicles In Handbuch der mikroskopischen Anatomie des Menschen, Vol 7, pt 6 A Oksche, L Vollrath (eds) Berlin Springer, 1979
25 Ban Y, Wang MC, Watt KWK, Loor R, Chu TM The proteolytic activity of human prostate-specific antigen Biochem Biophys Res Commun 123 482–488, 1984
26 Baumgarten HG, Falck B, Holstein AF, Owman C, Owman T Adrenergic innervation of the human testis, epididymis, ductus deferens and prostate Z Zellforsch 90 81–95, 1968
27 Bazer BT Basal cell proliferation and differentiation in regeneration of the rat ventral prostate Invest Urol 17 470–473, 1980
28 Beksac MS, Khan SA, Eliasson R, Skaekkeback NE, Shet AR, Diczfalusy E Evidence for the prostatic origin of immunoreactive inhibin-like material in human seminal plasma Int J Androl 7 389–397, 1984
29 Berry SJ, Strandberg JD, Saunders WJ, Coffey DS Development of canine benign prostatic hyperplasia with age Prostate 9 363–373, 1986
30 Bettuzzi S, Zoli M, Ferraguti F, Ingletti MC, Agnati LF, Corti A Regional and cellular distribution within the rat prostate of two mRNA species undergoing opposite regulation by androgens J Endocrinol 132 361–367, 1992
31 Biagini G, Preda P, Loligno M, Soli M, Bercovich E Ultrastructural aspects of human prostate in benign prostatic hyperplasia Prostate 3 99–108, 1982
32 Blacklock NJ The morphology of the parenchyma of the prostate Urol Res 5 155–158, 1977
33 Bonkhoff H, Wernert N, Dhom G, Remberger K Relation of endocrine-paracrine cells to cell proliferation in normal, hyperplastic, and neoplastic human prostate Prostate 19 91–98, 1991
34 Brandes D (ed) Male Accessory Sex Organs Structure and Function in Mammals New York Academic Press, 1974
35 Brandes D, Kirchheim D, Scott WW Ultrastructure of the human prostate Normal and neoplastic Lab Invest 13 1541–1560, 1964
36 Brawer MK, Peehl DM, Stamey TA, Bostwick DG Keratin immunoreactivity in the benign and neoplastic human prostate Cancer Res 35 3663–3667, 1985
37 Brendler CB, Berry SJ, Ewing LL, McCullogh AR, Cochran RC, Strandberg JD, Zirkin BR, Coffey DS, Wheaton LG, Hiler ML, Bordy MJ, Niswender GD, Scott WW, Walsh PC Spontaneous benign prostatic hyperplasia in the beagle Age-associated changes in serum hormone levels, and the morphology and secretory function of the canine prostate J Clin Invest 71, 1114–1123, 1984
38 Brenner RM, West N, McClellan M Estrogen and progestin receptors in the reproductive tract of male and female primates Biol Reprod 42 11–19, 1990
39 Breuer W Histologische, histochemische und feinstrukturelle Untersuchungen der postnatalen Entwicklung von dorsaler Prostata, Koagulations- und Samenblasendruse der mannlichen Albinoratte (*Mus rattus norvegicus albinus*) Vet Med Thesis, University of Munich, 1987
40 Brody I, Ronquist G, Gottfries A, Stegmayr B Abnormal deficiency of both Mg^{2+} and Ca^{2+}-dependent adenosine triphosphatase and secretory granules and vesicles in human seminal plasma Scand J Urol Nephrol 15 85–90, 1981
41 Brody I, Ronquist G, Gottfries A Ultrastructural localization of the prostasome An organelle in human seminal plasma Upsala J Med Sci 88 63–80, 1983
42 Brolin J, Skoog L, Ekman P Immunohistochemistry and biochemistry in detection of androgen, progesterone, and estrogen receptors in benign and malignant human prostatic tissue Prostate 20 281–295, 1992
43 Bruchovsky N, Lesser B, van Dooren E, Craven S Hormonal effects on cell proliferation in rat prostate In Vitamins and Hormones PL Munson, E Diczfalusy, G Glover, RE Olsom (eds) New York Academic Press, 1975, pp 61–102
44 Bruchovsky N, McLoughlin MG, Rennie PS, Ito MP Partial characterization of stromal and epithelial forms of 5α-reductase in human prostate In The Prostatic Cell Structure and Function GP Murphy, AAS Sandberg, JP Karr (eds) New York Alan R Liss, 1981, Part A, pp 161–175
45 Buttyan R, Olsson CA, Pintar J, Chang C, Bandyk M, Ng PY, Sawczuk IS Induction of the TRPM-2 gene in cells undergoing programmed death Mol Cell Biol 9 3473–3481, 1989
46 Carter BC, Coffey DS The prostate An increasing medical problem Prostate 16 39–48, 1990
47 Carter BS, Beaty TH, Steinberg GD, Childs B, Walsh PC Mendelian inheritance of familial prostate cancer Proc Natl Acad Sci USA 89 3367–3371, 1992
48 Chai LS, Karr JP, Murphy GP, Sandberg AA Effects of DES on the morphology of the lobes of the baboon prostate Invest Urol 19 202–208, 1981
49 Chan L, Wong YC Localization of prostatic glyco conjugates by the lectin-gold method Acta Anat 134 27–40, 1992
50 Chandler JA, Timms BG The effect of cadmium administration on the lateral prostate in organ culture Virchows Arch Pathol Anat Histopathol 25 17–33, 1977
51 Chang C, Chodak G, Sarac E, Takeda H, Liao S Prostate androgen receptor Immunohistochemical localization and mRNA characterization J Steroid Biochem 34 311–313 1989
52 Chang SM, Chung LWK Interaction between prostatic fibroblast and epithelial cells in culture Role of androgen Endocrinology 125 2719–2726, 1989
53 Chow PH, Pang SF Ultrastructure of secretory cells of male accessory sex glands of golden hamster (*Mesocricetus auratus*) and effect of melatonin Acta Anat 134 327–340, 1989

54 Chung LWK, Anderson NG, Neubauer BL, Cunha GR, Thompson TC, Rocco AK Tissue interactions in prostate development Roles of sex steroids In The Prostate Cell Structure and Function GP Murphy, AA Sandberg, JP Karr (eds) New York Alan R Liss, 1981, Part A, pp 177–203

55 Chung LWK, Gleave ME, Hsieh JT, Hong SJ, Zhau HE Reciprocal mesenchymal-epithelial interaction affecting prostate tumour growth and hormonal responsiveness Cancer Surv 11 91–121, 1991

56 Chung LWK, Matsura J, Runner MN Tissue interactions and prostatic growth I Induction of adult mouse prostatic hyperplasia by fetal urogenital sinus implants Biol Reprod 31 155–163, 1984

57 Cleary KR, Choi HY, Ayala AG Basal cell hyperplasia of the prostate Am J Clin Pathol 80 850–854, 1983

58 Crabb JW, Armes LG, Carr SA, Johnson CM, Roberts GD, Bordoli RS, McKeehan WL Complete primary structure of prostatropin, a prostate epithelial cell growth factor Biochemistry 25 4988–4993, 1986

59 Cunha GR, Donjacour AA, Sugimura Y Stromal-epithelial interactions and heterogeneity of proliferative activity within the prostate Biochem Cell Biol 64 608–614, 1986

60 Cunha GR, Reese BA, Sekkingstad M Induction of nuclear androgen-binding sites in epithelium of the embryonic urinary bladder by mesenchyme of the urogenital sinus of embryonic mice Endocrinology 107 1767–1770, 1980

61 Cunha GR, Shannon JM, Neubauer BL, Sawyer LM, Fujii H, Taguchi O, Chung LWK Mesenchymal-epithelial interactions in sex differentiation Hum Genet 58 68–77, 1981

62 Cunha GR Epithelial-stromal interactions in development of the urogenital tract Int Rev Cytol 47 137–194, 1976

63 Dahl E, Kjaerheim A, Tveter KJ The ultrastructure of the accessory sex organs of the normal male rat I Normal structure Z Zellforsch 137 345–359, 1973

64 Damjanov I, Mildner B, Knowles BB Immunohistochemical localization of the epidermal growth factor receptor in normal human tissues Lab Invest 55 588–592, 1986

65 Davies P, Eaton CL Regulation of prostate growth J Endocrinol 131 5–17, 1991

66 Davis NS, Di Sant'Agnese PA, Ewing JF, Mooney RA The neuroendocrine prostate Characterization and quantitation of calcitonin in the human gland J Urol 142 884–888, 1989

67 De Klerk DP, Human HJ, De Klerk JN The effect of 5α-androstane-3α, 17β-diol, and 17β-estradiol on the adult and immature Chacma baboon prostate Prostate 7 1–12, 1985

68 De Voogt HJ, Rao BR, Geldof AA, Gooren LJG, Bouman FG Androgen action blockade does not result in reduction in size but changes histology of the normal prostate Prostate 11 305–313, 1987

69 Del Fiacco M Enkephalin-like immunoreactivity in the human male genital tract J Anat 135 649–656, 1982

70 Dermer GB Basal cell proliferation in benign prostatic hyperplasia Cancer 41 1857–1862, 1978

71 Di Sant'Agnese PA, De Mesy Jensen KL, Churukian CJ, Agarwal MM Human prostatic endocrine-paracrine (APUD) cells Arch Pathol Lab Med 109 607–612, 1985

72 Di Sant'Agnese PA Neuroendocrine differentiation in carcinoma of the prostate Cancer 70(Suppl) 254–268, 1992

73 Djakiew D, Delsite R, Pflug B, Wrathall J, Lynch JH, Onoda M Regulation of growth by a nerve growth factor-like protein which modulates paracrine interactions between a neoplastic epithelial cell line and stromal cells of the human prostate Cancer Res 51 3304–3310, 1991

74 Djakiew D, Pflug B, Delsite R, Lynch JH, Onoda M Density dependent polarized secretion of a prostatic epithelial cell line Prostate 20 15–27, 1992

75 Djakiew D, Tarkington MA, Lynch JH Paracrine stimulation of polarized secretion from monolayers of a neoplastic prostatic epithelial cell line by prostatic stromal cell proteins Cancer Res 50 1966–1974, 1990

76 Doctor UM, Sheth AR, Simba MM, Arbatti NJ, Aaveri JP, Sheth NA Studies on immunocytochemical localization of inhibin-like material in human prostatic tissues Comparison of its distribution in normal, benign and malignant prostates Br J Cancer 53 547–554, 1986

77 Dube JY, Pelletier G, Gagnon P, Tremblay RR Immunohistochemical localization of a prostatic secretory protein of 94 amino acids in normal prostatic tissue in primary prostatic tumors and in their metastases J Urol 138 883–887, 1987

78 Elbadawi A, Goodman DC Autonomic innervation of accessory male genital glands In Male Accessory Sex Glands ESE Hafez, E Spring-Mills (eds) Amsterdam Elsevier/North Holland, 1980, pp 101–128

79 English HF, Drago JR, Santen RJ Cellular response to androgen depletion and repletion in the rat ventral prostate Autoradiography and morphometric analysis Prostate 7 41–51, 1984

80 English HF, Drago JR, Santen RJ Cellular response to androgen depletion and repletion in the rat ventral prostate Autoradiography and morphometric analysis Prostate 7 41–52, 1985

81 English HF, Santen RJ, Isaacs JT Response of glandular versus basal rat ventral prostatic epithelial cells to androgen withdrawal and replacement Prostate 11 229–243, 1987

82 Erdos EG, Schulz WW, Gafford JT, Defendini R Neutral metalloendopeptidase in human male genital tract Lab Invest 52 437–447, 1985

83 Evans GS, Chandler JA Cell proliferation studies in the rat prostate II The effects of castration and androgen-induced regeneration upon basal and secretory cell proliferation Prostate 11 339–352, 1987

84 Evans GS, Chandler JA Cell proliferation studies in the rat prostate II The effects of castration and androgen induced regeneration upon basal and secretory cell proliferation Prostate 11 339–352, 1987

85 Feitz WFJ, Debruyne FMJ, Vooijs GP, Herman CJ, Ramaekers FCS Intermediate filament proteins as tissue

specific markers in normal and malignant urological tissues J Urol 136 922–932, 1986

86 Fetissof F, Bruandet P, Arbeille B, Penot J, Marboeuf Y, Le Roux J, Guilloteau D, Beaulieu JL Calcitonin-secreting carcinomas of the prostate Am J Surg Pathol 10 702–710, 1986

87 Fetissof F, Dubois MP, Arbeille-Brassart B, Lanson Y, Boivin F, Jobard P Endocrine cells in the prostate gland, urothelium and Brenner tumors Cell Pathol 42 53–64, 1983

88 Feyrter F Uber das urogenitale Helle-Zellen-System des Menschen Z Mikrosk-Anat Forsch 42 324–326, 1951

89 Flickinger CJ Protein secretion in the rat ventral prostate and the relation of Golgi vesicles, cisternae and vacuoles, as studied by electron microscopic radioautography Anat Rec 180 427–447, 1974

90 Flickinger CJ The fine structure and development of the seminal vesicles and prostate in the fetal rat Z Zellforsch 109 1–14, 1970

91 Flickinger CJ The fine structure of the Wolffian duct and cytodifferentiation of the epididymis in fetal rats Z Zellforsch 96 344–360, 1969

92 Flickinger CJ Ultrastructural observations on the postnatal development of the rat prostate Z Zellforsch 113 157–173, 1971

93 Franks LM Benign prostatic hyperplasia of the prostate A review Ann Coll Surg Engl (Lond) 14 92–106, 1954

94 Franks LM Prostatic cancer In Prostatic Cancer RJ Ablin (ed) New York Dekker, 1981, pp 3–7

95 Frazier HA, Humphrey PA, Burchette JL, Paulson DF Immunoreactive prostatic specific antigen in male periurethral glands J Urol 147 246–248, 1992

96 Fritz FJ, Pabst R Numbers and heterogeneity of mast cells in the male genital tract of the rat Int Arch Allergy Appl Immunol 88 360–362, 1989

97 Fritz FJ, Westermann J, Pabst R The mucosa of the male genital tract, part of the common mucosal secretory system? Eur J Immunol 19 475–479, 1989

98 Garde SV, Sheth AR Immunoperoxidase localization of prostatic inhibin peptide in human, monkey, dog, and rat prostates Anat Rec 223 181–184, 1989

99 Gaytan F, Aceitero J, Lucena C, Aguilar E, Pinilla L, Garnelo P, Bellido C Simultaneous proliferation and differentiation of mast cells and Leydig cells in the rat testis Are common regulatory factors involved? J Androl 13 287–397, 1992

100 Gleason DF Histologic grading of prostate cancer Hum Pathol 23 273–279, 1992

101 Golz R, Schubert GE Prostatic specific antigen Immunoreactivity in urachal remnants J Urol 141 1480–1484, 1989

102 Gordon WL, Liu WK, Akiyama K, Tsuda R, Hara M, Schmid K, Ward DN Beta-microseminoprotein (β-MSP) is not an inhibin Biol Reprod 36 829–835, 1987

103 Graham CW, Lynch JH, Djakiew D Distribution of nerve growth factor-like protein and nerve growth factor receptor in human benign prostatic hyperplasia and prostatic adenocarcinoma J Urol 147 1444–1447, 1992

104 Grignon DJ, Ro JY, Srigley JR, Troncoso P, Raymond K, Ayala AG Sclerosing adenosis of the prostate gland Am J Surg Pathol 16 383–391, 1992

105 Gupta RK Mast cell variations in prostate and urinary bladder Arch Pathol 89 302–305, 1970

106 Gutman AB, Gutman EB An "acid" phosphatase occuring in the serum of patients with metastatic carcinoma of the prostate gland J Clin Invest 17 473–478, 1938

107 Habenicht UF, Schwarz K, Neumann F, El Etreby MF Induction of estrogen-related hyperplastic changes in the prostate of the cynomolgus monkey (*Macaca fascicularis*) by androstenedione and its antagonization by the aromatase inhibitor 1-methyl-androsta- 1,4-diene-3,17-dione Prostate 11 313–326, 1987

108 Hamilton DW Structure and function of the epithelium lining the ductuli efferentes, ductus epididymidis and ductus deferens in the rat In Handbook of Physiology, Section 7, Vol 5, Male Reproduction System Washington, D C American Physiological Society, 1975, pp 359–301

109 Hawkins WE, Geuze JJ Secretion in the rat coagulating gland (anterior prostate) after copulation Cell Tissue Res 181 519–529, 1977

110 Helminen HJ, Ericsson JLE On the mechanism of lysosomal enzyme secretion J Ultrastruct Res 33 528–549, 1970

111 Herr JC, Summers TA, McGee RS, Sutherland WM, Sigman M, Evans RJ Characterization of a monoclonal antibody to a conserved epitope on human seminal vesicle-specific peptides A novel probe/marker system for semen identification Biol Reprod 35 773–784, 1986

112 Heyns W, Peeters B, Mous J, Rombauts W, De Moor P Purification and characterization of prostatic binding protein and its subunits Eur J Biochem 89 181–186, 1978

113 Hierowski MT, McDonald MW, Dunn L, Sullivan JW The partial dependency of human prostatic growth factor on steroid hormones in stimulating thymidine incorporation into DNA J Urol 138 909–912, 1987

114 Ho KC, Quarmby VE, French FS, Wilson EM Molecular cloning of rat prostate transglutaminase complementary DNA J Biol Chem 267 12660–12667, 1992

115 Hoffer AP The ultrastructure of the ductus deferens in man Biol Reprod 14 425–443, 1976

116 Hohbach C Ultrastructural and histochemical studies of the prostate of the dog under cyproterone acetate Invest Urol 15 117–123, 1977

117 Hohbach Ch, Ueberberg H Ultrastructural and histochemical aspects of prostatic secretion in dog Pathol Res Pract 173 225–235, 1982

118 Holterhus PM, Zhao GQ, Aumuller G Effects of androgen deprivation and estrogen treatment on the structure and protein expression of the rat coagulating gland Anat Rec, 1993, in press

119 Horn R Histochemische, histologische und feinstrukturelle Untersuchungen zur postnatalen Entwicklung der Ventral- und Laterallappen der Prostata der Ratte (*Mus rattus norvegicus albinus*) Vet Med Thesis, University of Munich, 1987

120 Horton R Editorial Benign prostatic hyperplasia New

insights J Clin Endocrinol Metab 74 504A–504C, 1992
121 Huggins C, Hodges CV Studies on prostate cancer II The effects of castration on advanced carcinoma of the prostate Arch Surg 43 209–223, 1941
122 Huttunen E, Romppanen T, Helminen HJ A histoquantitative study of the effects of castration on the rat ventral prostate lobe J Anat 132 357–370, 1981
123 Ichihara I, Kawamura H The fine structure of ventral prostatic secretory epithelial cells in older rats Cell Tissue Res 203 181–188, 1979
124 Isaacs JT, Barrack ER, Isaacs WB, Coffey DS The relationship of cellular structure and function The matrix system In The Prostatic Cell Structure and Function GP Murphy, AA Sandberg, JP Karr (eds) New York Alan R Liss, 1981, Part A, pp 1–24
125 Isaacs JT Antagonistic effect of androgens on prostatic cell death Prostate 5 545–557, 1984
126 Isaacs JT Control of cell proliferation and cell death in the normal and neoplastic prostate A stem cell model In Benign Prostatic Hyperplasia II CH Rodgers, DS Coffey, G Cunha, JT Grayhack, F Hinman, R Horton (eds) Bethesda, MD NIH, 1987, pp 85–94
127 Jacobs SC, Story MT, Sasse J Lawson RK Characterization of growth factors derived from the rat ventral prostate J Urol 139 1106–1110, 1988
128 James K, Hargreave TB Immunosuppression by seminal plasma and its possible clinical significance Immunol Today 5 357–363, 1984
129 Jones EG, Harper ME Studies on the proliferation, secretory activities, and epidermal growth factor receptor expression in benign prostatic hyperplasia explant cultures Prostate 20 133–149 1992
130 Kachar B Pinto da Silva P Freeze-fracture study of rat ventral prostate Secretory mechanism in the epithelial cell Anat Rec 198 549–565, 1980
131 Kachar B, Pinto da Silva P Freeze fracture study of rat ventral prostate The columnar epithelial cell Am J Anat 161 49–69 1981
132 Kamushida S, Tsutsumi Y Extraprostatic localization of prostatic acid phosphatase and prostate specific antigen Distribution in cloacogenic glandular epithelium and sex dependent expression in human anal gland Human Pathol 21 1108–1113, 1990
133 Kastendieck H Ultrastrukturpathologie der menschlichen Prostatadruse Cyto- und Histomorphogenese von Atrophie Hyperplasie Metaplasie, Dysplasie und Carcinom Stuttgart Fischer, 1977
134 Kawai N Aumuller G Immuno electron microscopical localization of α-actinin and actin in microvilli of prostatic epithelial cells J Anat 161 125–132, 1988
135 Kawamura H Ichihara I Primary culture of epithelial cells derived from the rat ventral prostate Formation of three-dimensional acinus like structure in collagen gel Prostate 10 153–161, 1987
136 Kellokumpu-Lehtinen P Santti R Pelliniemi LJ Correlation of early cytodifferentiation of the human fetal prostate and Leydig cells Anat Rec 196 263–273, 1980
137 Kellokumpu-Lehtinen P Santti R, Pelliniemi LJ Role of mesenchyme in the early cytodifferentiation of human prostate In Endocrinological Cancer, Ovarian Function and Disease H Adlercreutz, RD Bullbrook, HY van der Molen, A Vermeulen, F Sciorro (eds) Amsterdam Excerpta Medica, Elsevier North Holland, 1979, pp 114–119
138 Kellokumpu-Lehtinen P, Santti RS, Pelliniemi LJ Development of human fetal prostate in culture Urol Res 9 89–98, 1981
139 Kellokumpu-Lehtinen P Localization of acid phosphatase activity in testosterone-treated prostatic urethra of human fetuses Prostate 4 265–270, 1983
140 Kellokumpu-Lehtinen P The histochemical localization of acid phosphatase in human fetal urethral and prostatic epithelium Invest Urol 17 435–440, 1980
141 Knabbe C, Lippmann ME, Wakefield LM, Flanders KC, Kasid A, Derynck R, Dickson RB Evidence that the transforming growth factor β is a hormonally regulated negative growth factor in human breast cancer cells Cell 48 417–428, 1987
142 Koenig H, Knight R, Nayyar R, Hughes C Testosterone induced changes in lysosomes of rat ventral prostate and seminal vesicle J Cell Biol 67 220, 1975
143 Koutsilieris M, Rabbani SA, Bennett HPJ, Goltzman D Characteristics of prostate-derived growth factors for cells of the osteoblast phenotype J Clin Invest 80 941–946, 1987
144 Koutsilieris M, Rabbani SA, Goltzman D Effects of human prostatic mitogens on rat bone cells and fibroblasts J Endocrinol 115 447–454, 1987
145 Kurihara H, Uchida K Distribution of microtubules and microfilaments in exocrine (ventral prostatic epithelial cells and pancreatic exocrine cells) and endocrine cells (cells of the adenohypophysis and islets of Langerhans) Histochemistry 87 223–227, 1987
146 Kutscher W, Wolbergs H Prostataphosphatase Z Physiol Chem 236 237–240, 1935
147 Lam KW, Lee P, Estlund T, Yam LY Antigenic and moleuclar relationship of human prostatic acid phosphatase isoenzymes Invest Urol 18 209–211, 1980
148 Leav J, Merk FB, Ofner P, Goodrich G, Kwan PWL, Stein BM, Sar M, Stumpf WE Bipotentiality of response to sex hormones by the prostate of castrated, or hypophysectomized dogs Direct effects of estrogen Am J Pathol 93 69–91, 1978
149 Lee C, Sensibar JA, Dudek SM, Hipakka RA, Liao S Prostatic ductal system in rats Regional variation in morphological and functional activities Biol Reprod 43 1079–1086 1990
150 Lee C Sensibar JA Proteins of the rat prostate II Synthesis of new proteins in the ventral lobe during castration-induced regression J Urol 138 903–908, 1987
151 Leong ASY, Gilham P, Milios J Cytokeratin and vimentin intermediate filament proteins in benign and neoplastic prostatic epithelium Histopathology 13 435–442, 1988
152 Li HC, Chernoff J, Chen LB, Kierszenbaum A A phosphotyrosyl-protein phosphatase activity associated with acid phosphatase from human prostate gland Eur J Biochem 138 45–51, 1984

153 Lilja H, Abrahamsson PA Three predominant proteins secreted by the human prostate gland Prostate 12 29–38, 1988

154 Lilja H, Oldbring H, Rannevik G, Laurell CB Seminal vesicle-secreted proteins and their reactions during gelation and liquefaction of human semen J Clin Invest 80 281–285, 1987

155 Lilja H A kallikerein-like serine protease in prostatic fluid cleaves the predominant seminal vesicle protein J Clin Invest 76 1899–1903, 1985

156 Lin MF, Clinton GM Human prostatic acid phosphatase has phosphotyrosyl protein-phosphatase activity Biochem J 235 351–357, 1986

157 Lowsley DS The development of the human prostate gland with reference to the development of other structures at the neck of the urinary bladder Am J Anat 13 299–349, 1912

158 Lubahn DB, Joseph DR, Sullivan PM, Willard F, French FS, Wilson EM Cloning of human androgen receptor complementary DNA a localization to the x chromosome Science 240 327–330, 1988

159 Lundwall A, Lilja H Molecular cloning of human prostate specific antigen cDNA FEBS Lett 214 17–22, 1987

160 Maddy SQ, Chisholm GD, Busuttil A, Habib FK Epidermal growth factor receptors in human prostate cancer Correlation with histological differentiation of the tumour Br J Cancer 60 41–44, 1989

161 Maddy SQ, Chisholm GD, Hawkins RA, Habib FK Localization of epidermal growth factor receptors in the human prostate by biochemical and immunocytochemical methods J Endocrinal 113 147–153, 1987

162 Maehama S, Li D, Nanri H, Leykam JF, Deuel TF Purification and partial characterization of prostate-derived growth factor Proc Natl Acad Sci USA 83 8162–8166, 1986

163 Mann T, Lutwak-Mann C Male Reproductive Function and Semen — Themes and Trends in Physiology, Biochemistry and Investigative Andrology Berlin Springer, 1981

164 Mansson PE, Adams P, Kan M, McKeehan WL Heparin-binding growth factor gene expression and receptor characteristics in normal rat prostate and two transplantable rat prostate tumors Cancer Res 49 2485–2494, 1989

165 Mariotti A, Mawhinney M Preliminary studies of the hormonal control of male accessory sex organ epithelial collagen In The Prostatic Cell Structure and Function GP Murphy, AA Sandberg, JP Karr (eds) New York Alan R Liss, 1981, Part A, pp 133–136

166 Maygarden SJ, Strom S, Ware JL Localization of epidermal growth factor receptor by immunohistochemical methods in human prostatic carcinoma, prostatic intraepithelial neoplasia, and benign hyperplasia Arch Pathol Lab Med 116 269–273, 1992

167 McKeehan WL Growth factor receptors and prostate cell growth Cancer Surv 11(Prostate Cancer) 165–175, 1991

168 McNeal JE Cancer volume and site of origin of adenocarcinoma in the prostate Hum Pathol 23 258–266, 1992

169 McNeal JE Regional morphology and pathology of the prostate Am J Clin Pathol 49 347–357, 1968

170 McNeal JE The prostate and prostatic urethra A morphological synthesis J Urol 107 1008–1016, 1972

171 McTigue JT, van Etten RL Isolation, characterization, and spontaneous interconversion of two forms of human prostatic acid phosphatase Prostate 3 165–181, 1982

172 Merchant DJ, Clarke SM, Harris S Primary explant culture An in vitro model of the human prostate Prostate 4 523–542, 1983

173 Merk FB, Kwan PWL, Leav I Gap junctions in the myometrium of hypophysectomized estrogen treated rats Cell Biol Int Rep 4 287–293, 1980

174 Merk FB, Ofner P, Kwan PWL, Leav I, Vena RL Ultrastructural and biochemical expression of divergent differentiation in prostates of castrated dogs treated with estrogen and androgen Lab Invest 47 437–450, 1982

175 Merk FB, Warhol MJ, Kwan PWL, Leav I, Alroy J, Ofner P, Pinkus GS Multiple phenotypes of prostatic glandular cells in castrated dogs after individual or combined treatment with androgen and estrogen — Morphometric, ultrastructural, and cytochemical distinctions Lab Invest 54 442–456, 1986

176 Moerman P, Fryns JP, Goddeeris P, Lauweryns JM Pathogenesis of the Prune-Belly Syndrome A functional urethral obstruction caused by prostatic hypoplasia Pediatrics 73 470–475, 1984

177 Montpetit L, Lawless KR, Tenniswood M Androgen repressed messages in the rat ventral prostate Prostate 8 25–36, 1986

178 Montpetit M, Abrahams P, Clark AF, Tenniswood M Androgen-independent epithelial cells of the rat ventral prostate Prostate 12 13–28, 1988

179 Mori H, Maki M, Oishi K, Jaye M, Igarashi K, Yoshida O, Hatanaka M Increased expression of genes for basic fibroblast growth factor and transforming growth factor type β_2 in human benign prostatic hyperplasia Prostate 16 71–79, 1990

180 Mori K, Wakasugi C Immunocytochemical demonstration of prostatic acid phosphatase Different secretion kinetics between normal, hyperplastic and neoplastic prostates J Urol 133 877–883, 1985

181 Morre DJ, Cline GB, Coleman R, Evans WH, Glaumann H, Headon DR, Reid E, Siebert G, Widnell CC Markers for membranous cell components Eur J Cell Biol 20 195–199, 1979

182 Morris GL, Dodd JG, Epidermal growth factor receptor mRNA levels in human prostatic tumors and cell lines J Urol 143 1272–1274, 1990

183 Muntzing J, Sufrin G, Murphy GP Prostatitis in the rat Scand J Urol Nephrol 13 17–22, 1979

184 Muntzing J Collagen synthesis and breakdown in the rat ventral prostate In The Prostatic Cell Structure and Function GP Murphy, AA Sandberg, JP Karr (eds) New York Alan R Liss, 1981, Part A, pp 137–144

185 Murphy BC, Pienta KJ, Coffey DS Effects of extracellular matrix components and dihydrotestosterone on the

structure and function of human prostate cancer cells Prostate 20 29–41, 1992

186 Nadji M, Tabei SZ, Castro A, Chu TM, Morales AR Prostatic-specific antigen An immunohistologic marker for prostatic neoplasms Cancer 48 1229–1232, 1981

187 Nagle RB, Ahmann FR, McDaniel KM, Paquin ML, Clark VA, Celniker A Cytokeratin characterization of human prostatic carcinoma and its derived cell lines Cancer Res 47 281–286, 1987

188 Nowels K, Kent E, Rinso K, Oyasu R Prostate specific antigen and acid phosphatase-reactive cells in cystitis cystica and glandularis Arch Pathol Cancer Med 112 734–738, 1988

189 Ostrowski W, Wasyl Z, Weber M, Guminska M, Luchter E The role of neuraminic acid in the heterogeneity of acid phosphomonoesterase from the human prostate gland Biochim Biophys Acta 221 297–306, 1970

190 Owman C, Sjostrand NO Short adrenergic neurons and catecholamine-containing cells in vas deferens and accessory male genital glands of different mammals Z Zellforsch 66 300–320, 1965

191 Peehl DM Searching for suppressor genes in prostate cancer Cancer Surv (Prostate Cancer) 11 25–34, 1991

192 Pegg AE, Williams-Ashman HG Biosynthesis of putrescine in the prostate gland of the rat Biochem J 108 533–539, 1968

193 Pekary AE, Hershman JM, Friedman S, Dekernion J Human semen and human prostate contain thyrotropin-releasing hormone (TRH) Fertil Steril 36 429–430, 1981

194 Pekary AE, Sharp B, Briggs J, Carlson HE, Hershman JM High concentration of p-Glu-His-Pro-NH_2 (thyrotropic releasing hormone) occurs in rat prostate Peptides 4 915–919, 1983

195 Pelttari A, Helminen HJ The effects of various fixatives on the relative thickness of cellular membranes in the ventral lobe of the rat prostate Histochem J 11 599–611, 1979

196 Pollen JJ, Dreilinger A Immunohistochemical identification of prostatic acid phosphatase and prostate specific antigen in female periurethral glands Urology 23 303–306, 1984

197 Pretlow T, Brattain MG, Kreisberg JI Separation and characterization of epithelial cells from prostates and prostatic carcinomas Cancer Treat Rep 61 157–160, 1977

198 Prins GS, Cooke PA, Birch L, Donjacour AA, Yalcinkaya TM, Siiteri PK, Cunha GR Androgen receptor expression and 5α-reductase activity along the proximal-distal axis of the rat prostatic duct Endocrinology 130 3066–3073, 1991

199 Prins GS Neonatal estrogen exposure induces lobe-specific alterations in adult rat prostate androgen receptor expression Endocrinology 130 3703–3714, 1992

200 Purnell DM, Heatfield BM, Anthony RL, Trump BF Immunohistochemistry of the cytoskeleton of human epithelium Evidence for disturbed organization in neoplasia Am J Pathol 126 384–395, 1987

201 Pylkkanen L, Santti R, Maentausta O, Vihko R Distribution of estradiol-17β hydroxysteroid oxidoreductase in the urogenital tract of control and neonatally estrogenized male mice Immunohistochemical, enzymehistochemical, and biochemical study Prostate 20 59–72, 1992

202 Pylkkanen L, Santti R, Newbold R, McLachlan JA Regional differences in the prostate of the neonatally estrogenized mouse Prostate 18 117–129, 1991

203 Qiu SD, Young CYF, Bilhartz DL, Prescott JL, Farrow GM, He WW, Tindall DJ In situ hybridization of prostate-specific antigen mRNA in human prostate J Urol 144 1550–1556, 1990

204 Rabl R Architekturstudien bei sog Prostatahypertrophien Virchows Arch Pathol Anat Histopathol 305 1–19, 1939

205 Reese JH, McNeal JE, Redwine EA, Samloff IM, Stamey TA Differential distribution of pepsinogen II between the zones of the human prostate and the seminal vesicle J Urol 136 1148–1151, 1986

206 Reese JH, McNeal JE, Redwine EA, Stamey TA, Freiha FS Tissue plasminogen activator as a marker for functional zones within the human prostate gland Prostate 12 47–54, 1988

207 Reid WA, Vongsorasak, Savasti J, Valler MJ, Kay J Identification of the acid proteinase in human seminal fluid as a gastricsin originating in the prostate Cell Tissue Res 236 597–600, 1984

208 Riva A, Usai E, Scarpa R, Cossu M, Lantini MS Fine structure of the accessory glands of the human male genital tract In Developments in Ultrastructure of Reproduction Progress in Clinical and Biological Research, Vol 296 PM Motta (ed) New York Alan R Liss, 1989, pp 233–240

209 Robel P, Eychenne B, Blondeau JP, Picard-Groyer MT, Baulieu EE, Bruner-Lorand J, Hechter O Characteristics of separated epithelial and stromal subfractions of prostate II Human prostate Prostate 5 255–268, 1984

210 Ronquist G, Brody I The prostasome Its secretion and function in man Biochem Biophys Acta 822 203–218, 1985

211 Ronquist G Effect of modulators on prostasome membrane-bound ATPase in human seminal plasma Eur J Clin Invest 17 231–236, 1987

212 Rowlatt C, Franks LM Myoepithelium in mouse prostate Nature 202 707–708, 1964

213 Rowley DR Characterization of a fetal urogenital sinus mesenchymal cell line U4F Secretion of a negative growth regulatory activity In Vitro Cell Dev Biol 28A 29–38, 1992

214 Samuel LH, Flickinger CJ Incorporation of ^{3}H-fucose and the secretion of glycoproteins in the coagulating gland of the mouse Anat Rec 214 53–60, 1986

215 Samuel LH, Flickinger CJ Intracellular pathway and kinetics of protein secretion in the coagulating gland of the mouse Biol Reprod 34 107–117, 1987

216 Sandberg AA, Karr JP, Muntzing J The prostates of dog, baboon and rat In Male Accessory Sex Glands E Hafez, E Spring-Mills (eds) Amsterdam Elsevier, 1980, pp 565–608

217 Sar M, Lubahn DB, French FS, Wilson EM Immunohistochemical localization of the androgen receptor in rat and human tissues Endocrinology 127 3180–3186, 1990

218 Schulze H, Barrack ER Immunocytochemical localiza-

tion of estrogen receptors in spontaneous and experimentally induced canine benign prostatic hyperplasia Prostate 11 145–162, 1987
219 Schuurmans ALG, Bolt J, Mulder E Androgens stimulate both growth rate and epidermal growth factor receptor activity in the human prostate tumor cell LNCaP Prostate 12 55–63, 1988
220 Secchi J, Bonne C Mitoses des cellules basales de l' épithélium prostatique survenant après la castration chez le rat puberé C R Soc Biol 167 1331–1334, 1973
221 Seitz J, Aumuller G Electrophoretic studies on the heterogeneity of acid phosphatases from human prostate, seminal fluid, and leukocytes Prostate 7 73–90, 1985
222 Seitz J, Aumuller G Secretory proteins from male accessory sex glands Isolation, biochemical and functional characterization In Reproductive Biology and Medicine AF Holstein, KD Voigt, D Grasslin (eds) Berlin Diesbach, 1989, pp 112–118
223 Seitz J, Keppler C, Rausch U, Aumuller G Immunohistochemistry of secretory transglutaminase from rodent prostate Histochemistry 93 525–530, 1990
224 Seitz J Biochemie, Cytochemie und Immunohistochemie saurer Phosphatasen Marburg Habilitationsschrift, 1985
225 Sinha AA, Bentley MD The relationship of epithelial cell types in the ventral prostate glands of castrated mice treated with testosterone Anat Rec 208 533–544, 1984
226 Sinha AA, Hagen KA, Sibley RK, Wilson MJ, Limas C, Reddy PK, Blackard CE, Gleason DF Analysis of fixation effects on immunohistochemical localization of prostatic specific antigen in human prostate J Urol 136 722–727, 1986
227 Smith JK, Whitby LG The heterogeneity of prostatic acid phosphatase Biochim Biophys Acta 151 607–618, 1967
228 Song GX, Lin CKT, Wu JY, Lan KW, Li CY, Yam LT Immunoelectron microscopic demonstration of prostatic acid phosphatase in human hyperplastic prostate Prostate 7 63–72, 1985
229 Sporn MD, Todaro GJ Autocrine secretion and malignant transformation of cells N Engl J Med 303 878–880, 1980
230 Srigley JR, Dardick I, Warren R, Hartwick J, Klotz L Basal epithelial cells of human prostate gland are not myoepithelial cells Am J Pathol 136 957–966, 1990
231 Stegmayr B, Brody I, Ronquist G A Biochemical and ultrastructural study on the endogenous protein kinase activity of secretoiy granule membranes of prostatic origin in human seminal plasma J Ultrastruct Res 78 206–214, 1982
232 Steiner MS, Barrack ER Transforming growth factor-β_1 overproduction in prostate cancer Effects on growth in vivo and in vitro Mol Endocrinol 6 15–25, 1992
233 Steinhoff M, Seitz J, Dammshauser I, Aumuller G Hormonabhangiger intrazellularer Transport bei der apokrinen Sekretion in der Koagulationsdruse der Ratte Anat Anz 174(Suppl 87) 210, 1992
234 Stiens R, Helpap B Histologische und proliferationskinetische Untersuchungen zum Wachstum der Rattenprostata in verschiedenen Lebensaltern Acta Anat 109 79–88, 1981
235 Story MT, Esch F, Shimasaki S, Sasse J, Jacobs SC, Lawson RK Amino-terminal sequence of a large form of basic fibroblast growth factor isolated from human benign prostatic hyperplastic tissue Biochem Biophys Res Commun 142 702–709, 1987
236 Story MT, Esch F, Shimasaki S, Sasse J, Jacobs SC, Lawson RK Amino-terminal sequence of a large form of basic fibroblast growth factor isolated from human benign prostatic hyperplastic tissue Biochem Biophys Res Commun 142 702–709, 1987
237 Story MT Polypeptide modulators of prostatic growth and development Cancer Surv (Prostate Cancer) 11 123–146, 1991
238 Sugimura Y, Cunha GR, Donjacour AA, Bigsby RM, Brody JR Whole-mount autoradiography study of DNA synthetic activity during postnatal development and androgen-induced regeneration in the mouse prostate Biol Reprod 34 985–995, 1986
239 Sugimura Y, Cunha GR, Donjacour AA Morphogenesis of ductal networks in the mouse prostate Biol Reprod 34 961–971, 1986
240 Sugimura Y, Cunha GR, Donjacour AA Morphological and histological study of castration-induced degeneration and androgen-indued regeneration in the mouse prostate Biol Reprod 34 973–983, 1986
241 Swinnen K, Cailleau J, Heyns W, Verhoeven G Stromal cells from the rat prostate secrete androgen-regulated factors which modulate Sertoli cell function Mol Cell Endocrinol 62 147–152, 1989
242 Swinnen K, Cailleau J, Heyns W, Verhoeven G Stromal cells from the rat prostate secrete androgen-regulated factors which modulate Sertoli cell function Mol Cell Endocrinol 62 147–152, 1989
243 Swinnen K, Deboel L, Cailleau J, Heyns W, Verhoeven G Morphological and functional similarities between cultured prostatic stromal cells and testicular peritubular myoid cells Prostate 19 99–111, 1991
244 Tackett RE, Heston LWDW, Parnish RF, Pletscher LS, Fair WR Mitogenic factors in prostatic tissue and expressed prostatic secretion J Urol 133 45–48, 1985
245 Tan J, Joseph DR, Quarmby VE, Lubahn DB, Sar M, French FS, Wilson EM The rat androgen receptor Primary structure, autoregulation of its messenger ribonucleic acid, and immunocytochemical localization of the receptor protein Mol Endocrinol 12 1276–1285, 1988
246 Tenniswood M Role of epithelial-stromal interactions in the control of gene expression in the prostate An hypothesis Prostate 9 375–385, 1986
247 Thompson TC, Kadmon D, Timme TL, Merz VW, Egawa S, Krebs T, Scardino PT, Park SH Experimental oncogene-induced prostate cancer Cancer Surv (Prostate Cancer) 11 55–71, 1991
248 Timms BG, Chandler JA, Sinowatz F The ultrastructure of basal cells of rat and dog prostate Cell Tissue Res 173 543–554, 1976
249 Timms BG, Chandler JA, Sinowatz F The ultrastructure of basal cells of rat and dog prostate Cell Tissue Res 173 543–554, 1976
250 Tisell LE, Salander H The lobes of the human prostate Scand J Urol Nephrol 9 185–191, 1975
251 Toma JG, Buzzell GR Fine structure of the ventral and

dorsal lobes of the prostate in the young adult Syrian hamster, *Mesocricetus auratus* Am J Anat 181 132–140, 1988

252 Traish AM, Wotiz HH Prostatic epidermal growth factor receptors and their regulation by androgens Endocrinology 121 1461–1467, 1987

253 Tunn VW, Schuring B, Senge T, Neumann F, Schweikert U, Rohr HP Morphometric analysis of prostates in castrated dogs after treatment with androstanediol, estradiol, and cyproterone acetate Invest Urol 18 289–292, 1980

254 Tuohimaa P, Niemi M Cell renewal and mitogenic activity of testosterone in male accessory sex glands In Male Accessory Sex Organs — Structure and Function in Mammals D Brandes (ed) New York Academic Press, 1974, pp 329–347

255 Tuohimaa P Control of cell proliferation in male accessory sex glands In Male Accessory Sex Glands E Spring-Mills, ESE Hafez (eds) Amsterdam Elsevier, 1980, pp 131–154

256 Vaalasti A, Hervonen A Innervation of the ventral prostate of the rat Am J Anat 154 231–244, 1979

257 Vaalasti A, Linnoila I, Hervonen A Immunohistochemical demonstration of VIP, [Met^5] and [Leu^5]-enkephalin immunoreactive nerve fibres in the human prostate and seminal vesicles Histochemistry 66 89–98, 1980

258 Vaalasti A, Tainio H, Pelto-Huikko M, Hervonen A Light and electron microscope demonstration of VIP and enkephalin-immunoreactive nerves in the human genitourinary tract Anat Rec 215 21–27, 1986

259 Vaalasti A Autonomic innervation of the prostate Acta Universitatis Tamperensis Ser A 13 1–30, 1980

260 Verhagen APM, Aalders TW, Ramaekers FCS, Debruyne FMJ, Schalken JA Differentiation process in the prostatic epithelium on basis of intermediate filament expression Prostate 13 25–47, 1988

261 Vihko P, Kontturi M, Korhonen LK Purification of human prostatic acid phosphatase by affinity chromatography and isoelectric focusing Part I Clin Chem 24 466–471, 1978

262 Vihko P Characterization of the principal human prostatic acid phosphatase isoenzyme purified by affinity chromatography and isoelectric focusing Part II Clin Chem 24 1783–1789, 1978

263 Vilches J, Lopez A, De Palacio L, Munoz C, Gomez J SEM and x-ray microanalysis of human prostatic calculi J Urol 127 371–373 1982

264 Vittoria A, Cocca T, La Mura E, Cecio A Immunocytochemistry of paraneurons in the female urethra of the horse, cattle, sheep, and pig Anat Rec 233 18–24 1992

265 Walsh PC, Wilson JD The induction of prostatic hypertrophy in the dog with androstenediol J Clin Invest 57 1093–1097, 1976

266 Wang MC, Loor RM, Li SL, Chu TM Physico-chemical characterization of prostate gland and seminal plasma IRCS Med Sci 11 327–328, 1983

267 Wang MC, Valenzuela LA, Murphy GP, Chu TM Purification of a human prostate specific antigen Invest Urol 17 159–163, 1979

268 Ware JL Prostate tumor progression and metastasis Biochim Biophys Acta 907 279–298, 1987

269 Warhol MJ, Longtine JA The ultrastructural localization of prostatic specific antigen and prostatic acid phosphatase in hyperplastic and neoplastic human prostates J Urol 134 607–616, 1985

270 Watt KWK, Lee PJ, M Timukulu T, Chan WP, Loor R Human prostate-specific antigen Structural and functional similarity with serine proteases Proc Natl Acad Sci USA 83 3166–3170, 1986

271 Weaver MG, Abdul-Karim FW, Srigley J, Bostwick DG, Ayala AG Paneth cell-like change of the prostate gland Am J Surg Pathol 16 62–68, 1992

272 Weiber H, Andersson C, Murne A, Rannevik G, Lindstrom C, Lilja H, Fernlund P β-microseminoprotein is not a prostate-specific protein Am J Pathol 137 593–604, 1990

273 Weiss G Relaxin in the male — Minireview Biol Reprod 40 197–200, 1989

274 Wernert N, Gerdes J, Loy V, Seitz G, Scherr O, Dhom G Investigations of the estrogen (ER-ICA-test) and the progesterone receptor in the prostate and prostatic carcinoma on immunohistochemical basis Virchows Arch Pathol Anat Histopathol 412 387–391, 1988

275 Wernert N, Seitz G, Achtstatter T Immunohistochemical investigation of different cytokeratins and vimentin in the prostate from the fetal period up to adulthood and in prostate carcinoma Pathol Res Pract 182 617–626, 1987

276 Williams-Ashman HG Transglutaminases and the clotting of mammalian seminal fluids Mol Cell Biochem 58 51–61, 1984

277 Wilson EM, French FS Biochemical homology between dorsal prostate and coagulating gland J Biol Chem 255 10946–10953, 1980

278 Wilson MJ, Whitaker JN, Sinha AA Immunocytochemical localization of cathepsin D in rat ventral prostate Evidence for castration-induced expression of cathepsin D in basal cells Anat Rec 229 321–333, 1991

279 Witorsch RJ Immunohistochemical studies of prolactin binding in sex accessory organs of the male rat J Histochem Cytochem 26 565–580, 1978

280 Wong YC, Tse MKW Fine structural and functional study of the prostatic complex of the guinea pig Acta Anat 109 289–312, 1981

281 Yam LT, Janckila AJ, Li CY, Lam WKW Presence of "prostatic" acid phosphatase in human neutrophils Invest Urol 19 34–38 1981

282 Zhao GQ, Bacher M, Friedrichs B, Schmidt W, Rausch U, Goebel HW, Tuohimaa P, Aumuller G Functional properties of isolated stroma and epithelium from rat ventral prostate during androgen deprivation and estrogen treatment Exp Clin Endocrinol, 1993, in press

283 Zirkin BR, Strandberg JD Quantitative changes in the morphology of the aging canine prostate Anat Rec 208 207–214, 1984

284 Zondek T, Mansfield MD, Attree SL, Zondek LH Hormone levels in the foetal and neonatal prostate Acta Endocrinol 112 447–456, 1986

CHAPTER 6

Female Prostatic Glands: *A Comparative Study*

LIBERATO J.A. DI DIO & SYLVIA CORRER

1. Introduction

Since Virchow [42] in 1853 pointed out the homology between female urethral glands and the male prostate [26,29], supported by Tourneaux [41] almost four decades later, and by Evatt [4] in 1911, investigators have searched for the presence of prostatic glands in female animals.

A well-developed female prostate was found in *Arvicanthis cinereus* by Rauther [33] in 1903, and several authors [17–20,27,45], based upon homologous glands, kept on recognizing prostatic glands in several species. On the other hand, embryological investigations [4,5,41] attempted to recognize in humans the counterpart of the prostate in females.

In rats [31], the female prostatic gland, considered to be Skene's paraurethral glands by Price [30] in 1936, appeared at 19 days and 19 hours, a few hours later than in the male. Resorting to inbreeding, Witschi and Riley [44] in 1936 were able to develop a strain of rats that presented a female prostate in a very high percentage of animals (83%).

Male hormonal stimulation resulted in the appearance of rudimentary prostatic glands in female rats [14], thus leading to several investigations [8,21–25,32,34,35,43] and the publication of numerous papers relating to this new line of scientific research.

A landmark in the study of female prostate was set in 1940 [1], when the presence of this gland was discovered in all normal females of *Mastomys erithroleucus* Temm. This rodent, and a few other species of the same genus [3], were bound to become an excellent experimental animal model for physiological and pathological studies concerning the prostate and other organs. In fact [37], the female prostatic gland developed spontaneously, along with, in some cases, adenocarcinoma and proliferative hyperplasia. Almost at the same time, Oettle [28] described hypertrophy of the ventral prostate in the female during the luteal phase, persisting through gestation.

Spontaneus hyperplasia and neoplasia were found [15] after testing the effects of aging and hormones in female *Praomys* prostate. After several experiments [6,7], involving labeling the ventral prostate and ovariectomy, it was concluded that the mechanism of androgen action in female *Praomys* is similar to that occurring in the male and the rat. Under normal conditions, the prenatal development of this gland is the same in either sex and resembles that of the male rat in time of appearance, location, and structure. These observations led our group [9,11] to undertake investigations on the development of *Praomys* prostate, with reference to its subcellular structure in different ages and functional phases of either sex, including a comparative study of the gland in pregnant and nonpregnant animals, and a histochemical determination of carbohydrates in the female and male prostatic gland.

2. Female Prostate of *Praomys*

The prostate of female *Praomys* begins its development at 19.5 days of gestation (Fig. 1) as

Riva, A., Testa Riva, F., and Motta, P.M., (eds.), Ultrastructure of Male Urogenital Glands: Prostate, Seminal Vesicles, Urethral, and Bulbourethral Glands. *ISBN 0-7923-2800-0.*

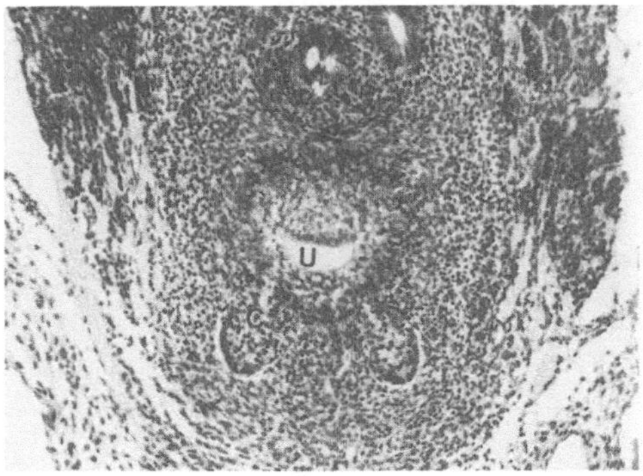

Fig. 1. Photomicrograph of a transverse section through the pelvis of a 19.5-day embryo of a female *Praomys* (*Mastomys*) *Natalensis* showing two prostatic cords (C) budding from the (urethral) epithelium lining the urogenital sinus (U). The buds grow into a stromal condensation ventrally to the urethra (H & E, ×200). From Gross et al. [12], with permission.

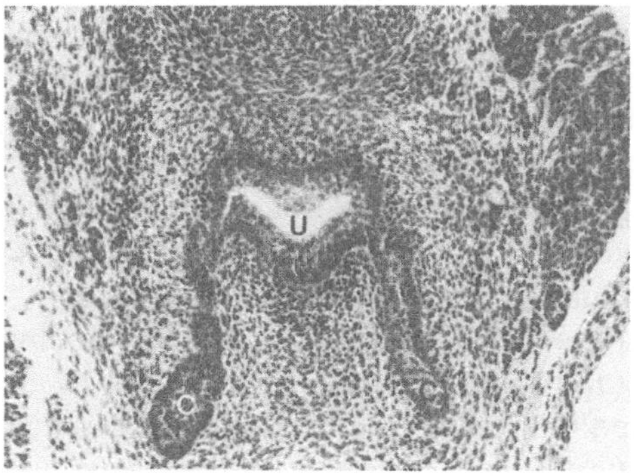

Fig 2 Photomicrograph of a transverse section through the pelvis of a 20-day embryo of a female *Praomys*. The prostatic cords (C), originating from the urogenital sinus (U), increased their length when compared to those seen in the preceding figure (H & E, ×200) From Gross et al [12], with permission

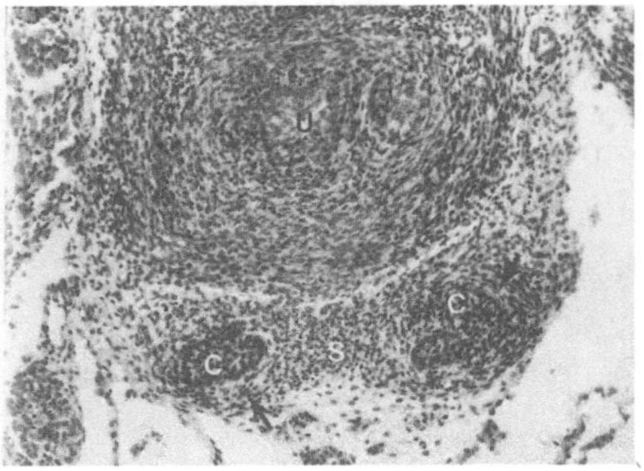

Fig. 3. Photograph of a transverse section through the pelvis of a 20.5-day embryo of a female *Praomys*. Prostatic clusters (C), surrounded by concentrically oriented cells of the stroma (S). These cells form a primitive capsule around the clusters (arrows) (H & E, ×200) From Gross et al. [12], with permission.

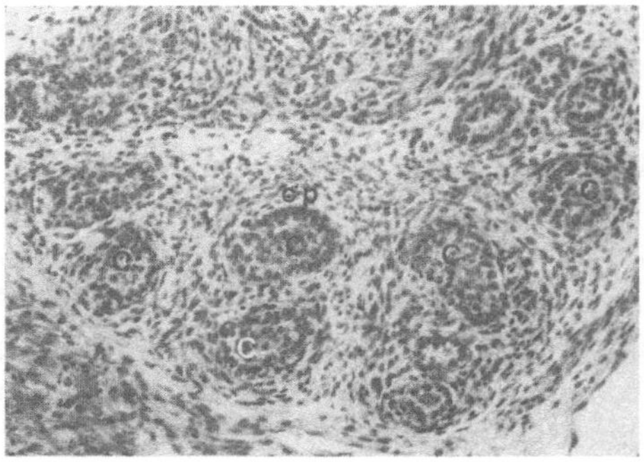

Fig 4. Photomicrograph of a cross section of a prostate of a newborn female *Praomys* showing the increase in number and size of the cell clusters (C), surrounded by a capsule (cp) The cell clusters represent cross sections of prostatic cords (H & E, ×290). From Gross et al. [12], with permission.

two cellular cords that bud from the urethral epithelium and grow into a stromal condensation ventrally to the urethra [12]. These cords increase in length, branch, and coil (Figs. 2 and 3), and then soon after birth the cords, increased in number (Fig. 4), present lumina (Fig. 5), thus becoming tubules and making up the larger component of the prostate. The diameter of the lumina of the tubules increases, whereas the peritubular cellular layers decrease. By 12 days the tubules become acini, and are larger, irregular in shape, and lined by one coat of columnar cells. By 18 days (Fig. 6), the epithelium forms villi or folds, prominent in the lumen, where a secretion is noted. It is, however, only after 30 days that supranuclear light areas become evident (Fig. 7) and the morphology of the prostate acquires the appearance of the adult (Fig. 8): The principal cells are columnar, resting on a basal lamina, surrounded by layers of capsular flattened cells, some of which are smooth myocytes and fibroblasts, occasionally separated by capillaries. Basal cells are wedged between the bases of principal or secreting cells and the basal lamina. The cytoplasm of basal cells is lighter than that of principal cells,

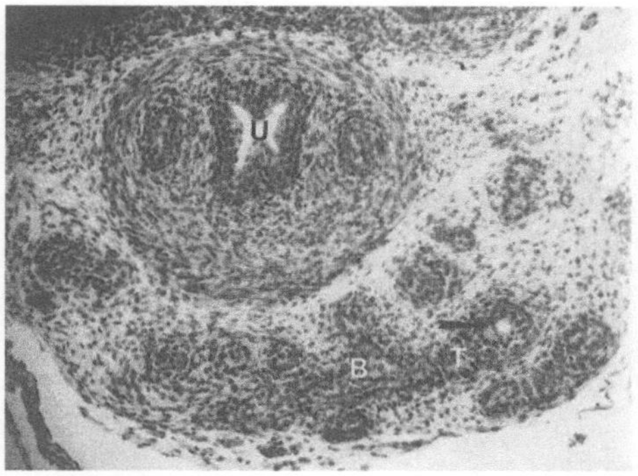

Fig 5 Photomicrograph of a cross section of a prostatic gland of a 2-day female *Praomys* showing the appearance of the first lumina (arrow) within prostatic cords, which become then tubules (T) These run through the stroma for a long distance before they branch (B), turn, or coil U = urethra (H & E, ×155) From Gross et al [12], with permission

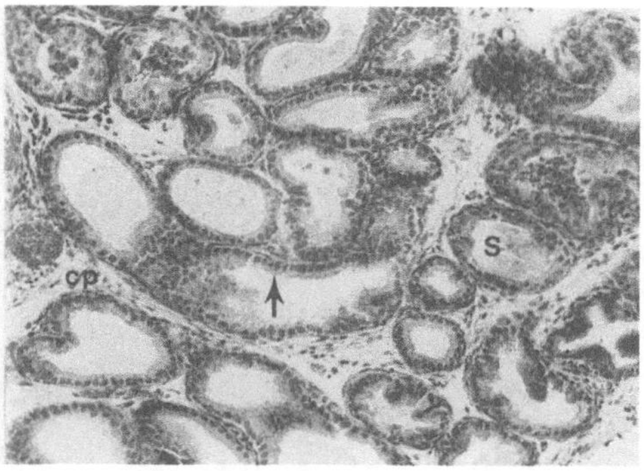

Fig 7 Photomicrograph of a section of the prostate in a 1-month-old female *Praomys* The prostatic gland consists of large acini, lined by epithelial cells and surrounded by a capsule (cp) The apical area of the epithelial cells shows light areas (arrow) and a secretory product (S) can be seen within the acinar lumen (H & E, ×195) From Gross et al [12], with permission

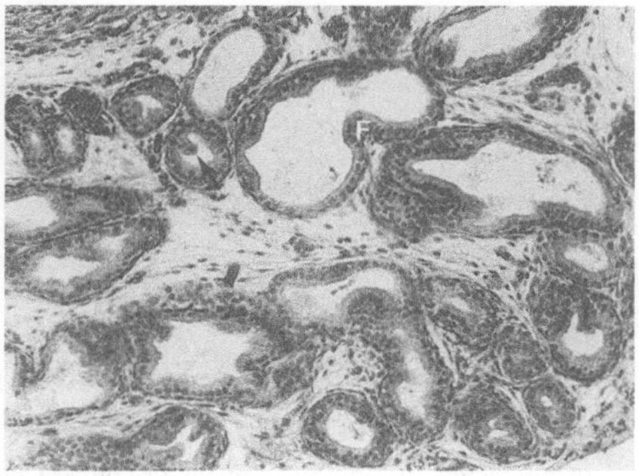

Fig 6 Photomicrograph of a section of the prostate of an 18-day female *Praomys* Many cross and oblique sections of large acini are seen, the walls of which are made up mainly by epithelium, surrounded by a thin capsule The columnar epithelial cells contain basal nuclei and homogeneous cytoplasm The epithelium may form large folds (F) or broad, short villi (arrow) that project into the lumina (H & E, ×195) From Gross et al [12], with permission

containing a large, irregular nucleus. The polarity of the organelles in each principal cell shows endoplasmic reticulum in the basal area and a large nucleus that invades the middle area. The supranuclear area contains a well-developed Golgi complex, lysosomal and residual bodies, and secretion granules. The apical area contains endoplasmic reticulum and secretion granules. Mitochondria and clear membrane-bound vacuoles are scattered throughout the cytoplasm.

The prenatal development of the ventral prostate in the male *Praomys* closely resembles that of the female, as described above, and that of the male rat in terms of time of appearance, location, and structure [9]. Electron micrographs of the prostate in newborn female *Praomys* display the details of the simple epithelium, surrounded by numerous stroma cells, the nuclei of which are mostly smaller than those of epithelial cells (Fig. 9).

The demonstration and localization of carbohydrates (associated with proteins) in the ventral lobes of the prostate of female and male *Praomys* (*Mastomys*) *Natalensis* were determined histochemically [13]. A weakly PAS-positive material appeared in the secretory product along with secretion granules of epithelial cells of the ventral lobes of both female and male prostates. This reaction was unaffected by diastase (ruling out glycogen) and was completely blocked by acetylation (indicating that the secretory cells contain little or no lipid). Alcian blue, toluidine blue, and methylene blue stains demonstrated metachromasia only after sulphation. All reactions indicated the presence of neutral carbohydrates (whether neutral mucopolysaccarides or mucoproteins or both) or mucosubstances in the secretion and secretion granules of the principal cells of the prostatic ventral lobe in both sexes. In short, the nature and mode of secretion of the

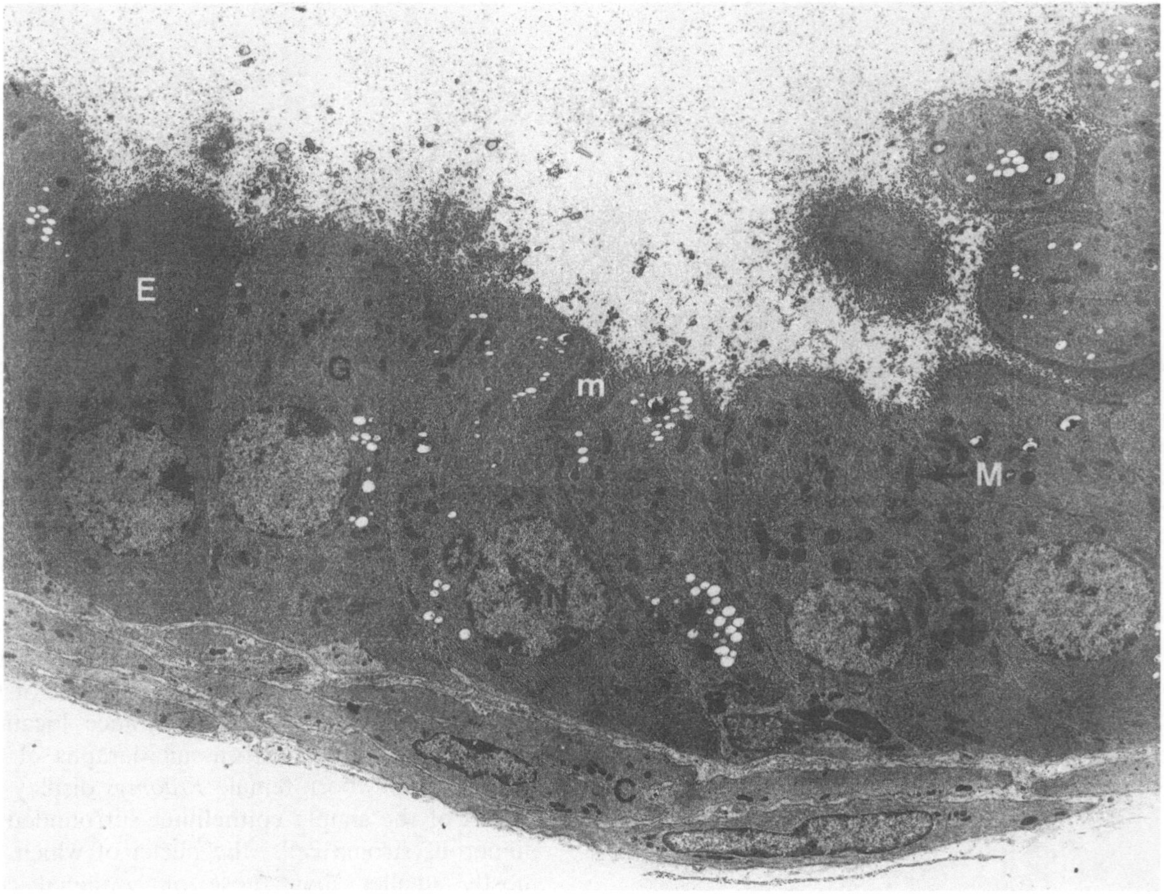

Fig 8 Transmission electron micrograph of a portion of the wall of a prostatic acinus of an adult female *Praomys* Columnar principal cells (E) rest on a basal lamina and on a capsule (C) of flat cells the major axis of which is perpendicular to the major axis of the principal cells The epithelial cells have basal nuclei (N) a supranuclear Golgi complex (G) mitochondria (arrow M) microvilli (m) and vacuoles (V) B = basal cell (Uranyl acetate lead citrate ×4800) From Gross et al [12] with permission

ventral prostate of the female and male *Praomys* are very similar

A study of the morphology of the prostatic gland in adult female and male *Praomys* (*Mastomys*) *natalensis* [10] indicated only small sexual differences The female prostate is less active than the male one, as judged by a smaller amount of secretion and fewer supranuclear light areas in the former At the subcellular level, there is less rough endoplasmic reticulum and a lower number of secretion granules in the female prostate The cellular arrangement, subcellular organization, and mechanism of secretion, however, are similar in both sexes

The prostatic gland of the pregnant *Praomys* appears more active than that of nonpregnant animals [11] Epithelium of the prostatic acini in the nonpregnant *Praomys* is made up of cuboidal or columnar secreting (principal) cells (Fig 10) and small, flat basal cells These cells display relatively large nuclei at their base, and their apex does not reach the lumen, which is usually filled with a fine, granular secretion The prostatic epithelium of the pregnant *Praomys* has taller and narrower principal cells than those of the nonpregnant animal The nucleus of the cells in pregnant rodents is located between the basal and middle third of each cell (Fig 11) and is

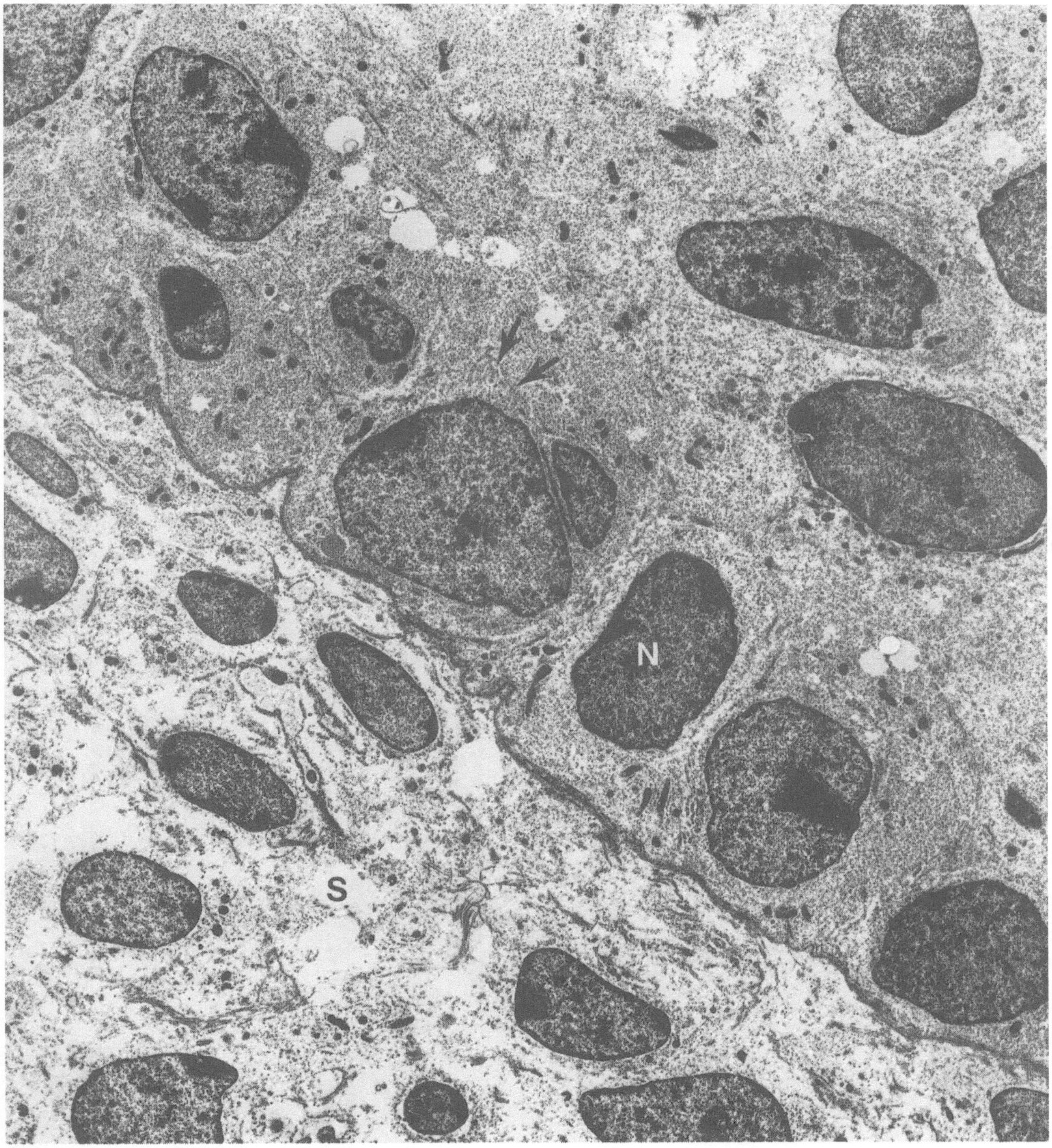

Fig. 9. Transmission electron micrograph of the prostate of a newborn female *Praomys* (see Fig. 4). A portion of a cluster of cells shows both the epithelial and capsular cells, the nuclei of the former (N), being larger than those of the latter. The plasmalemma between adjacent cells appears as finely filamentous lines (arrows). S = stroma (Uranyl acetate-lead citrate, ×5435). From Gross et al. [12], with permission.

surrounded by a flocculent cytoplasm. The cellular apex is prominently convex into the lumen, which contains abundant secretions.

The plasmalemma of the secreting epithelial cell in nonpregnant *Praomys* shows interdigitations with adjacent cells and at its bottom surface contacts an amorphous basal lamina (Fig. 12). The apical plasmalemma displays microvilli that vary in length and prominently extend into the lumen.

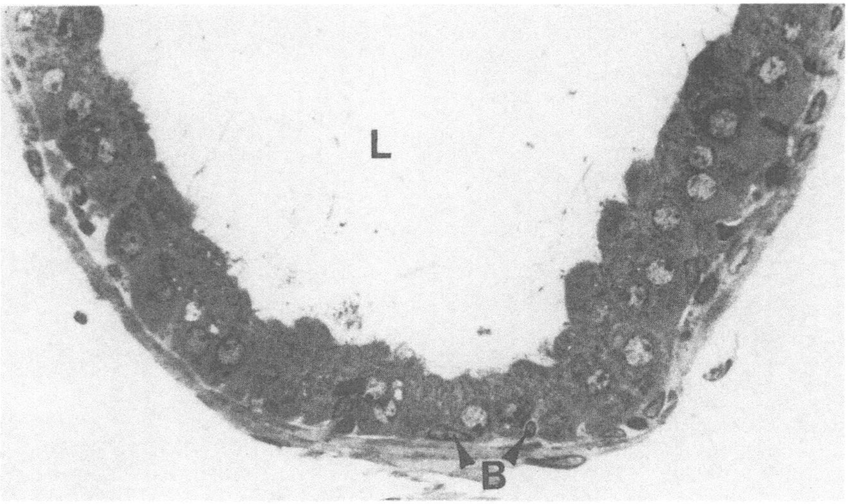

Fig 10 Photomicrograph of a section of the acinar wall of the prostate of the nonpregnant *Praomys*, showing cuboidal and columnar principal cells, their apex facing the lumen (L), and small basal cells (arrows B) (Toluidine blue ×520) From Gross et al [11], with permission

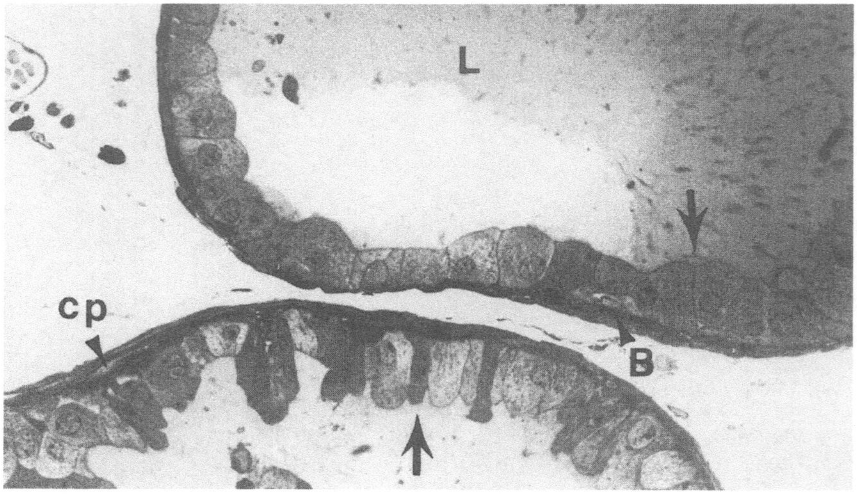

Fig 11 Photomicrograph of a section through the prostate of the pregnant female *Praomys* The wall of the acinus is made up of columnar cells (large arrows), some of which have convex apical areas The nucleus is located between the basal and middle third of the epithelial cells Secretory product is seen in the lumen (L) of the acinus A few basal cells (arrowhead B) appear next to the capsule (arrowhead cp) (Toluidine blue, ×430) From Gross et al [11], with permission

In the pregnant *Praomys* the plasmalemma of the principal cells of the prostate appear more complex and exhibit more interdigitations than in the nonpregnant animal. The secreting epithelial cells of the nonpregnant *Praomys*, present numerous vacuoles, some of which contain flocculent material. Large nuclei are usually located in the basal third of the cells of nonpregnant *Praomys*, whereas in pregnant *Praomys* they occupy the middle third of each cell.

The basal and perinuclear areas of the cells in the nonpregnant rodent contain rough endo-

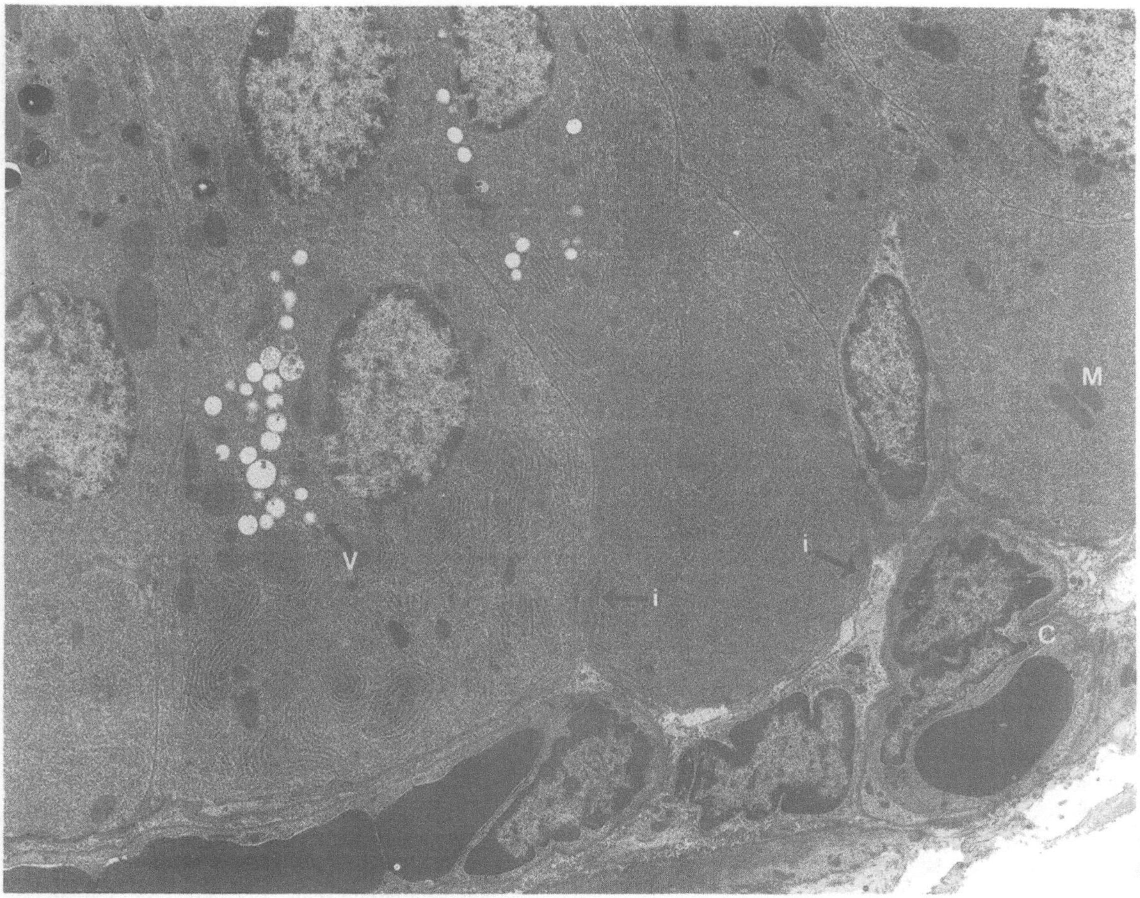

Fig 12 Transmission micrograph of a section taken through the prostate of a nonpregnant *Praomys*, showing epithelial cells and part of the capsule There are sections of nuclei, surrounded by whorls of endoplasmic reticulum and the plasmalemma, with interdigitations (arrow i) Vacuoles (V, arrow) form clusters next to the nucleus or are scattered Mitochondrion (M) and a cross section of a capillary (C) are indicated (Uranyl acetate-lead citrate, ×7990) From Gross et al [11], with permission

plasmic reticulum (Fig. 13), made up of short, parallel, narrow cisternae. In pregnant *Praomys* (Fig. 14), the basal cisternae are long and dilated, and some of them are filled with electron-dense material. Variable-sized secretion granules are scattered in the basal area of the pregnant animal.

In nonpregnant *Praomys* a well-developed Golgi complex is evident, with narrow vesicles, occasional dense onionoid bodies, or corpora cepiformia (Fig. 15), and the apical area is devoid of organelles and granules. In the pregnant animal the vesicles of the Golgi complex area are very dilated (Fig. 16), the onionoid bodies are in different stages of development, and the apical secretion granules are numerous, sometimes located between microvilli, on the surface of the microvilli, or in the lumen.

The histological aspects of the *Praomys* prostate in the last days of gestation may be interpreted as expressions of stimuli received by the prostatic gland during pregnancy. In fact, the lumina of prostatic acini contain more secretion in the pregnant than in the nonpregnant animal. Stimulation of the gland was evident under the electron microscope (increase and dilation of the granular endoplasmic reticulum, higher number of secretion granules, and larger Golgi complex). These subcellular and cytological variations, indicative of glandular increased activity, may be due to direct or indirect effects of androgenic stimulation

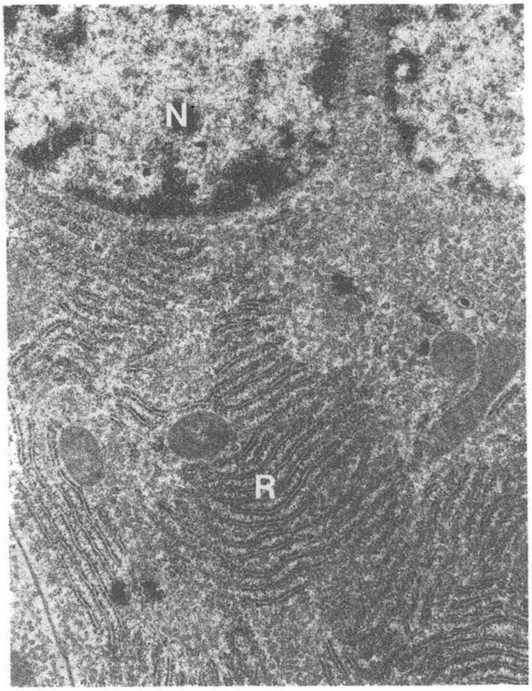

Fig 13 Transmission electron micrograph of the basal area of a principal cell of the prostate in a nonpregnant *Praomys* Part of the nucleus (N) and the rough endoplasmic reticulum (R), made up of parallel, short, narrow cisternae, is seen (Uranyl acetate-lead citrate, ×18,030) From Gross et al [11], with permission

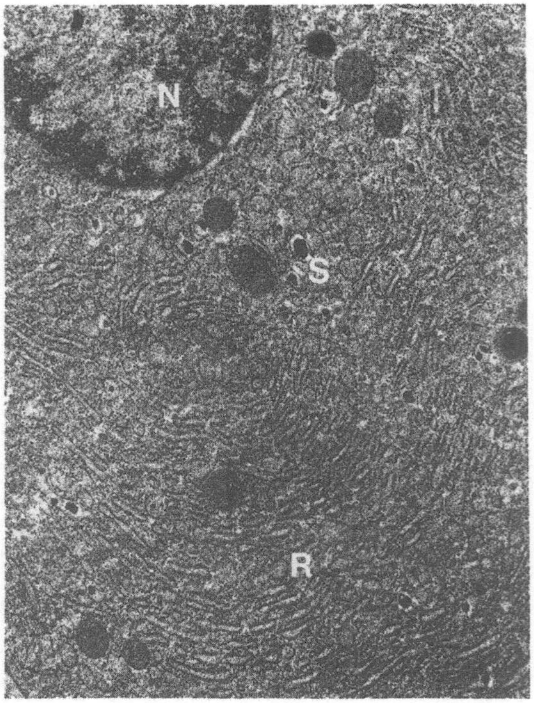

Fig 14 Transmission electron micrograph of the basal area of a pregnant *Praomys* prostatic principal cell Parts of the nucleus (N), rough endoplasmic reticulum (R), and secretion granules (S) are shown The rough endoplasmic reticulum consists of long and dilated cisternae (Uranyl acetate-lead citrate stain, ×17,280) From Gross et al [11], with permission

Prostatic bud formation from the rat urogenital sinus appears to be induced by a critical surge of testosterone production between 16.5 and 19 days of gestation [40]. Differential exposure to androgen levels, as a consequence of intrauterine position, in Sprague-Dawley rats contributes to the occurrence of female prostatic bud development. A study of this phenomenon is being carried out in *Mastomys coucha* [39].

3. Concluding Remarks

Review of the literature indicates that the primitive multimammate rodent *Praomys* (*Mastomys*) *natalensis* has a large and well-developed prostatic gland in both sexes [1,2]. This unique feature makes this animal a useful experimental model for investigations on the prostate, as this rodent provides the opportunity for study of the gland in two separate hormonal environments. The prostate of female *Praomys* develops at 19.5 days of gestation [12], almost coinciding with Price's findings [30]. By 18 days after birth, a secretion appears and by 30 days light supranuclear areas are clearly seen.

Histochemical study of the prostatic ventral lobe in both sexes of *Praomys* demonstrated the presence of PAS-positive material in the secretion [13], containing neutral carbohydrates of mucosubstances but no glycogen and little or no lipid. Only small sexual differences were noted in the adult *Praomys* prostatic gland [10]. This gland is more active in the pregnant *Praomys* than in the nonpregnant animal [11].

After demonstration in Sprague-Dawley rats [21] that differential exposure to androgen levels, as a consequence of embryo and fetal intrauterine

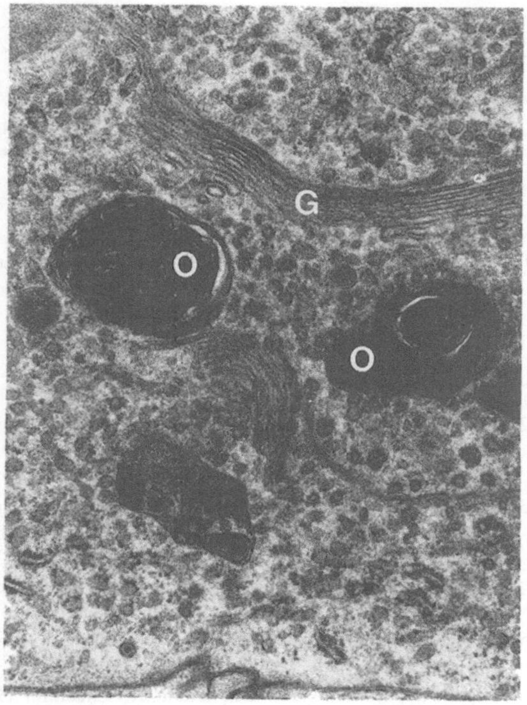

Fig 15 Transmission electron micrograph of the supra nuclear area of nonpregnant *Praomys* prostatic principal cell Next to a well developed Golgi complex (G) two onionoid bodies or corpora cepiformia (O) are evident (Uranyl acetate lead citrate ×28 930) From Gross et al [11] with permission

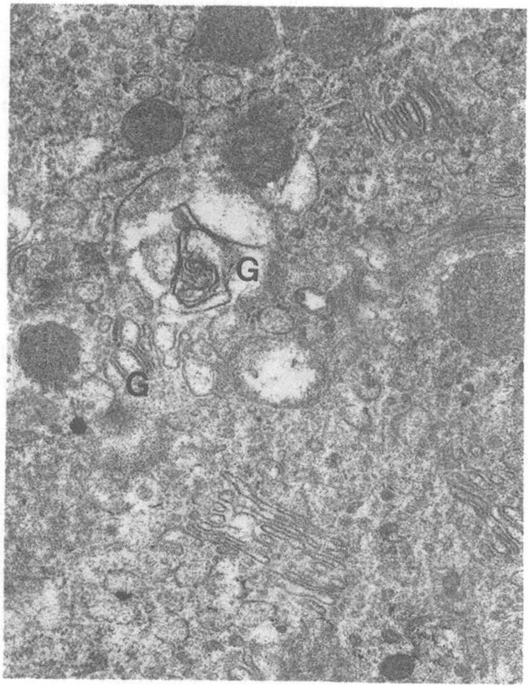

Fig 16 Transmission electron micrograph of the supranuclear area of a pregnant *Praomys* prostatic principal cell illustrating the Golgi complex (G) with dilated vesicles containing dense material and occasional membranous whorls (Uranyl acetate lead citrate ×32 370) From Gross et al [11] with permission

positions, contributes to the occurrence of female prostatic bud development, Timms et al [39] are now carrying out the same study in *Mastomys coucha*

The homology of *Praomys* adult, female prostate [16,36] with the ventral lobe of the male prostate enhances the importance of this rodent as an experimental animal model that can be used to verify changes, both natural and not, induced in the other sex

In addition, the fact that the female prostate may spontaneously develop adenocarcinoma and hyperplasia [15], as well as aging alterations, namely, papillary formation, hyperchromatism, cell enlargement, and broadening and flattening of papillae [37], increases the scientific value of this animal model for normal and pathologic comparative studies In addition, *Praomys* is also a very promising model for geriatric studies because it both presents a variety of age-associated neoplastic and non-neoplastic lesions and develops pathologic processes that are suggestive of autoimmune diseases [38]

References

1 Brambell FWR Davis DHS The normal occurrence structure and homology of prostate glands in adult female *Mastomys erythroleucus* Temm J Anat 75 64–74 1940

2 Burrill MW Greene RR Androgenic production during pregnancy and lactation in the rat Anat Rec 83 209–227 1942

3 Davis DHS Oettle AG The multimammate mouse *Rattus* (*Mastomys*) *Natalensis* Smith A laboratory adapted African wild rodent Proc Zool Soc Lond 131 293–299 1958

4 Evatt EJ A contribution to the development of the pros tate gland in the human female and a study of the homologies of the urethra and vagina of the sexes J Anat Physiol 45 122–130 1911

5 Felix W The development of the urogenital organs In Manual of Human Embryology F Keibel FP Mall (eds) Philadelphia JB Lippincott 1912

6 Ghanadian R, Holland JM, Chisholm GD Identification of a prostate in female *Praomys* (*Mastomys*) *Natalensis* using ^{3}H-steroids Br J Urol 47 77–82, 1975
7 Ghanadian R, Smith CB, Chisholm GD Receptor protein for dihydrotestosterone in nuclei of the female prostate of *Praomys* (*Mastomys*) *Natalensis* Invest Urol 16 119–122, 1978
8 Greene RR, Burrill MW, Ivy AC Masculinization of female rats by postnatal administration of male sex hormones Proc Soc Exp Biol Med 38 4–5, 1938
9 Gross SA, Didio LJA Prenatal development of the prostate in male *Praomys* (*Mastomys*) *Natalensis* Arch Ital Anat Embriol 91 21–28, 1986
10 Gross SA, DiDio LJA Comparative morphology of the prostate in adult male and female *Praomys* (*Mastomys*) *Natalensis* studied with electron microscopy J Submicrosc Cytol 19 77–84, 1987
11 Gross SA, DiDio LJA The prostate in pregnant and non-pregnant *Praomys* (*Mastomys*) *Natalensis* at the subcellular level J Submicrosc Cytol Pathol 20 101–107, 1988
12 Gross SA, DiDio LJA, Morse DE, Allen DJ Development of the prostate in female *Praomys* (*Mastomys*) *Natalensis* J Submicrosc Cytol 16 521–531, 1984
13 Gross SA, Sirigu P, DiDio LJA Histochemical determination of carbohydrates in the prostate of male and female *Praomys* (*Mastomys*) *Natalensis* Basic Appl Histochem 30 367–373, 1986
14 Hamilton JB, Wolfe JM Prostatic type of paraurethral glands induced in female rats by administration of male sex hormones Proc Soc Exp Biol Med 36 465–468, 1937
15 Holland JM Prostatic hyperplasia and neoplasia in female *Praomys* (*Mastomys*) *Natalensis* J Natl Cancer Inst 45 1229–1236, 1970
16 Ichihara I The fine structure of the epithelium of prostate glands in adult female *Mastomys erythroleucus* Temm Anat Anz 140 477–484, 1976
17 Johnson FP The homologue of the prostate in the female J Urol 8 13–27, 1922
18 Korenchevsky V Homology of the female periurethral glands and prostate Nature 136 185, 1935
19 Korenchevsky V The female prostatic gland and its reaction to male sexual compounds J Physiol 10 371–476, 1937
20 Lehmann I Quoted from [1]
21 Mahoney JJ The embryonic and postnatal development of the female prostate gland in the albino rat Anat Rec 75 122, 1939
22 Mahoney JJ The embryology and postnatal development of the prostate gland in the female rat Anat Rec 77 375–395, 1940
23 Mahoney JJ Relative influence of genetic and hormonal factors in the development of the female prostate gland Anat Rec 79 45–46, 1941
24 Mahoney JJ Genetic and hormonal determination of prostate development in the female rat J Exp Zool 90 413–419, 1942
25 Mahoney JJ, Witschi E Genetics of the female prostate in rats Genetics 32 369–378, 1947
26 Mansell-Moullin CM A contribution to the morphology of the prostate J Anat Physiol 29 201–204, 1894
27 Marx L Zur anatomie der prostata weiblicher ratten Zeit Zellforsch Mikr Anat 16 48, 1932
28 Oettle AG The multimammate mouse In The UFAW Handbook The Care and Management of Laboratory Animals London E S Livingstone, 1967, pp ••–••
29 Pallin G Beitrag zur anatomie und embryologie der prostata und der samenblasen Arch Anat Entw •• 135–176, 1901
30 Price D Normal development of the prostate and seminal vesicles of the rat with a study of experimental post-modifications Am J Anat 60 79–127, 1936
31 Price D Normal development and regression of the prostate gland of the female rat Proc Soc Exp Biol Med 41 580–583, 1939
32 Price D A comparison of the reactions of male and female rat prostate transplants Anat Rec 82 93–113, 1942
33 Rauther M Ueber den Genitalapparat einiger Nager und Insektivoren, insbesondere die akzessorischen Genitaldrusen derselben Jen Zeit Naturw 31 377, 1903
34 Shehata R Female prostate in the house rat *Rattus rattus* Acta Anat 83 426–434, 1972
35 Shehata R Female prostate in *Arvicanthis Niloticus* and *Meriones Libycus* Acta Anat 92 513–523, 1975
36 Smith AF, Landon GV, Ghanadian R, Chisholm GD The ultrastructure of the male and female prostate of *Praomys* (*Mastomys*) *Natalensis* I Normal, castrated, and ovariectomized animals Cell Tissue Res 190 539–552, 1978
37 Snell KC, Stewart HL Adenocarcinoma and proliferative hyperplasia of the prostate gland in female *Rattus* (*Mastomys*) *Natalensis* J Natl Canc Inst 35 7–14, 1965
38 Solleveld HA *Praomys* (*Mastomys*) *Natalensis* in Aging Research Rijswyk, The Netherlands Institute for Experimental Gerontology TNO, 1981
39 Timms BG, Bezuidenhout AJ, DiDio LJA Intrauterine position of fetuses of *Mastomys coucha* and occurrence of female prostate In preparation
40 Timms BG, DiDio LJA The effect of intrauterine position on the occurrence of female prostatic bud development 103rd Annual Meeting of the American Association of Anatomy, Philadelphia, Pennsy lvania, April 22–25, 1990 Anat Rec 226 104A, 1990
41 Tourneux F Sur le developpement et l'evolution du tubercule genital chez la foetus humain dans deux sexes J Anat Physiol (Paris) 175 229–263, 1889
42 Virchow R Prostata-concretionen beim Weib Arch Path Anat 5 403–404, 1853
43 Witschi E, Mahoney JJ, Riley GM Occurrence of prostatic lobes in the female rat Biol Zentralbl 58 455–464, 1938
44 Witschi E, Riley GM Effect of inbreeding and selection on frequency of prostates in female rats Genetics 24 90–91, 1936
45 Young HH quoted in Moore T The female prostate Bladder-neck obstruction in women Lancet 1 1305–1309, 1960

CHAPTER 7

Histochemistry and Electron Microscopy for Diagnosis of Prostatic Cancer

CARLO CAPELLA, BRUNO FRIGERIO, GIOVANNA FINZI, MAURIZIO SALVADORE, & ALDO BONO

1. Introduction

The treatment and prognosis of prostatic carcinomas (PCs) depend on the spread, differentiation, and exact histological type [24,28]. Although the histopathological differential diagnosis between various tumor types and benign conditions in most cases is fairly easy, at times unequivocal diagnosis of malignancy or definition of tumor type is exceedingly difficult or even impossible [57]. To overcome this, special staining or electron microscopy can be used to show the presence of cellular components such as enzymes, intermediate filaments, oncofetal proteins, or peculiar ultrastructural findings. Histochemical, immunohistochemical, and electron microscopy techniques can confirm or exclude a previously assumed histopathological diagnosis; in addition, they are capable of demonstrating functional heterogeneity or of clarifying the histogenetic origin of a neoplasm. The purpose of this review is to investigate existing methodologies that meet the above criteria and to recognize the methods that enable a complete pathological evaluation of PCs.

2. Histochemistry and Immunohistochemistry

2.1. Prostate-Specific Antigen and Prostatic Acid Phosphatase

Prostate-specific antigen (PSA) was first identified by Wang et al. [63] and is a 33 kD glycoprotein that has the characteristics of a kallicreinlike serine protease [32]. The cDNA for PSA has been cloned and sequenced [34]. PSA is considered to be a specific marker of both benign and malignant prostatic epithelia. It is now considered a serum marker for PCs that is more specific and sensitive than prostatic acid phosphatase (PAP). The serum values are higher in PCs than in benign hyperplasias and correlate with the volume of tumor [59].

Immunohistochemical localization of PSA in the normal prostate is uniform and strong in both the central and peripheral zones. Positive staining is granular and is observed in all ductal and acinar secretory cells, but not in basal cells. At the ultrastructural level PSA is localized by the immunogold technique within the clear matrix of supranuclear secretory vesicles of secretory cells (Fig. 1).

Prostatic acid phosphatase (PAP) is probably the best characterized prostate marker available for routine study. It was firstly identified in the prostate, urine, and seminal fluid by Demuth [12] and Kutscher and Wolberg [30]. PAP is a sialoglycoprotein with a molecular mass of approximately 90 kD and is produced, under the regulation of androgens, by both benign and malignant prostatic epithelia. The atrophy of benign or malignant prostatic tissue induced by castration or estrogen therapy can be reversed by androgen therapy. Serum levels of PAP can be measured more precisely by immunologic than by enzymatic techniques. Serum PAP is mainly used for the staging and monitoring of patients with PCs.

Riva, A., Testa Riva, F., and Motta, P.M., (eds.), Ultrastructure of Male Urogenital Glands: Prostate, Seminal Vesicles, Urethral, and Bulbourethral Glands. *ISBN 0-7923-2800-0.*

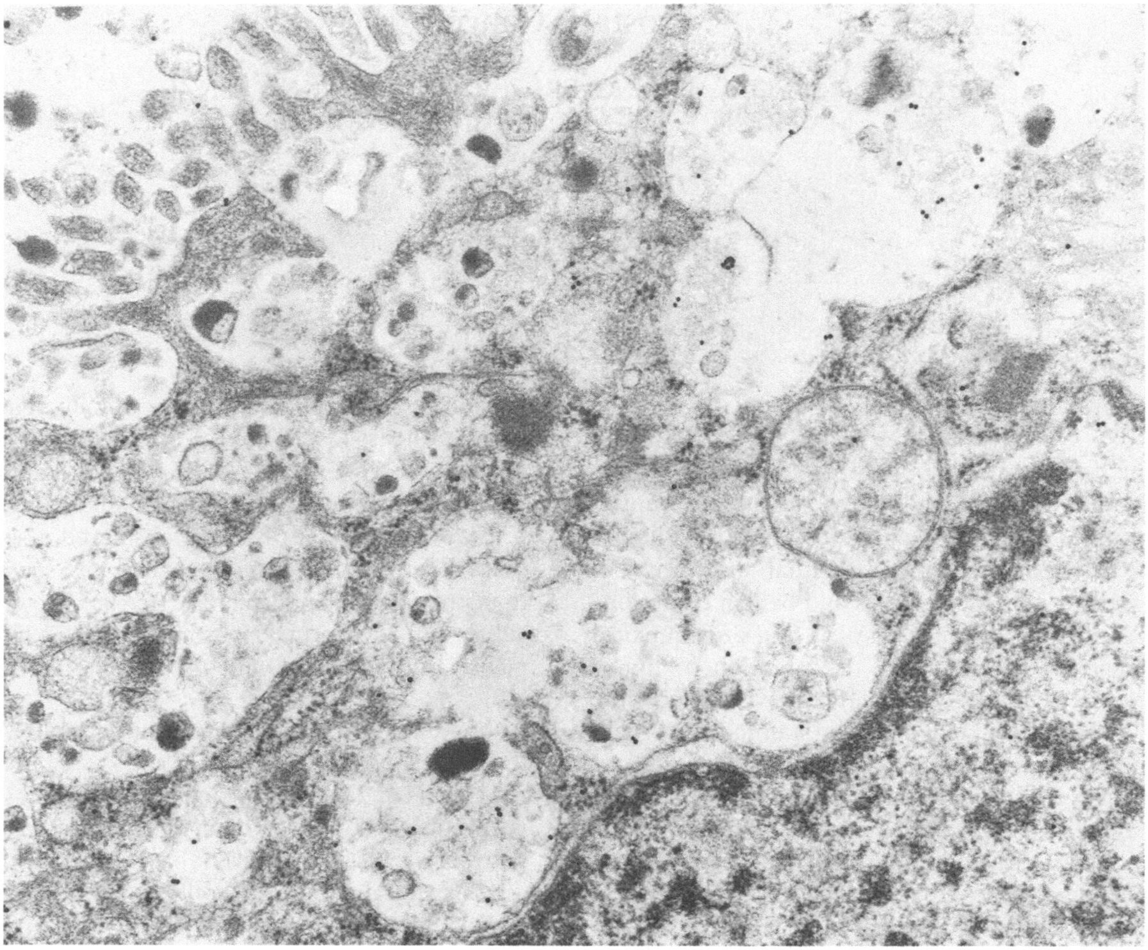

Fig 1 PSA immunoreactivity in secretory vesicles of a vesicular granule glandular (VGG) cell of the peripheral normal prostate (immunogold ×45 000)

On tissue sections direct histochemical localization of PAP has generally been replaced by immunohistochemistry [39] The distribution and pattern of positivity for PAP in the normal prostate mirrors both the light and electron microscopic level analysis of PSA (Fig 2) Staining of PCs for both PSA and PAP is less than observed in benign prostatic tissue [23 25] In addition, within a given tumor great variation in staining intensity for both PSA and PAP of individual cells occurs and a relationship between staining heterogeneity and increasing tumor grade has been observed [9,62] In high grade tumors PAP staining has been reported to be generally stronger than PSA staining [23] In contrast to the majority of PCs, which are positive for both PAP and PSA, some high grade tumors stain only for PAP or PSA, or occasionally, neither stain is positive Decreased PSA staining has been correlated with progression in stage A_2 prostatic carcinoma [14], while PAP staining, which reflects the number of androgen sensitive cells, has shown some correlation with responsiveness to hormonal therapy [25]

PSA is considered an immunohistochemical marker more specific than PAP, since false-positive staining for PSA is rarer than that for PAP Positive staining for PAP has been demonstrated in some tumors such as carcinoid tumors [54], with special emphasis on rectal carcinoids

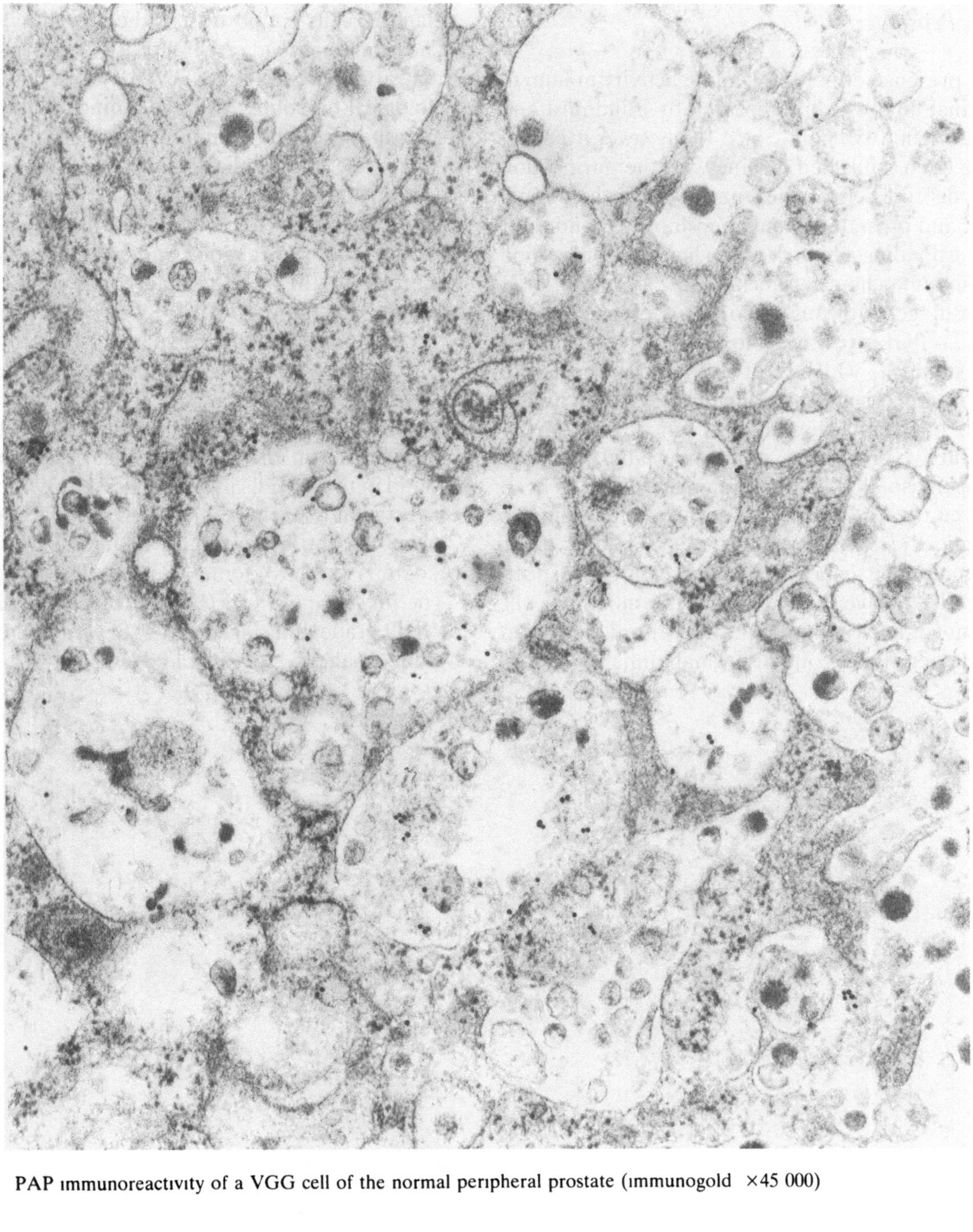

Fig 2 PAP immunoreactivity of a VGG cell of the normal peripheral prostate (immunogold ×45 000)

[3], and occasionally, islet cell tumors [10], breast cancers, and primary bladder adenocarcinoma [16] In addition, immunoreactivity for PAP and PSA has been shown in Skene glands, which represent the female equivalent of the prostate, and in related tumors [44,60] With the exception of these tumors, the practical contribution of PSA and PAP immunohistochemistry is mainly in identification of metastatic PC and in differentiating a PC invading the urinary bladder from a

primary transitional cell carcinoma arising in this site [16].

2.2. Pepsinogen II

The presence of pepsinogenlike activity in human seminal fluid was first reported by Lundquist and Seedorf in 1952 [33]. Since then, several papers have been published dealing with the purification and distribution of the enzyme in both seminal fluid and prostate. In man pepsinogens (and their corresponding active pepsins) have been classified by immunochemical techniques as either PGI (pepsinogen 1 through 5) or PGII (pepsinogens 6 and 7). PGI is restricted to the oxyntic mucosa of the stomach, while PGII is found in the entire gastric mucosa and in duodenum [11,51]. Whether PGII plays any physiological function in the reproductive process has not been established. Pepsinogen isolated in the seminal fluid has been proven to be electrophoretically and immunochemically identical to gastric PGII [50].

Immunohistochemical studies employing specific antisera have shown that PGII-containing cells are much more common in the central zone than in the peripheral zone of normal human prostate, and that they are also present in seminal vesicles [45]. In the central zone more than 50% of glandular cells are positive for PGII, while no more than 5% cells are positive in the peripheral zone. These findings lead researchers to suggest that the central and peripheral zones may serve different biological functions, and that a functional kinship exists between the seminal vesicle and the central zone. The biochemical similarity between the central zone and the seminal vesicle lends support to the theory of a common Wolffian duct origin for both the central zone and seminal vesicle, in contrast to the endodermal origin of the peripheral zone [37,45].

Using an immunoperoxidase method, Reid et al. [46] were able to localize the gastric acid proteinase gastricsin (pepsin II) in prostate. However, they did not notice any regional distribution of gastricsin in the prostate. Gastricsin was also found in tumor cells in 21 of 54 cases (39%) of PC investigated. We have studied 89 PCs with specific anti-PGII antiserum (kindly donated by Dr. I.M. Samloff) and have found 48 positive cases (54%). The presence of PGII (Fig. 3) correlated with the WHO grade and stage of PCs. Seventy percent of grade I and 54% of grade II PCs were PGII

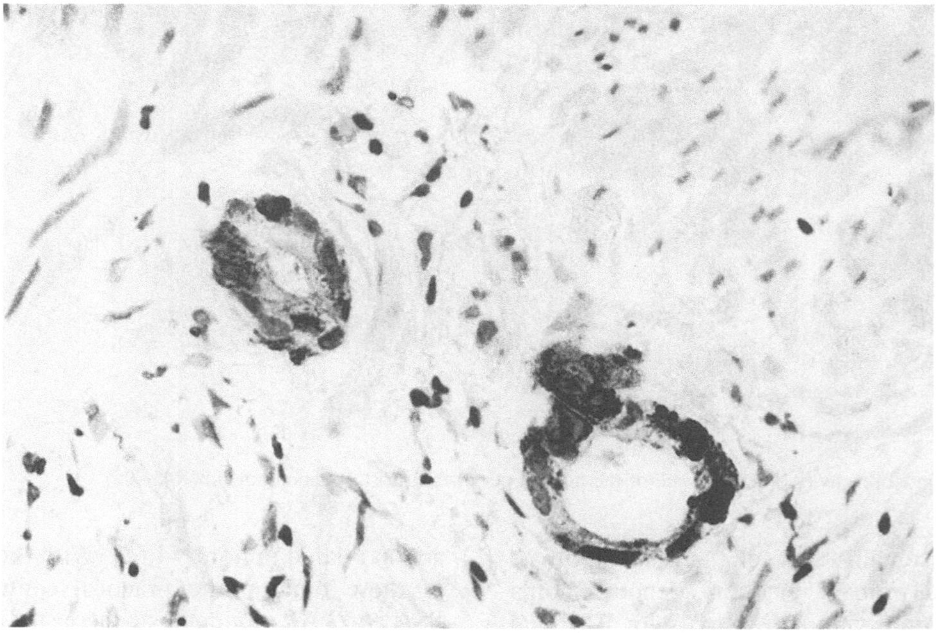

Fig 3 Intense immunoreactivity for PGII in a microglandular PC (immunoperoxidase, hematoxylin conterstain, ×400)

positive, while all grade III PCs were devoid of PGII. PGII was expressed in 66% of cases treated with radical prostatectomy, which were mainly at Stages A and B, and in 41% of the cases treated with transurethral resection (TUR), which were mainly at Stages C and D.

2.3. *Mucins*

The presence of mucins in normal and pathological prostate has been described by many authors [13,15,19,21,27,31,40,43,48,49]. Mucins are of three types: *neutral mucins*, which stain purple red with the PAS method; *sialomucins*, which stain blue with Alcian blue PAS technique at pH 2.5; *sulphomucins*, which stain brown to black with the HID-AB method [56]. The normal prostate and benign prostatic hyperplasia (BPH) produce only neutral mucins, whereas PC is characterized by both sulphated and sialomucins. Therefore, the demonstration of acid mucins is helpful in differentiating PC from other non-malignant glandular proliferations and is of utmost importance when dealing with small samples of prostatic tissue, such as those extracted with prostate needle biopsy [2].

Although most PCs produce mucins, there is great variation in the number of mucus secreting cells within a given tumor. Pinder and McMahon [43] studied a series of PCs that showed 60% of cases with less than 5% mucus-secreting cells, 20% with 5–25%, and 20% with more than 25% mucus-secreting cells. The tumors produced sialomucins and/or sulphomucins. Our studies (unpublished data), based on a series of PCs, have confirmed the expression of sialomucins in the majority of cases (about 70%), whereas sulphomucins were present in only 15% of cases. The presence of acid mucins, however, was not related to tumor grading and did not show any prognostic value.

Mucinous and signet ring cell PCs are rare and clinically aggressive tumors that are easily identified by their strong staining for sialomucins [43, 48,49]. According to Epstein and Lieberman [15], a PC may be defined as mucinous if it contains no less than 25% mucin lakes.

2.4. *Lectins*

Lectin binding is quite similar in normal prostate and benign prostatic hyperplasia (BPH) [2]. Dif-

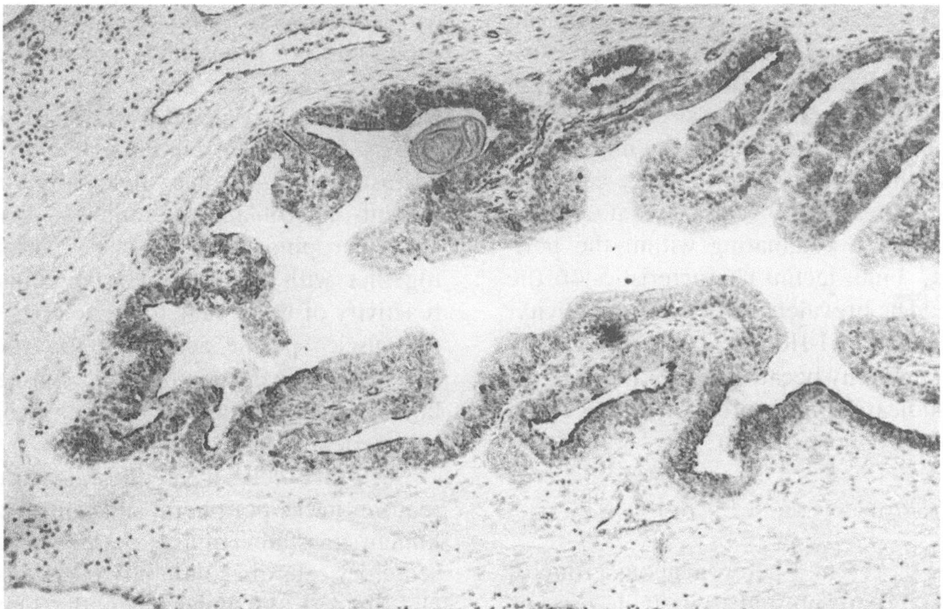

Fig 4 Intense reactivity to UEA lectin of a gland of the central zone of the normal prostate (×100)

ferences in lectin binding, however, have been demonstrated between benign prostatic lesions and PCs [36,55]. A different qualitative and quantitative lectin pattern has also been found between primary and metastatic PCs [1,20], suggesting the existence of cell subpopulations in PCs with a different metastatic potential.

McNeal et al. [38] demonstrated that the central and peripheral zones of human prostate show different lectin binding patterns. Secretory cells of the central zone are selectively stained by three lectins: J-WGA, PNA, and UEA-I (Fig. 4), whereas the peripheral zone is unreactive to them. However, both zones are stained by LCA, Con-A, WGA, and PNA-N lectins. Dysplastic foci within the prostate are characterized by reduction or absence of lectin binding, and areas of peripheral zone adjacent to dysplastic foci abnormally bind the lectins, which are typical of the central zone. This "ectopic" lectin pattern of "normal adjacent areas" may be regarded as a histochemical lesion that precedes the development of a morphologically identifiable dysplasia.

In our studies (unpublished data) we have found positive staining for UEA-I in 69% and for Con-A in 71% of 45 PCs that were in an early tumor stage and were treated by radical prostatectomy. The reactive cases were 45% for UEA-I and 39% for Con-A in a group of 44 patients who were in more advanced stages and were treated by trans-urethral resection prostatectomy (TURP). In addition, in the radical prostatectomy group reactivity was expressed in a higher proportion of tumor cells, while in the TURP group the percentage of positive cells was much lower. These data indicate that a large proportion of PCs, originating within the peripheral zone, bind lectin characteristic of the central zone. The prevalence of UEA-I reactivity, which parallels PGII-IR, in cases undergoing radical prostatectomy because of an early stage of the tumor, indicates that expression of this lectin is a favorable prognostic factor.

2.5. *Cytokeratins*

Cytokeratins represent a heterogeneous group of polypeptides and are present in variable proportions and associations in various types of epithelial cells. They can be selectively identified by immunohistochemistry using specific monoclonal antibodies [2].

Studies of the pathology of the prostate have taken advantage of the use of "basal cell specific" (high molecular weight) cytokeratin antibodies for differential diagnosis of well-differentiated PC from other nonmalignant lesions. The presence of basal cells is generally considered to be a marker for a benign lesion; in fact, there are no basal cells in PC and thus the immunohistochemical demonstration of basal cells is a helpful tool to rule out PC [7,8]. In studies on the histogenesis of PC, it has been observed [26] that in lesions preceding invasive PC, the so-called prostatic intraepitelial neoplasia (PIN), the number of basal cells demonstrated immunohistochemically decreases progressively with an increasing grade of PIN.

3. Ultrastructure

The fine structure of the human prostate has been studied both in normal and neoplastic conditions by many authors [4,5,29,35,61]. The normal glandular exocrine epithelium is represented by two cell types: basal cells and secretory cells.

The basal cells have an elongated shape and lie in close contact with the basement membrane [4]. They are located in a triangular space between two adjacent secretory cells, their nuclei are round and not prominent, and their cytoplasmic matrix is dense and shows many mitochondria. Neither secretory vesicles nor signs of secretory activity have been demonstrated in basal cells. Ultrastructural studies also show an absence of thin microfilament bundles, dense bodies, and micropinocytotic vesicles. These findings, together with the lack of immunohistochemical reactivity of these cells to monoclonal antibodies to muscle specific actin, and on the contrary, specific positive staining with cytokeratin antibodies, demonstrate that basal epithelial cells are not myoepithelial cells [58].

Secretory cells have different ultrastructural features in the peripheral and central zones of the human prostate. In the peripheral zone, most secretory cells are columnar. The apical portion is club-shaped and bulges into the lumen so that elongated pits, filled with secretory material, form between adjacent apical protrusions (Fig.

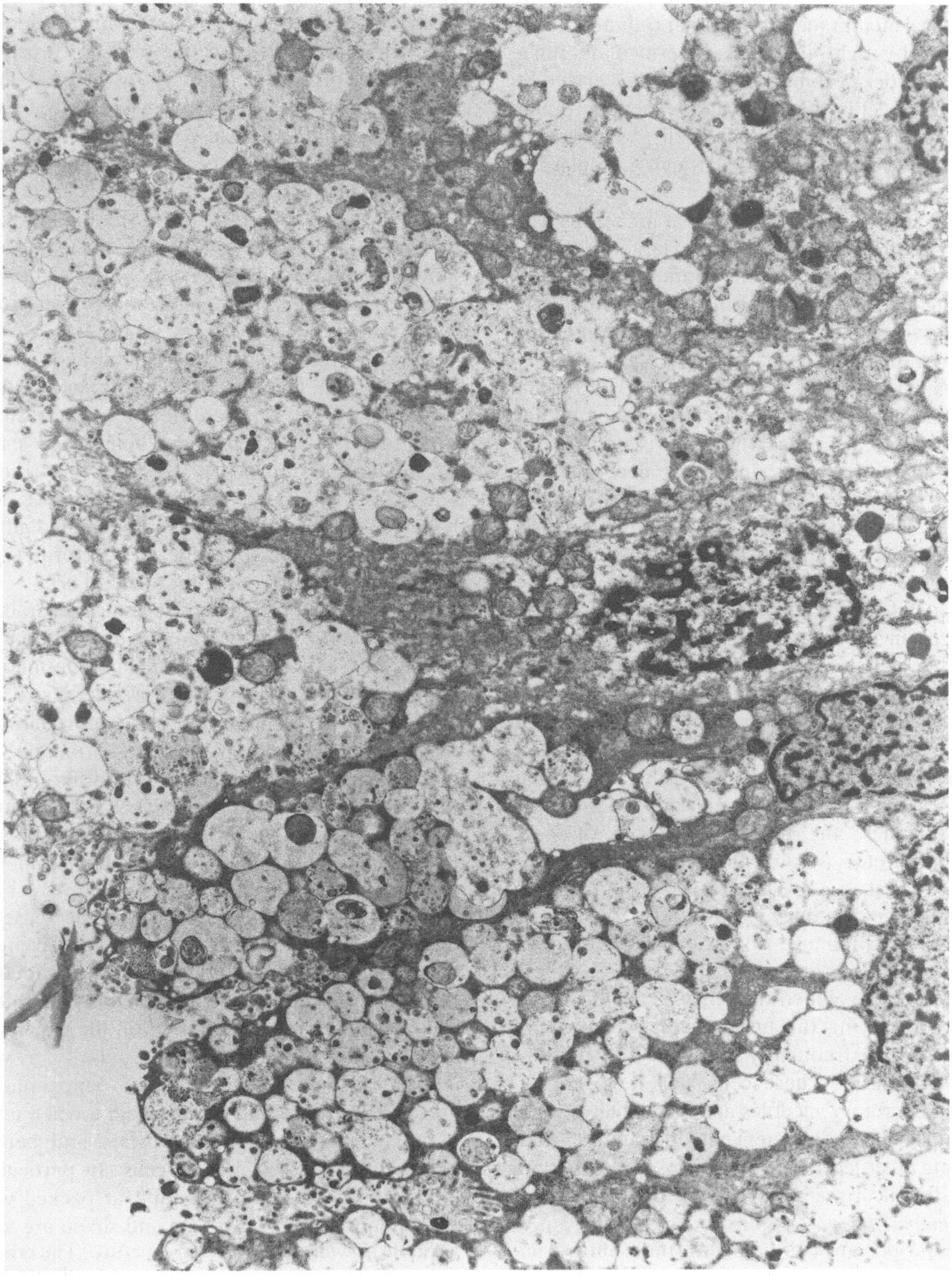

Fig 5 Electron micrograph of secretory cells of the peripheral normal prostate (×8800)

5). The apical surface shows quite numerous microvilli. In the subapical part of the cytoplasm, the lateral membranes of columnar cells are joined together by tight junctions, intermediate junctions, and desmosomes. The nuclei are placed at the same level in the epithelium. They are round and located at the base of the cells, where many mitochondria and profiles of rough endoplasmic reticulum are also present.

The Golgi apparatus consists of numerous flattened saccules, small vesicles, and larger vacuoles, and is situated mainly in the supranuclear part of the cell. The apical pole of the cell is occupied by secretory vacuoles, which are often in contact or fuse with the luminal plasmalemma. The secretory vacuoles are large, measuring 200–700 nm in diameter, and are bound by a simple membrane. They appear mostly as empty cavities, some of which contain small, round dense cores or flocculent, nondense material floating in the empty vesicles. Due to this characteristic ultrastructural feature, we call these cells *vesicular granule glandular* (VGG) cells of the prostate. By the immunogold technique both PSA and PAP are localized in the clear part of the secretory vacuoles, but not in their dense small cores (Figs. 1 and 2). While some authors [18] suggest that these PAP containing vacuoles are lysosomes, no other hydrolytic enzymes have been demonstrated within them. The absence of other lysosomal enzymes, such as β-glucoronidase [64], in secretory vacuoles, the high optimal pH of 5–7, and its secretory nature all suggest that PAP is nonlysosomal.

In the central zone, most secretory cells (Fig. 6) are low columnar, and have less prominent apical protrusions and microvilli. The Golgi apparatus is less developed than in VGG cells. Dense bodies displaying the fine structural features of lysosomes are frequently found in the supranuclear cytoplasm. These cells lack large empty-looking secretory vacuoles and instead have small (about 200 nm in diameter) haloed granules, often showing an eccentric core, and closely resembling those found in secretory cells of human seminal vesicles [47].

We propose to call cells with these ultrastructural characteristics *seminal vesicle-like glandular* (SVLG) cells of the prostate. Although we have not been able to localize PGII within these cells by the immunogold technique applied on plastic embedded material (including London White and Lowicryl), we think that, due to the coincidence of distribution of SVLG cells and PGII-IR cells in the central prostate and the ultrastructural similarity of SVLG cells and principal cells of the seminal vesicles, which also contain PGII, SVLG cells could be the source of production of PGII within the prostate. By the immunogold technique PAP and PSA do not appear to be localized within the small secretory granule of SVGB cells, although some labelling for both of these antigens is observed in empty vesicles and in the apical cytoplasm [17].

Several studies have been published on the ultrastructural features of PCs. Some of these studies have stressed the difference in ultrastructural features between tumor cells of PCs and cells of normal prostate [4,18,35]. Other studies have classified different cells types in PCs and have related the types of cells identified ultrastructurally to the different architectural types and degree of differentiation of PCs [29].

The most important ultrastructural characteristics of tumor cells in PCs are the nucleus, plasma membrane, mitochondria, and endoplasmic reticulum. The nucleus is quite variable in size and shape, with convoluted and lobulated contours, margination, and clumping of the chromatin and prominence of nucleoli. In poorly differentiated tumor cells, the nucleus shows round, regular contours and low electron density. The plasma membrane is equipped with a variable number of junctions on the lateral cell surface. By both TEM [35] and SEM [22,52,61], a decrease in desmosomes, resulting in a lack of cohesiveness, has been observed, and this has been regarded as responsible for the infiltrative activity of tumor cells. Gaeta et al. [22] reported on the paucity or absence of microvilli and the irregularity, as well as interruptions in the basal lamina. Mitochondria are increased in number and swollen when compared to those in normal prostate and benign prostatic hyperplasia (BPH) cells. In particular, undifferentiated tumor cells appear packed with mitochondria [35]. Their size and shape are very variable as well as their inner structure. The cristae are irregular in length and show a longitudinal or transverse disposition; the mitochondrial matrix appears dark to pale to finely granular.

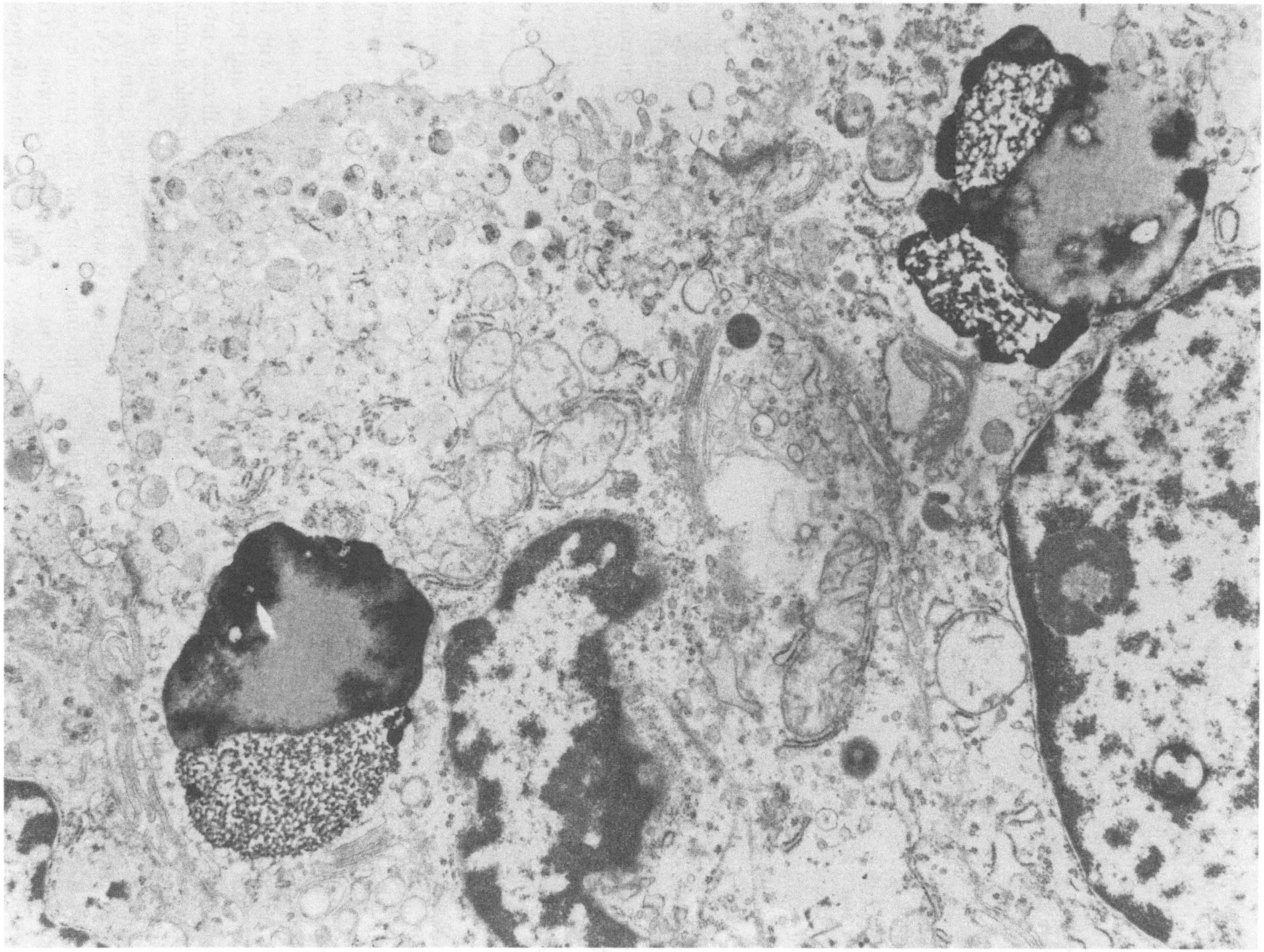

Fig 6 Electron micrograph of secretory cells (seminal vesicle like glandular cell) of the central zone of normal prostate (×22 400)

The rough endoplasmic reticulum of well-differentiated cells of PCs is distributed in an orderly fashion, as in normal cells, while in poorly differentiated PCs it appears abundant, with irregular dilatations and tubular forms [35]. Secretory vacuoles and granules are located at the apical portion of the cell in well-differentiated PCs and are similar to those of normal prostate cells. In poorly differentiated PCs, the secretory vacuoles tend to fuse with larger vesicles that do not contain secretory material and appear to represent, according to Brandes et al. [4], "pathologic vacuolation." Lipid droplets of variable morphology, randomly distributed in the cytoplasm of the acinar cells, are a frequent finding in PCs [35]. These droplets have been tentatively related to androgenic metabolites or androgenic hormones. However, this possibility has not been supported by experimental data. An increased amount of lipid in prostatic cancer cells may represent "stuffing" of tumor cells unable to gain access to an excretory duct for secretion [6]. Alternatively, these droplets, which are heterogeneous in nature, may represent either raw material, secretion, degradation, or degenerative products [35].

Particles resembling type C virus particles, 90–130 nm in diameter, were observed in intracytoplasmic vacuoles in 5 of 32 cases of PCs and in 1 of 8 cases of BPH [41]. In addition, intracisternal viruslike particles, 150–200 nm in diameter, were found in epithelial cells of four carcinomas. In some of these particles, an electron-dense central core or two concentric layers were discernible. The observation of particles resembling virus particles in cells of PCs is of interest. However, further studies are needed to establish a relationship, if any, between the viruslike particles and the origin of hyperplastic and malignant changes in prostatic tissue.

Needlelike, rectangular; straight, rodlike; or irregular intraluminal crystalloids, showing high electron density and lacking a limiting membrane, have been described in PCs [42]. They are mostly less than 6 μm long and 2 μm wide, and are mostly homogeneous in internal structure; however, some reveal internal slits and annular ringlike structures. In light microscopy these crystals are strongly positive to phosphotungstic acid-hematoxilin (PTHA) and are epithelial membrane antigen (EMA) immunoreactive. Intraluminal crystals are present in 10–23% of PCs [42] and are considered as a good marker of malignancy.

Kastendieck and Altenähr [29] classified the PCs according to the ultrastructural characteristics of the cell types and their aggregation to form glandular, solid/cribriform, and anaplastic patterns of growth. The cell types identified are undifferentiated (type I), immature (type II), highly differentiated (type III), functionally deranged (type IV), and degenerative (type V) glandular tumor cells. These types represent different stages of maturation of tumor cells. Tumors with a glandular pattern are mainly composed of differentiated type III and type IV cells, which maintain cell polarity, but show signs of early stromal infiltration. The solid/cribriform pattern consists of a central part of less differentiated type II–IV cells, with or without lumen formation, and of a peripheral layer of basal cells. The anaplastic pattern consists of solid masses composed of mixed populations of tumor cells (type I–IV) with all stages of differentiation and progressive tumor cell degeneration.

Sinha et al. [53] have reported two distinct types of basal cells and have correlated these with behavior. Type I cells were characterized by round nuclei with many small aggregates of euchromatin and large nucleoli. Type II cells had highly pleomorphic nuclei, many small aggregates of heterochromatin, and large pleomorphic nucleoli. PCs that were or subsequently became refractory to estrogen therapy were richer in type II basal cells than those of responsive patients. Therefore, type II cells were regarded as endocrine nonresponsive cells and were considered responsible of proliferation, metastasis, and killing of the patient.

We have studied the fine structure of 16 cases of PCs and have correlated the tumor cell types, ultrastructurally identified according to the criteria used for the normal prostate, with the histologic pattern, cytological grade, and PGII-immunoreactivity. We detected in all cases investigated cells resembling vacuolar granule glandular (VGG) cells (Fig. 7) of the outer zone of the normal prostate (Table 1). On the contrary, cells similar to seminal vesiclelike glandular (SVLG) cells of the inner zone of the prostate were found only in cases (Fig. 8) showing PGII-immunoreactivity, a finding that indirectly proves PGII is produced by SVLG cells.

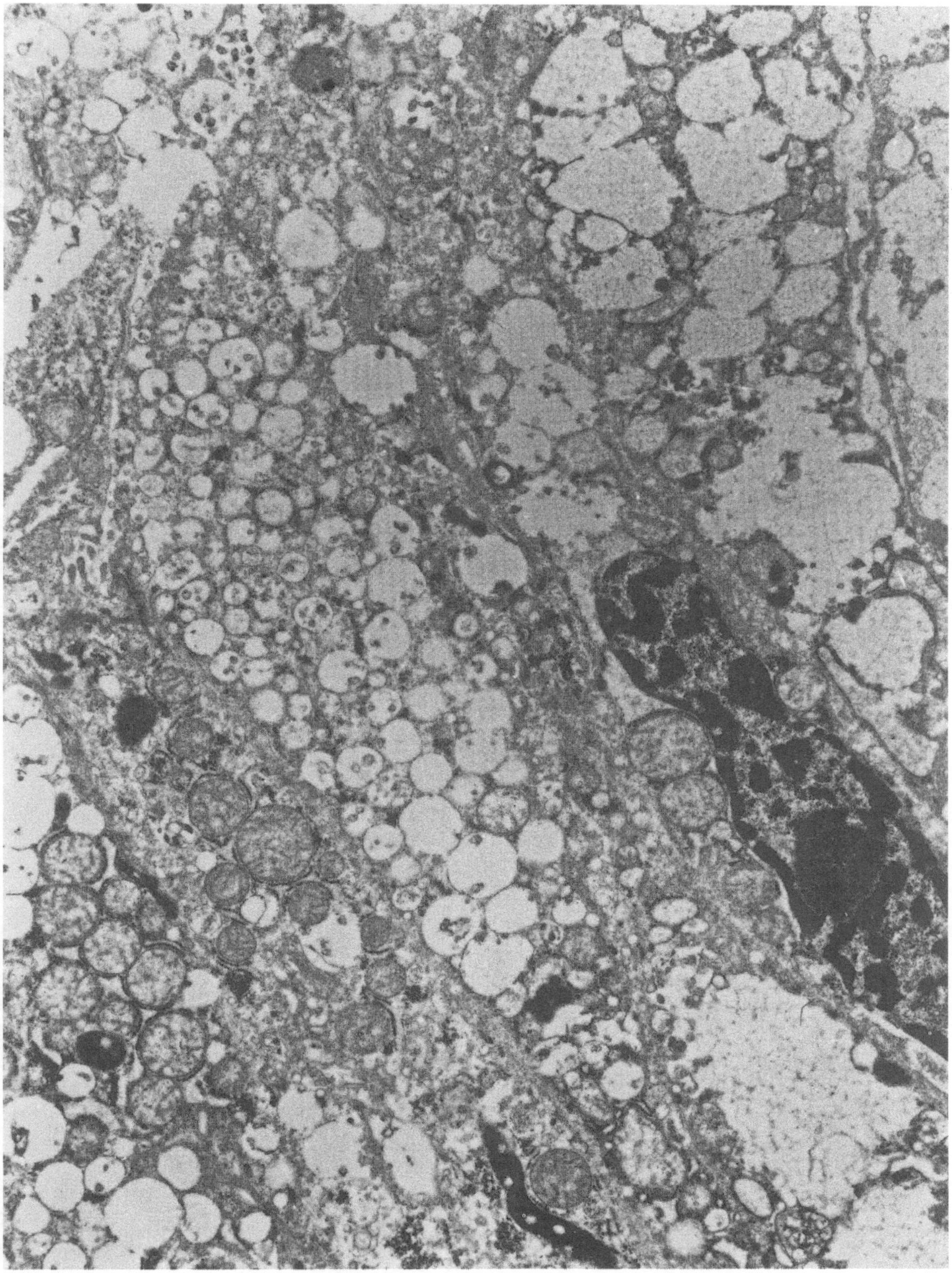

Fig 7 Ultrastructural features of cells of a PC resembling VGG cells of the normal peripheral zone (×14,000)

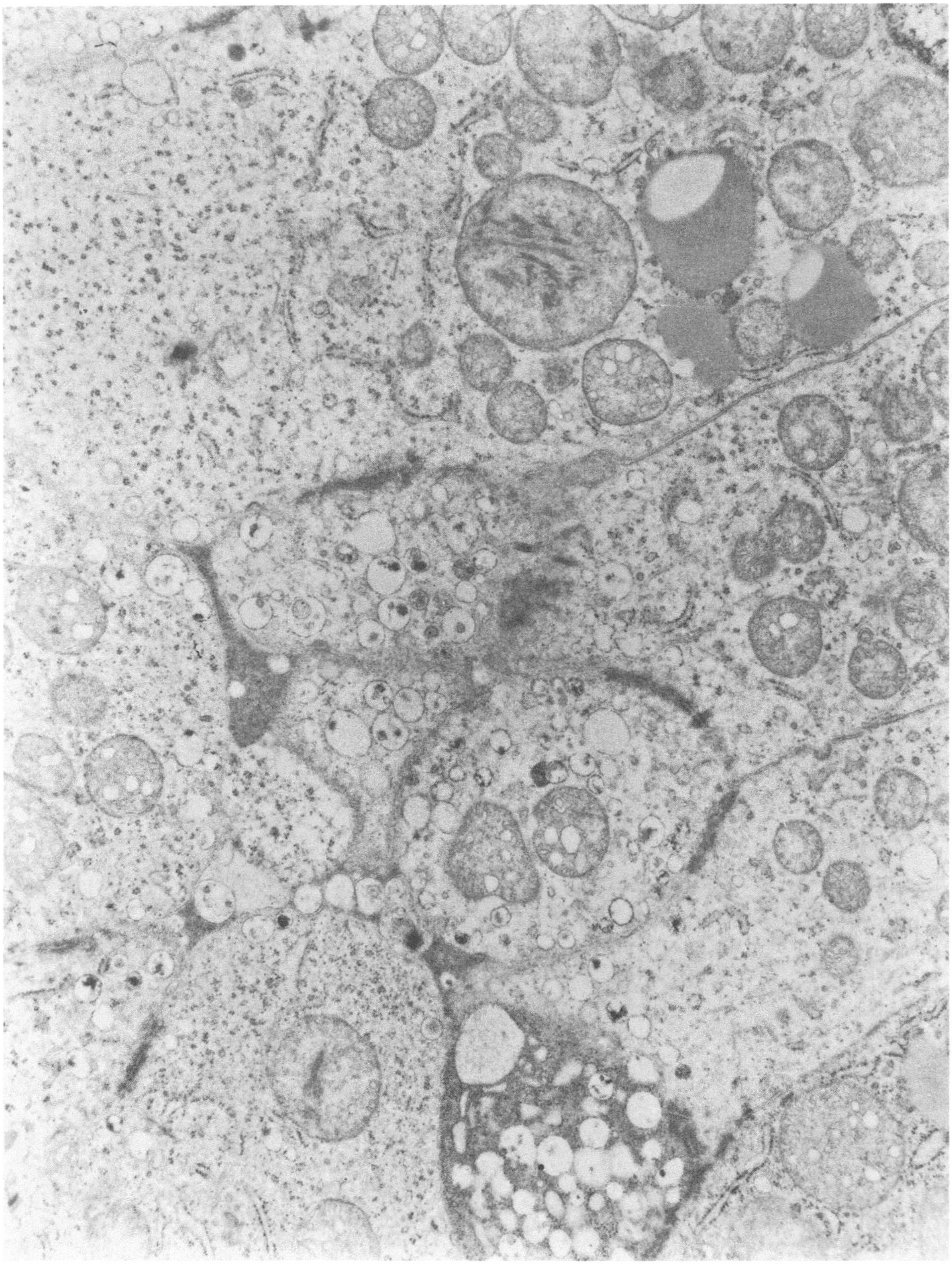

Fig 8 Electron micrograph of cells of a PC resembling seminal vesicle like glandular (SVLG) cells of the normal central zone (×22 000)

Table 1 Relationships between PGII immunoreactivity and ultrastructural cell types in PCs

Histological features					Ultrastructural features	
Case	Grade	Type	PGII-IR cells	SVLG cells	VGG cells	Endocrine cells
1	1	G	70%	+	+	+
2	1	G	50%	+	+	−
3	3	S	10%	+	+	+
4	2	G	10%	+	+	−
5	2	G	5%	+	+	−
6	1	G	2%	+	+	−
7	2	G	2%	+	+	−
8	2	G	10%	+	+	−
9	2	G/S	—	−	+	+
10	2	Cr	—	−	+	+
11	2	Cr	—	−	+	−
12	2	Cr	—	−	−	−
13	1	G	—	−	+	+
14	2	Cr	—	−	+	−
15	3	Cr/S	—	−	+	−
16	2	G	—	−	+	+

+ = present, − = absent, SVLG = seminal vesicle-like glandular, VGG = vesicular granule glandular, G = glandular, Cr = cribriform, S = solid

4. Concluding Remarks

The techniques used to demonstrate PAP, PSA, pepsinogen II, and lectins, and different ultrastructural features of tumor cells, are clearly capable of demonstrating the existence of functional heterogeneity within PCs. Combination of markers such as PSA and PAP is a good indicator of histogenetic origin. Special features of secretory granules at the ultrastructural level can also be of help in recognizing the prostatic origin of a tumor. Markers specific to the central zone of the prostate, such as PGII and Ulex E. lectin, are also expressed in PCs and seem to be useful prognostic indicators. Subdivision of existing grades of PCs becomes more plausible and clinically relevant when complemented by the addition of histochemical, immunohistochemical, and ultrastructural data demonstrating tumor heterogeneity.

References

1 Abel PD, Foster CS, Tebbutt S, Williams G Differences in expression of oligosaccharide determinants by phenotipically distinct sublines of the Dunning 3327 rat prostate cancer J Urol 144 760–765, 1990
2 Allsbrook WC, Simms WW Histochemistry of the prostate Hum Pathol 23 297–305, 1992
3 Azumi N, Trawcek ST, Battifora H Prostatic acid phosphatase in carcinoid tumors Am J Surg Pathol 15 785–790, 1991
4 Brandes D, Kirchheim D, Scott WW Ultrastructure of human prostate Normal and neoplastic Lab Invest 13 1541–1560, 1964
5 Brandes D The fine structure and histochemistry of prostate glands in relation to sex hormones Int Rev Cytol 20 207–276, 1966
6 Braunstein H Staining lipid in carcinoma of the prostate gland Am J Clin Pathol 41 44–48, 1964
7 Brawer MK, Peehl DM, Stamey TA, Bostwick DG Keratin immunoreactivity in the benign and neoplastic human prostate Cancer Res 45 3363–3367, 1985
8 Brawer MK, Nagle RB, Pitts W, Freiha F, Gamble SL Keratin immunoreactivity as an aid to the diagnosis of persistent adenocarcinoma in irradiated human prostates Cancer 63 454–460, 1989
9 Cho KR, Epstein JI Metastatic prostatic carcinoma to supradiaphragmatic lymph nodes Am J Surg Pathol 11 457–463, 1987
10 Cohen C, Bentz MS, Budgeon IR Prostatic acid phosphatase in carcinoid and islet cell tumors Arch Pathol Lab Med 107 277, 1983
11 Cornaggia M, Riva C, Capella C, Solcia E, Samloft IM Subcellular localization of pepsinogen II in stomach and duodenum by the immunogold technique Gastroenterology 92 585–593, 1987
12 Demuth F Uber Phosphatstoffwechsel I Uber Hexose-Phosphata-sen in menschlichen Organen und korperflussigkeiten Biochemz 159 415, 1925
13 Dolberg L Early prostatic carcinoma Hum Pathol 11 688–689, 1980
14 Epstein JI, Egglestone H Immunohistochemical localization of prostate specific acid phosphatase and prostate specific antigen in stage A_2 adenocarcinoma of the prostate Prognostic implications Hum Pathol 15 853–859, 1984
15 Epstein JI, Lieberman PH Mucinous adenocarcinoma of the prostate gland Am J Surg Pathol 9 299–308, 1985
16 Epstein JI, Kuhayada FP, Lieberman PH Prostate specific acid phosphatase in adenocarcinomas of the urinary bladder Hum Pathol 17 939–942, 1986
17 Finzi G, Frigerio B, Salvadore M, Capella C Unpublished observations 1992
18 Fisher ER, Sieraki JC Ultrastructure of human normal and neoplastic prostate In Pathology Annual SC Sommers (ed) New York Appleton-Century-Crofts, 1970, pp 1–26
19 Foster EA, Levine AJ Mucin production in metastatic carcinomas Cancer 16 506–509, 1963

20 Foster CS, McLoughlin J, Bashir I, Abel PD Markers of metastatic phenotype in prostate cancer Hum Pathol 23 381–394, 1992
21 Franks LM, O'Shea JD, Thompson AER Mucin in the prostate A histochemical study in normal gland, latent, clinical, and colloid cancers Cancer 17 983–991, 1964
22 Gaeta JF, Berger JE, Gamarra MC Scanning electron microscopic study of prostatic cancer Cancer Treat Rep 61 227–253, 1977
23 Gallee HPW, Vissez-diJong E, Van der Korput JHGH, Vanderkwast TH, Tenkate FJW, Schroeder FH Trapman J Variation of prostatic specific antigen expression in different tumor growth patterns present in prostatectomy patients Urol Res 18 181–187, 1990
24 Gleason DF, Mellinger GT The Veterans Administration Cooperative Research Group Prediction of prognosis for prostatic adenocarcinoma by combined histological grading and clinical staging J Urol 111 58–64, 1974
25 Hammond ME, Sause WT, Martz KI, Pilepich MV, Asbell SO, Rubin P, Myers RP, Farrow GM Correlation of prostate specific acid phosphatase and prostate specific antigen immunocytochemistry with survival in prostate carcinoma Cancer 63 461–466, 1989
26 Hendrik L, Epstein JI Use of keratin 903 as an adjunt in the diagnosis of prostate carcinoma Am J Surg Pathol 13 389–396, 1989
27 Hukill PB, Vidone RA Histochemistry of mucus and other polysaccharides in tumors Lab Invest 16 395–406, 1967
28 Jewett LA Prostatic carcinoma N Engl J Med 300 824–833, 1979
29 Kastendieck H, Altenahr E, Burchardt P Cyto- and histomorphogenesis of the prostate carcinoma A comparative light- and electron-microscopic study Virchows Arch A Pathol Anat Histopathol 370 207–224, 1976
30 Kutscher W, Wolberg H Prostatic phosphatase Hopper Seylers Z Physiol Chem 236 237–240, 1935
31 Levine AJ, Foster EA The relation of mucicarmine-staining properties of carcinomas of the prostate to differentiation, metastasis and prognosis Cancer 17 21–25, 1964
32 Lilja H A kallicrein-like serine protease in prostatic fluid cleaves the predominant seminal vesicle protein J Clin Invest 76 1899–1903, 1985
33 Lundquist F, Seedorf HH Pepsinogen in human seminal fluid Nature 170 1115–1116, 1952
34 Lundwall A Characterization of the gene for prostatic specific antigen, a human glandular kallicrein Biochem Biophys Res Commun 61 1151–1159, 1989
35 Mao P, Nakao K, Angrist A Human prostatic carcinoma An electron microscope study Cancer Res 26 955–973, 1966
36 McLoughlin J, Foster CS, Brawn P, Williams G, Abel PD Alteration in lectin binding between primary prostatic human carcinomas and their corresponding lymph nodes metastases J Urol 147 413, 1992
37 McNeal JE The prostate gland Morphology and pathology Monogr Urol 4 3–33, 1983
38 McNeal JE, Leav I, Alroy J, Skutelsky E Differential lectin staining of central and peripheral zone of the prostate and alterations in dysplasia Am J Clin Pathol 89 41–48, 1988
39 Nadji M, Morales AR Immunohistochemistry of prostatic acid phosphatase In Prostatic Acid Phosphatase Measurement Its Role in Detection and Management of Prostatic Cancer, Vol 390 LH Shaw, NA Romas, H Cohen (eds) New York New York Academy of Sciences, 1982, pp 133–141
40 Nagakura K, Hayakawa M, Mukai K, Aikawa A, Nakamura H Mucinous adenocarcinoma of the prostate A case report and review of the literature J Urol 135 1025–1028, 1986
41 Ohtsuki Y, Seman G, Maruyama K, Bowen JM, Johnson DE, Dmochowski L Ultrastructural studies of human prostatic neoplasia Cancer 37 2295–2305, 1976
42 Ohtsuki Y, Furihata H, Inone K, Iwata J, Manabe Y, Sonobe H, Ochi K, Seike H, Hashimoto H, Terao N Immunohistochemical and ultrastructural studies of intraluminal crystalloids in human prostatic carcinomas Virchows Arch A Pathol Anat Histopathol 421 421–425, 1992
43 Pinder SE, McMahon RFT Mucins in prostatic carcinoma Histopathology 16 43–46, 1990
44 Pollen JJ, Dreilinger A Immunohistochemical identification of prostatic acid phosphatase and prostate specific antigen in female periurethral glands Urology 23 303–304, 1984
45 Reese JH, McNeal JE, Redwine EA, Samloff IM, Stamey TA Differential distribution of the pepsinogen II between the zones of the human prostate and the seminal vesicle J Urol 136 1148–1152, 1986
46 Reid WA, Liddle CN, Svasti J, Kay J Gastricsin *in the* benign and malignant prostate J Clin Pathol 38 639–643, 1985
47 Riva A Fine structure of human seminal vesicle epithelium J Anat 102 71–86, 1967
48 Ro YI, Grignon DJ, Troncoso P, Ayala AG Mucin in prostatic adenocarcinoma Semin Diagn Pathol 5 273–283, 1988
49 Ro YI, El-Naggar A, Ayala AG, Mody DR, Ordoñez NG Signet-ring ring cell carcinoma of the prostate Electron microscopic and immunohistochemical studies of eight cases Am J Surg Pathol 12 453–460, 1988
50 Samloff IM, Liebman WM Purification and immunochemical characterization of group II pepsinogens in human seminal fluid Clin Exp Immunol 11 405–414, 1972
51 Samloff IM, Liebman WM Cellular localization of the group II pepsinogens in human stomach and duodenum by immunofluorescence Gastroenterology 65 36–42, 1973
52 Sinha AA, Bentley MD, Blackard CE Freeze-fracture observation on the membranes and junctions in human prostatic carcinoma and benign prostatic hypertrophy Cancer 40 1182, 1977
53 Sinha AA, Blackard CE, Seal US A critical analysis of tumor morphology and hormone treatments in the untreated and estrogen-treated responsive and refractory human prostatic carcinoma Cancer 40 2836–2850, 1977
54 Sobin LH, Hjermstad BM, Sesterhenn IA, Helwig EB

Prostatic acid phosphatase activity in carcinoid tumors Cancer 58 136–138, 1986
55 Soderstrom KO Lectin binding to prostatic carcinoma Cancer 60 1823–1831, 1987
56 Spicer SS Diamine methods for differentiating mucosubstances histochemically J Histochem Cytochem 13 211–234, 1965
57 Srigley JR Small-acinar patterns in the prostate gland with emphasis on atypical adenomatous hyperplasia and small acinar carcinoma Semin Diagn Pathol 5 254–272, 1988
58 Sringley JR, Dardick I, Hartwick RWJ, Klotz L Basal epithelial cells of the human prostate gland are not myoepithelial cells Am J Pathol 136 957–966, 1990
59 Stamey TA, Yang N, Hay AR, McNeal JE, Freiha FS, Redwine E Prostatic specific antigen as a serum marker for adenocarcinomas of the prostate N Engl J Med 317 909–916, 1987
60 Svanholm H, Andersen OP, Rohl H Tumor of female paraurethral duct Immunohistochemical similarity with prostatic carcinoma Virchows Arch A Pathol Anat Histopathol 411 395–398, 1987
61 Tannenbaum M, Tannenbaum S Ultrastructural pathology of human prostatic carcinoma In Diagnostic Electron Microscopy F Trump, T Jones (eds) New York John Wiley, 1980, pp 175–201
62 Vernon SF, Williams WD Pre-treatment and post-treatment evaluation of prostatic adenocarcinoma for prostatic specific acid phosphatase and prostatic specific antigen by immunohistochemistry J Urol 130 95–98, 1983
63 Wang HD, Valenzuela LA, Murphy GP, Chu TM Purification of a human prostatic specific antigen Invest Urol 17 159–163, 1979
64 Yanka-Perttula T, Nieun R, Helminen HJ Separate lysosomal and secretory acid phosphatase in the rat ventral prostate Invest Urol 9 345–352, 1972

CHAPTER 8

A Review of the Ultrastructure of Human Prostatic and Urethral Endocrine-Paracrine Cells and Neuroendocrine Differentiation in Prostatic Carcinoma

KAREN L. DE MESY JENSEN & P. ANTHONY DI SANT'AGNESE

1. Introduction

Endocrine-paracrine (EP) cells of the human prostate and urethra were first noted as a third epithelial cell type (in addition to basal and secretory cells) in 1944 by Pretl [51]. He designated them *clear cells* with an affinity for silver (argentaffin reaction). In 1951, Feyrter [35] further characterized these "clear" cells (Helle Zellen) in the prostate and urethra as being not only argentaffin (no reducing agent) but also argyrophilic (exogenous reducing agent added), including some of which were argyrophil only, indicating a heterogenous population of cells. The prostatic and urethral endocrine-paracrine cells are a component of a dispersed neuroendocrine regulatory system first proposed by Feyrter in 1938 [36]. He also coined the term *paracrine*, since he believed these cells exerted their action on nearby cells and tissues rather than a distant target.

In 1969 Pearse [49] elaborated on this concept naming this system the *diffuse neuroendocrine system*. Shared common cytochemical characteristics led to the acronym *APUD* (amine precursor uptake and decarboxylation) for cells of this system. These cells also shared common morphologic features, including dense core secretory granules. Elements of the peripheral diffuse neuroendocrine system include the gastro-entero-pancreatic (GEP) EP cells, pulmonary (Kultchitzky) cells, thyroid C-cells, urogenital [50] cells, and adrenal chromaffin [50] cells.

Endocrine-paracrine cells of the prostate and urethra are intraepithelial cells with hybrid neural and epithelial characteristics [22] and are distributed throughout the epithelium and urothelium [23], often adjacent to the basement membrane, either as single cells or in clusters (Figs. 1 and 2). These endocrine-paracrine cells are of the closed cell types with basally oriented granules (Figs. 3 and 4) or open cell (extensions to the lumen of the gland) types (Figs. 5 and 6). Long dendritic processes [21,22] originating from these cells extend between adjacent secretory and basal cells, as well as contacting other nearby endocrine-paracrine cells (Figs. 2 and 7).

Immunohistochemical studies have identified serotonin (Fig. 1) in most, if not all, endocrine-paracrine cells as well as a variety of peptides/hormones in subpopulations of these cells. These peptides/hormones include chromogranin A [4], calcitonin [26,32], calcitonin gene related peptide [20], somatostatin [24], bombesinlike peptides [26,58], and thyroid stimulating hormone (TSH)-like peptide [1,2], the latter having only partial homology of the beta-chain of thyroid stimulating hormone demonstrated [1,2]. Calcitonin is contained within a significant subpopulation of EP cells [21,26,32]. Smaller numbers of endocrine-paracrine cells contain bombesinlike peptide and somatostatin.

The functional role of endocrine-paracrine cells of the prostate and urethra is not known. One can only speculate on their role based on analogy with the other better studied EP cells of the diffuse neuroendocrine system. It is likely that these cells regulate both growth and differentiation, as well as exocrine secretory processes

Riva, A., Testa Riva, F., and Motta, P.M., (eds.), Ultrastructure of the Male Urogenital Glands: Prostate, Seminal Vesicles, Urethral, and Bulbourethral Glands. *ISBN 0-7923-2800-0.*

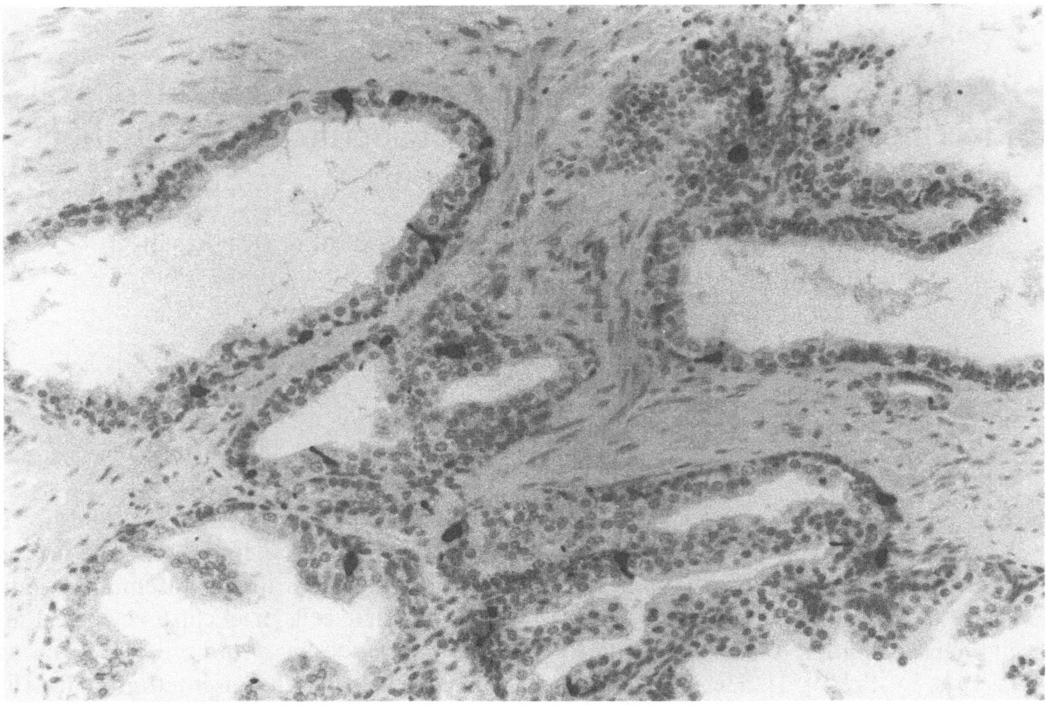

Fig 1 Serotonin immunoreactive endocrine-paracrine cells in normal prostatic epithelium demonstrating open and closed endocrine paracrine cell types (serotonin immunoperoxidase ×272)

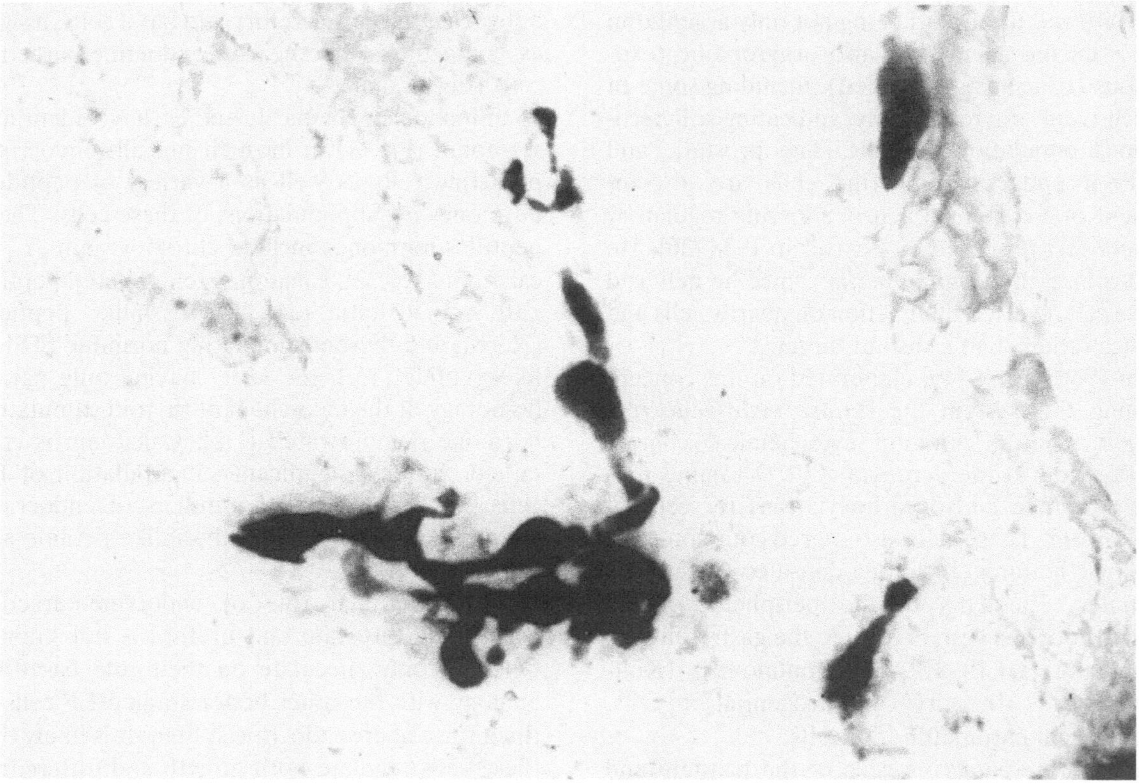

Fig 2 Serotonin immunolabeling of eight endocrine-paracrine cells in a thick (40 μm) frozen section Note the numerous cell processes extending to neighboring endocrine paracrine cells, demonstrating the paracrine relationship of endocrine paracrine cells to one another (serotonin immunoperoxidase ×575)

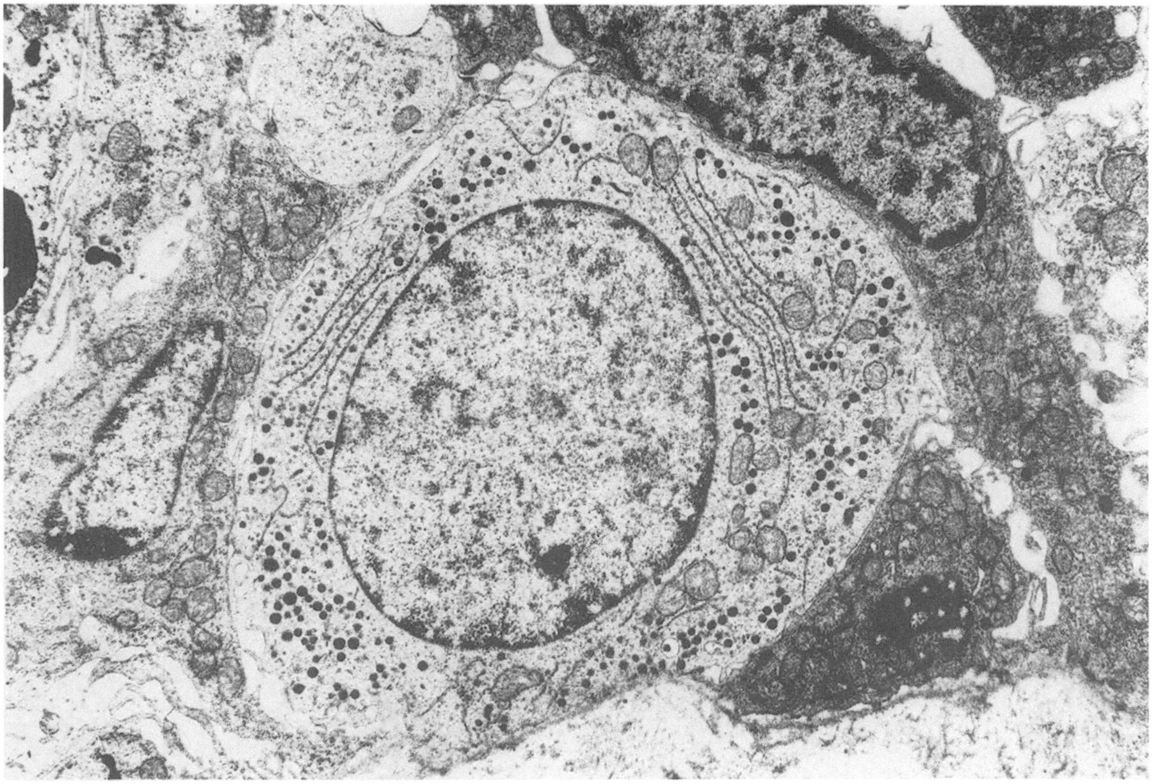

Fig. 3. An endocrine-paracrine cell with intermediate round (PR type 3) secretory granules. This is an example of a closed cell type with evenly distributed granules (×25,000).

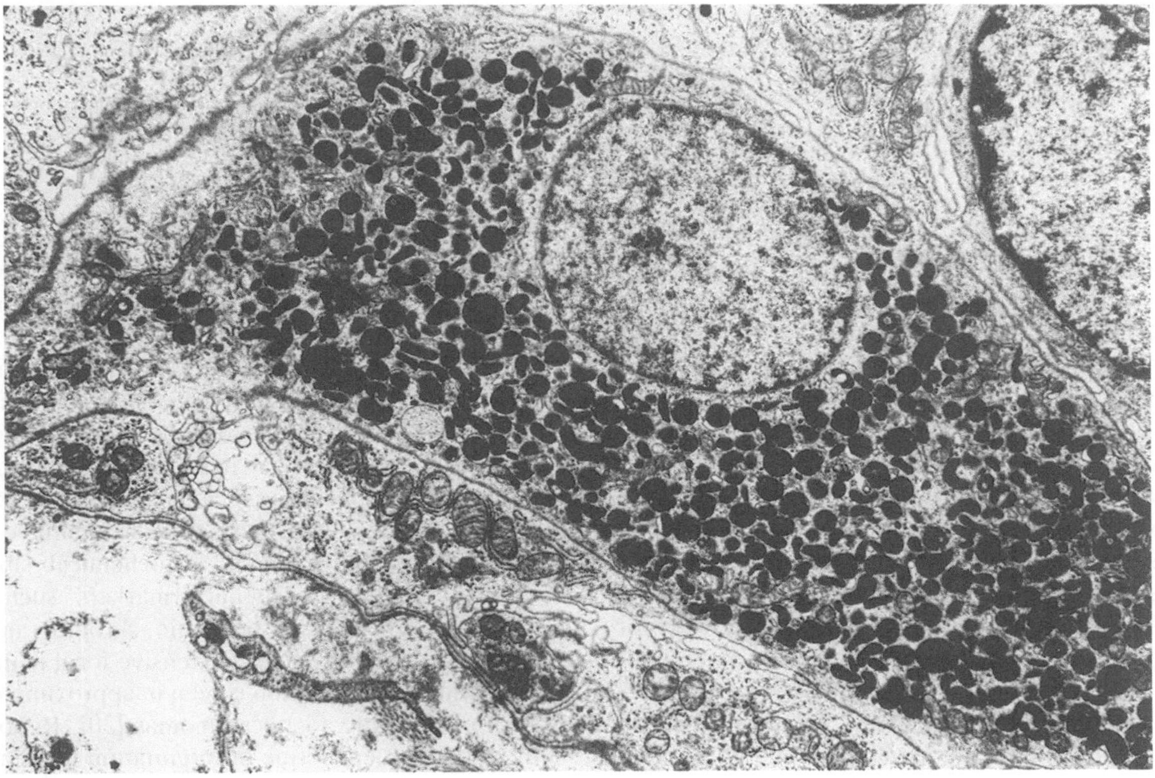

Fig. 4. An endocrine-paracrine cell with large pleomorphic (PR type 9) secretory granules (×25,000).

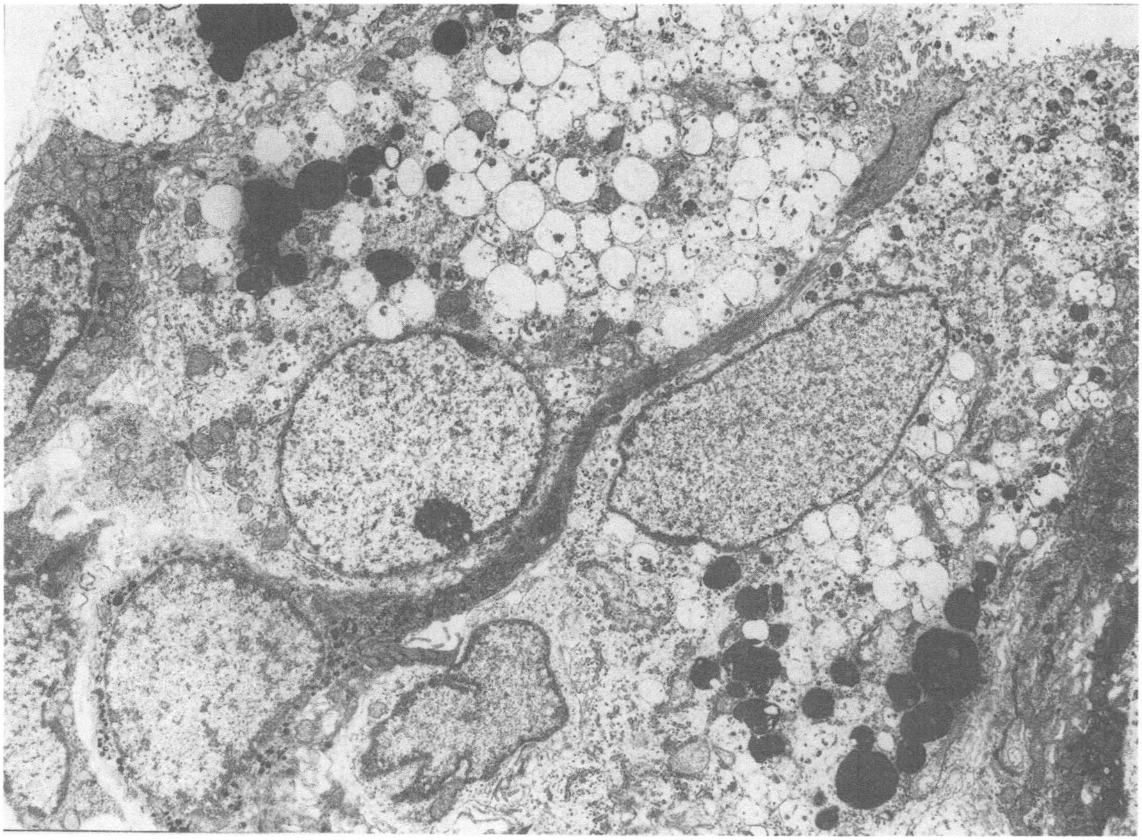

Fig 5 Electron micrograph of an open endocrine paracrine cell with cytoplasmic secretory granules and with a long cytoplasmic process extending to the lumen of the gland (×3300)

[15 40 43,67], through endocrine and paracrine functions Additionally, open prostatic endocrine-paracrine cell types may secrete in a lumencrine or exocrine fashion Many peptides have been found in relatively high concentrations in the ejaculate [6,38,53,55,62] Microvilli on the surface of the open endocrine-paracrine cell types are longer and more complex than those on neighboring secretory cells (Figs 5 and 6) These specialized microvilli may monitor the luminal contents enabling the endocrine paracrine cell to send regulatory messages via their dendritic processes to other endocrine-paracrine or secretory cells to regulate lumenal contents Closed endocrine-paracrine cell types may secrete in the classic endocrine manner Finally, an association between endocrine-paracrine cells and afferent and efferent nerves has been noted by various investigators [8,22,29] It is possible that endocrine-paracrine cells may also release their amines or peptides to regulate via neurocrine mechanisms or may be themselves regulated by nerves

In cancers of the prostate, focal neuroendocrine (NE) differentiation is a common phenomenon and may occur to some extent in all prostatic adenocarcinomas Focal neuroendocrine differentiation is defined as an adenocarcinoma with scattered individual or nests of cells identified as neuroendocrine by classic histochemical silver stains or immunocytochemical markers, such as neuron specific enolase, serotonin, chromogranin, or polypeptide hormones Extensive focal neuroendocrine differentiation is seen in approximately 10% of prostatic adenocarcinomas [30] Reports of focal neuroendocrine differentiation in adenocarcinomas have increased from an initial 10–47%

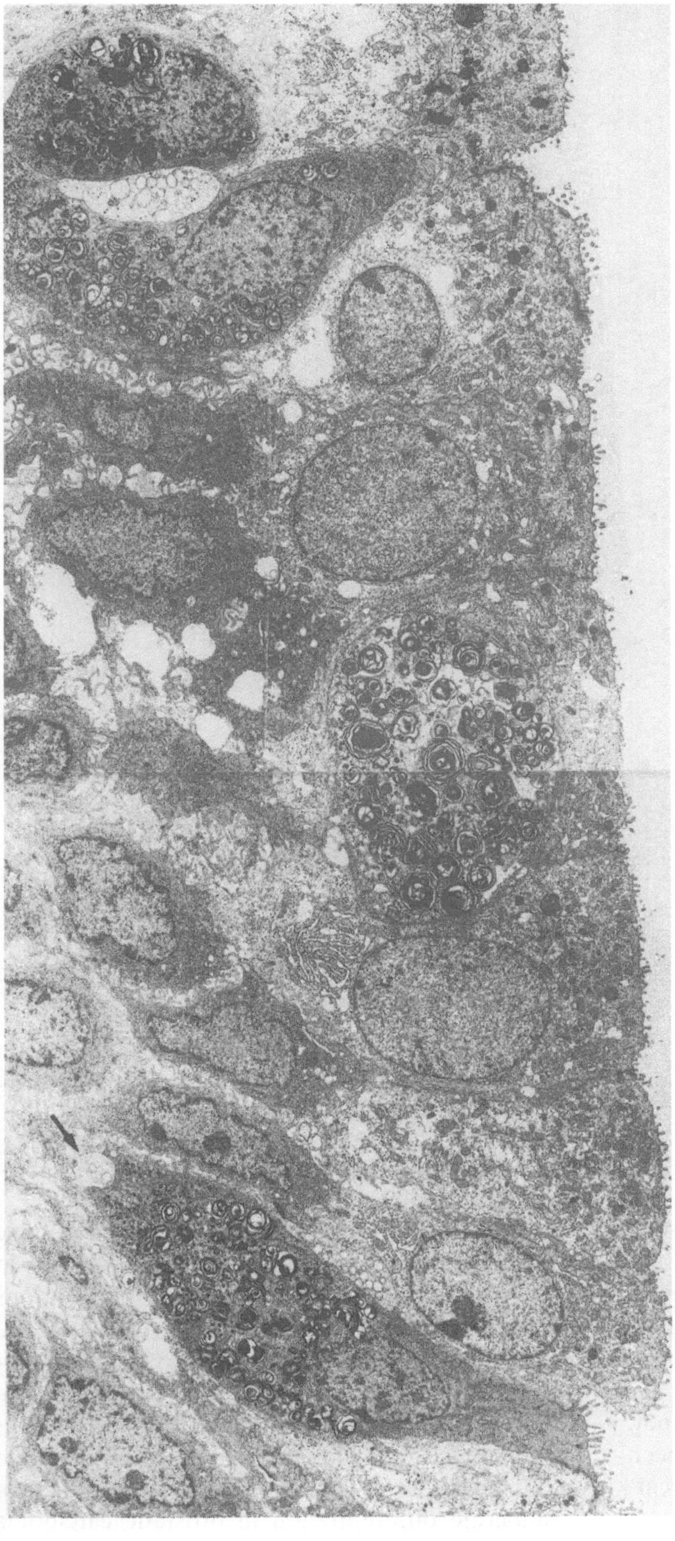

Fig. 6. Several periurethral endocrine-paracrine cells containing myelinoid bodies. An open endocrine-paracrine cell with specialized microvilli is at the bottom. If serial thin sections were examined, it probably could be demonstrated that the majority of these endocrine-paracrine cells are of the open cell type. Nerves are abutting the cytoplasmic membranes of several endocrine-paracrine cells (arrows) (composite electron micrograph, orig. mag. ×2000).

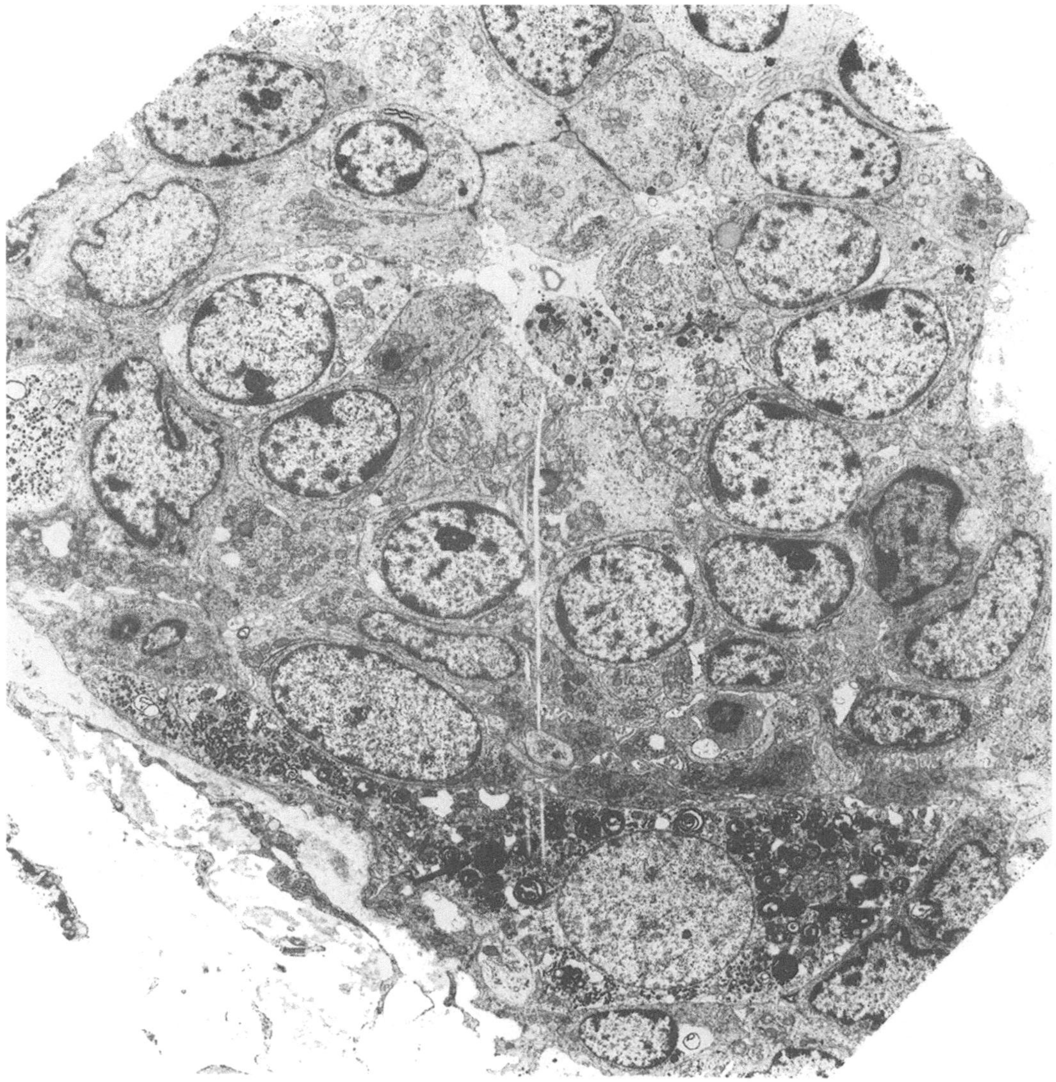

Fig. 7. Electron micrograph of a whole prostatic alveolus with a basally located endocrine-paracrine cell. Note the myelinoid bodies (arrows) and the dendritic process extending from the endocrine-paracrine cell body along the base of the gland (×1500).

[7,25,42] to 100% of cases [3]. This increase is probably due to the use of more sensitive immunocytochemical techniques with antibodies to various generic and specific (polypeptide hormones and serotonin) neuroendocrine markers. In addition, 1–2% of prostatic malignancies are small cell neuroendocrine carcinomas [13,59,60]. Finally, rare carcinoidlike tumors have also been described in the prostate but are not typical carcinoid tumors [5,16,33,57,63].

Recently, clinicopathologic investigations have indicated that neuroendocrine differentiation in prostatic carcinoma has prognostic implications that may be independent of, or be related to, the resistance of carcinomas to hormonal manipulation [3,4,14,16]. Serum studies of chromogranin A and neuron specific enolase (NSE) in patients with advanced prostatic carcinoma have tended to confirm the latter [41,61]. The presence of neuroendocrine differentiation in prostatic carcinoma raises the possibility of new avenues of therapeutic intervention [29], including the use of streptozotozin, long-acting somatostatin analogs, peptide analogs, (which may inhibit binding of peptides with growth activity such as bombesin analogs), and the use of monoclonal antibodies to these peptides. Conventional chemotherapy that has been developed and is relatively effective against small cell neuroendocrine carcinoma of the lung may also be effective against small cell carcinoma of the prostate.

The focus of this chapter is to present a review of the ultrastructural studies documenting the secretory granule morphology of prostatic and urethral endocrine-paracrine cells and of neuroendocrine differentiation in prostatic carcinoma.

2. Ultrastructural Studies of Normal Human Prostatic-Urethral EP Cells

Attempts to classify prostatic and urethral EP cells have resulted in numerous studies published in the medical literature. Table 1 lists many of these studies, which include morphologic descriptions of secretory granules found in normal prostatic and urethral endocrine-paracrine cells.

The first ultrastructural study of human male urethral endocrine-paracrine cells was reported by Casanova et al. in 1974 [11]. Two endocrine-paracrine cell types were described based on differences in the morphology of their secretory granules and ultrastructural silver staining properties. Type I cells (more common) contained "irregularly round" 100–170 nm secretory granules, some of which had prominent halos and were strongly argentaffin and argyrophil positive by ultrastructural histochemistry. Type II cells (less common) contained small round secretory granules measuring 80 nm and were argentaffin negative. The sparsity of these cells precluded agyrophil staining. An important final observation noted autonomic nerve endings "in close contact" with the basal portion of the granule containing (EP) cells.

The first ultrastructural study of endocrine-paracrine cells of the female urethra was reported by Lendon et al. in 1976 [44]. Autopsy tissue formed the basis of this study and revealed numerous yellow formaldehyde induced fluorescent (presumably serotonin containing) endocrine-paracrine cells, which contained small round secretory granules measuring 80–100 nm in diameter. These investigators concluded these endocrine-paracrine cells were similar to those previously described by Casanova et al. [11]. Indeed, the granules in these cells closely resemble those seen in the Type II cell.

Also in 1976, the first ultrastructural study of prostatic endocrine-paracrine cells was reported by Aumüller et al. [6]. Endocrine-paracrine cells with fluorescent serotonin content were seen in the *veru montanum* and the prostatic urethra. Only a single cell is illustrated with intermediate pleomorphic secretory granules, which were not measured. It was concluded by the authors that the cell's secretory granules were morphologically similar to the secretory granules of intestinal enterochromaffin cells.

In the early 1980s reports of prostatic and urethral EP cells became more numerous. In 1981 Capella et al. [10] reported a study of normal and hyperplastic prostatic tissue as well as neuroendocrine differentiation in malignant prostatic tissues. The findings related to prostate carcinoma will be detailed later. Normal and hyperplastic tissue was processed for routine electron microscopy. Although only a few endocrine-paracrine cells were found, ultrastructural examination identified two cell types based on the morphology of secretory granules. Type I cells, the most frequent, contained intermediate pleomorphic secretory granules measuring 248 ± 27 nm. Ultrastructural silver staining was positive for both argentaffin and argyrophil. Type II cells contained smaller oval to round secretory granules, some of which had eccentric halos, measuring 123 ± 27 nm. These cell's granules were argyrophil positive, but unfortunately, due to the scarcity of endocrine-paracrine cells, argentaffin status could not be determined. The investigators concluded that Type I cells closely resembled intestinal enterochromaffin cells and appeared to be the same as those described in Aumüller et al. [6]. They also concluded that Type II cells were the same as the Type I cells described by Casanova et al. [11].

In 1983 Fetissof et al. [34] evaluated endocrine-paracrine cells of the prostatic urethra and prostate as well as neuroendocrine differentiation in prostatic carcinoma. Endocrine-paracrine cells

Table 1 Ultrastructural studies of normal human prostatic-urethral endocrine-paracrine (EP) cells

Year	Authors	Region	Method, EP cell secretory granule description
1974	Casanova S, Corrado F, Vignoli G [66]	Male urethra	EM routine (two EP cells illustrated) Type I — small irregularly round granules, 100–170 nm (NOS) Type II — small round granules, 80 nm (NOS)
1976	Lendon RG, Dixon JS, Gosling JA [44]	Female urethra	EM routine from autopsy (one EP cell illustrated from female) Small round granules, 80–100 nm (NOS)
1976	Aumuller G, Metz W, Grube D [6]	Prostatic urethra colliculus seminalis	EM routine (two EP cells illustrated) Intermediate pleomorphic granules
1981	Capella C, Usellini L, Buffa R, Frigerio B, Solcia E [10]	Prostate gland	EM routine & paraffin retrieved tissue (two EP cells illustrated) Type I — intermediate pleomorphic granules, 248 ± 27 nm (NOS) Type II — small oval to round granules, 123 ± 27 nm (NOS)
1983	Fetissof F, Dubois MP, Arbeille-Brassart B, Lanson Y, Boivin F, Jobard P [32]	Prostatic urethra & prostate gland	EM routine (two EP cells illustrated) Large slightly pleomorphic to round granules, 160–450 nm (NOS) Intermediate round granules, 150–260 nm (NOS)
1984	di Sant'Agnese PA, de Mesy Jensen KL [22]	Prostatic urethra & prostate gland	EM large block, "pop-off" technique (nine EP cells illustrated) PR type 1 small round granules, avg 118 nm, 68–168 nm (range max dia) PR type 2 small pleomorphic granules, avg 125 nm, 66–204 nm PR type 3 intermediate round granules, avg 178 nm, 92–313 nm PR type 4 intermediate round granules, avg 188 nm, 99–271 nm PR type 5 intermediate pleomorphic granules, avg 220 nm 56–437 nm PR type 6 intermediate pleomorphic granules, avg 236 nm, 93–382 nm PR type 7 large pleomorphic granules, avg 343 nm, 136–512 nm PR type 8 large pleomorphic, avg 359 nm, 78–546 nm PR type 9 large pleomorphic, granules, avg 408 nm, 90–625 nm
1987	di Sant'Agnese PA, de Mesy Jensen KL [21]	Female urethra & periurethral ducts	EM large block, "pop-off" technique (three EP cells illustrated) Type I small round granules, 80–120 nm (range max dia) Type II intermediate round granules, 80–200 nm (range max dia) Type III large pleomorphic granules, 300 nm (avg max dia)
1989	di Sant'Agnese PA, de Mesy Jensen KL [20]	Prostate gland	EM large block, "pop-off" technique & large block immuno "pop-off" tech Two calcitonin immunoreactive EP cells illustrated — correlation of granule morphology with peptide hormone content Small round granules & intermediate pleomorphic granules
1989	di Sant'Agnese PA, de Mesy Jensen KL [28]	Prostate gland & prostatic urethra	EM large block, "pop-off" technique (six EP cells containing distinctive myelinoid bodies illustrated) Suggestive of a crinophagic form of secretory granules

NOS = not otherwise specified, PR = prostatic endocrine-paracrine cell, dia = diameter, max = maximum, avg = average, immuno = immunocytochemical, tech = technique

appeared to be Grimelius argyrophil positive and serotonin immunoreactive, with some argentaffin positive cells as well. Two cell types were defined based on granule morphology. The most frequent type was found in both the prostate and urethra, and contained intermediate-sized round to ovoid granules with dense inner cores and a less osmophilic periphery forming a "target-like pattern." These granules measured 150–260 nm. It was noted that these cells were similar to those described by Casanova et al. [11] and Lendon et al. [44]. It is assumed that they were comparing this cell to the Type I cell of Casanova et al. [11], but the granules here are larger and have dense inner cores not seen in the previous report. Lendon et al. [44] described a cell type with even smaller granules, similar to the Type II cell of Casanova et al. [11]. Therefore, this appears to be a description of a new cell type.

The other cell type found was present only in the prostate and more sparsely distributed. The granules were large in size and "round, ovoid, angular, or bean-shaped," measuring 160–450 nm in size. This also seems to be a new cell type in the intermediate to large granule category. The granules are somewhat larger and less pleomorphic than those seen by Aumüller et al. [6] and Capella et al. [10].

In 1984, an extensive study of normal human prostatic and urethral EP cells was published by di Sant'Agnese and de Mesy Jensen [22], which described the remarkable ultrastructural diversity of EP cells in prostatic urethral and glandular tissue. Over 200 endocrine-paracrine cells and their processes were examined ultrastructurally. Various endocrine-paracrine cells were somewhat arbitrarily categorized into nine types based on morphometric analysis of the secretory granules. These cells were then broadly classified into small granule, intermediate, and large granule types (Fig. 8). Listed below are the nine cell types with the secretory granule sizes and morphologic descriptions:

Small granule types

PR1. 118 nm mean diameter, 68–168 nm range
1. uniformly small and round
2. small indistinct central densities

PR2. 125 nm mean diameter, 66–204 nm range,
1. pleomorphic with round, oval, and elongated forms
2. some with large lucent halos or dense inner cores

Intermediate granule types

PR3. 178 nm mean diameter, 92–313 nm range
1. uniformally round, variable sizes and densities
2. central, poorly circumscribed dense cores surrounded with less dense moderate sized halos

PR4. 188 nm mean diameter, 99–271 nm range
1. 4a granule type, large round mucigenlike lucent granules containing loose, flocculent material
2. 4b granule type, round with central to eccentric dense cores

PR5. 220 nm mean diameter, 56–437 nm range
1. elongated dumbbell-shaped granules
2. uniform dense matrix

PR6. 236 nm mean diameter, 93–382 nm range
1. some granules similar to type 5 with an additional population of round granules
2. eccentric dense cores surrounded by slightly less dense matrix

Large granule types:

PR7. 343 nm mean diameter, 136–512 nm range
1. round to elongated granules
2. finely to coarsely matrix, rarely a uniform dense matrix

PR8. 359 nm mean diameter, 178–546 nm range
1. round to elongated granules
2. uniform dense matrix with eccentric moderate sized dense core

PR9. 408 nm mean diameter, 90–625 nm range
1. round to elongated granules
2. uniform dense core

The majority of endocrine-paracrine cells were of the intermediate granule type (PR types 3, 4, 5, and 6) with the small (PR types 1 and 2) and large (PR types 7, 8, and 9) granule types less frequent (Fig. 8). Very small granule types were easily distinguished from very large ones. Endocrine-paracrine cells with intermediate-sized granules were postulated to either represent different cell types or to form a continuum somewhere between small and large granules types. There was difficulty in separating intermediate cell types using primarily visual observations.

Several endocrine-paracrine cell types had luminal extensions with specialized microvilli on their surface (open cell type) and basally located granules (Figs. 5 and 6). However, the majority

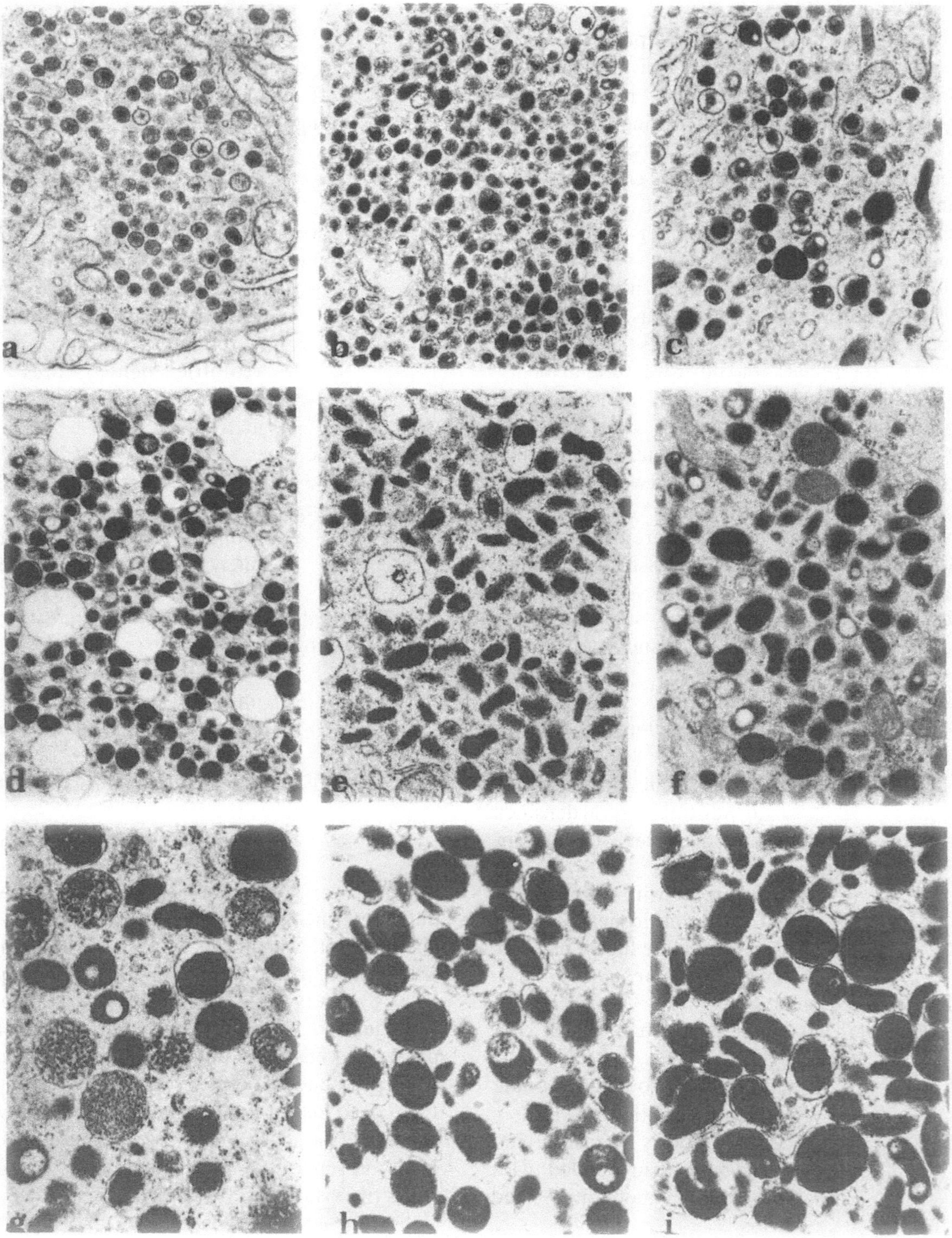

Fig 8 Composite of nine different endocrine-paracrine cells (a) PR type 1, (b) PR type 2, (c) PR type 3, (d) PR type 4, (e) PR type 5, (f) PR type 6, (g) PR type 7, (h) PR type 8, (i) PR type 9, all taken at the same magnification, demonstrating the wide range of secretory granule morphology from cell to cell (×25,000 orig mag) (Reprinted with permission from W B Saunders, Co , [22])

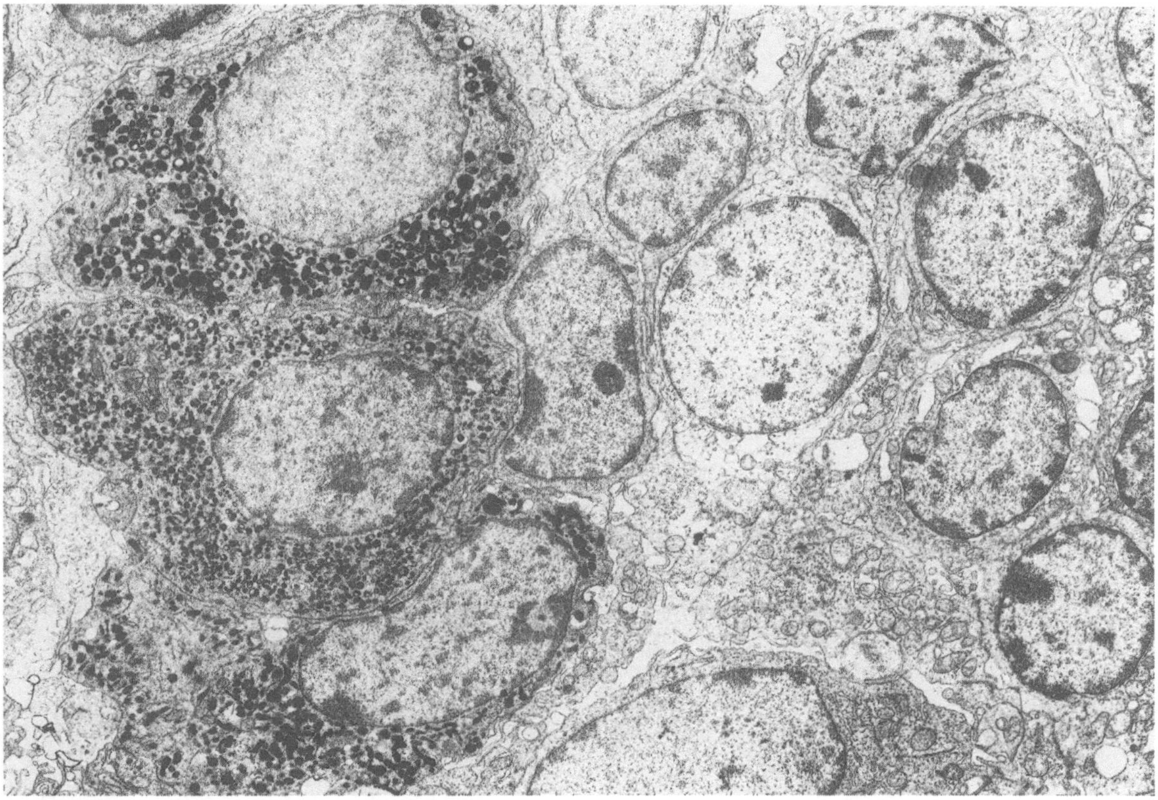

Fig 9 A low power electron micrograph of three prostatic endocrine paracrine cells The center endocrine paracrine cell contains intermediate (PR type 4) pleomorphic secretory granules which contrast with the large (PR type 9) pleomorphic secretory granules present in the top and bottom endocrine paracrine cells (×3300)

of the cells in this study appeared to be of the closed cell type with granules more uniformally distributed (Figs 3 and 4) The open cell types may have been underrepresented because of the thinness of the tissue sections, which increased the chance of not seeing the apical processes in the ultrastructural sections (Fig 6)

Additionally, endocrine-paracrine cells were shown to have one or more efferent autonomic nerve processes, appearing to be both adrenergic and cholinergic, intimately apposed to the endocrine-paracrine cell membrane No true synapses were seen, although occasional bimembranous densities were noted Some probable afferent nerve processes were also seen abutting on or near endocrine-paracrine cells (Fig 6)

Two or more endocrine-paracrine cells were at times seen lying next to each other with contiguous cell membranes (Fig 9) Usually different cell types were next to each other Also dendritic processes often made contact and were usually from cells of different granule types

Di Sant Agnese and de Mesy Jensen accomplished the above study by developing a new technique for finding and ultrastructurally examining widely scattered endocrine-paracrine cells [27] Standard methodology for electron microscopy involved the time-consuming sectioning of 1 mm^3 tissue blocks and infrequent localization of endocrine-paracrine cells A large block method, which utilized large Spurr Epoxy tissue blocks (10 mm × 10 mm × 1 mm thickness) and a "pop-off" technique allowed for direct thin sectioning without cutting down the original large tissue block Endocrine-paracrine cells in large plastic thick (2 5 μm) tissue sections were identified using

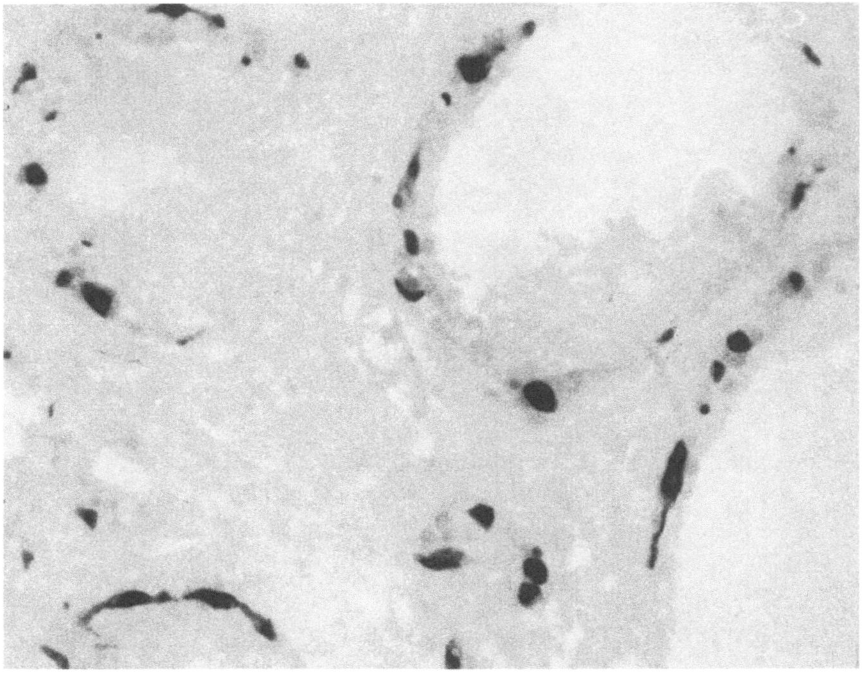

Fig 10 Calcitonin immunoreactive endocrine-paracrine cells in the human prostate demonstrating several calcitonin immunoreactive cells in an area of prostatic atrophy (Spurr plastic 2 0 μm section, calcitonin immunoperoxidase, ×575)

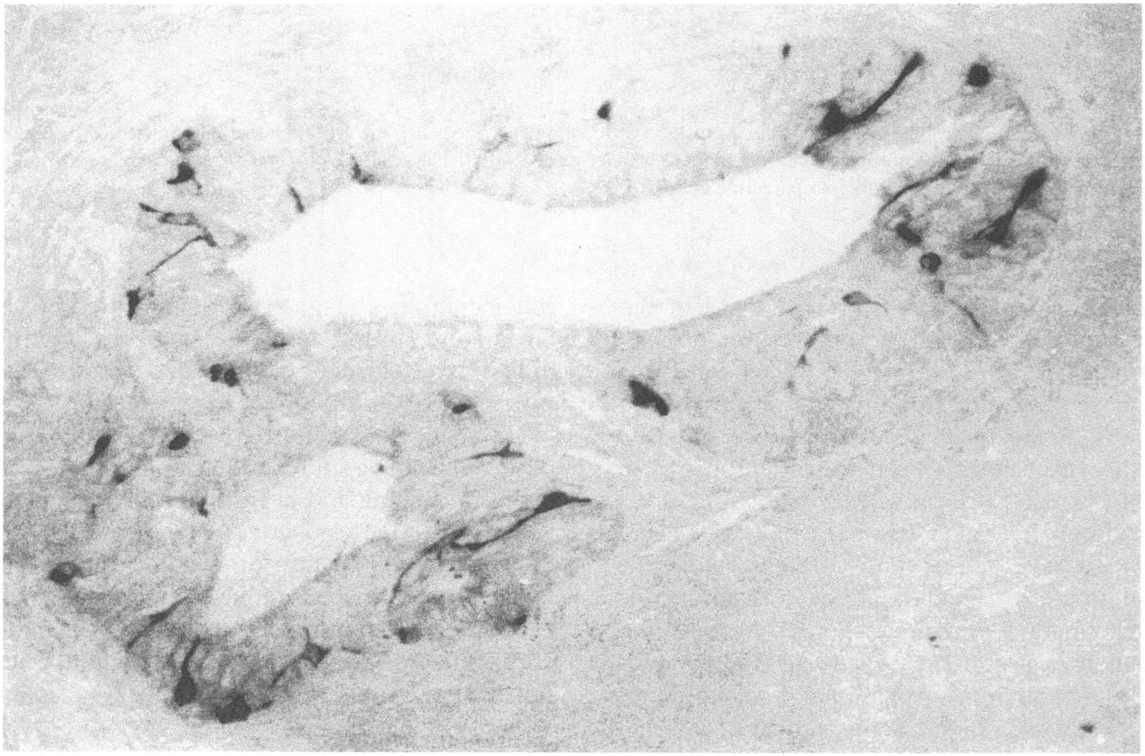

Fig 11 Female paraurethral duct with serotonin immunoreactive endocrine-paracrine cells with numerous dendritic processes (serotonin immunoperoxidase, ×480)

either a silver (argyrophil) stain or serotonin and/or calcitonin immunocytochemical localization [21] (Fig. 10). Large 1.5 × 1.0 mm thick tissue sections of prostate were scanned and individual or groups of endocrine-paracrine cells were selected for electron microscopic examination. Matched areas on adjacent unstained thick sections were "popped off," thin sectioned, and examined ultrastructurally.

This same method was used in an additional ultrastructural study of the female urethra and paraurethral ducts reported by di Sant'Agnese and de Mesy Jensen in 1987 [21]. Scattered endocrine-paracrine cells were observed along the length of the urethra, with more numerous cells present in the paraurethral ducts (Fig. 11). The majority of these endocrine-paracrine cells were argyrophil positive as well as positive for serotonin, chromogranin, and neuron specific enolase (NSE), with only a few cells positive for bombesin, and rarely calcitonin. Ultrastructurally, it was not possible to define discrete endocrine-paracrine cell types because of the relatively small numbers; however, three general types of endocrine-paracrine cells were defined based on secretory granule morphology and morphometry (Fig. 12): (a) endocrine-paracrine cells with small round granules ranging in size from 80 to 120 nm in diameter; (b) endocrine-paracrine cells with intermediate round granules ranging in size from 80 to 200 nm; and (c) endocrine-paracrine cells with intermediate to large pleomorphic granules averaging 300 nm in diameter. Again, the presence of nerve fibers abutting onto the endocrine-paracrine cells was noted.

The first immunoelectron microscopic study of calcitonin containing endocrine-paracrine cells was reported in 1989 by di Sant'Agnese and de

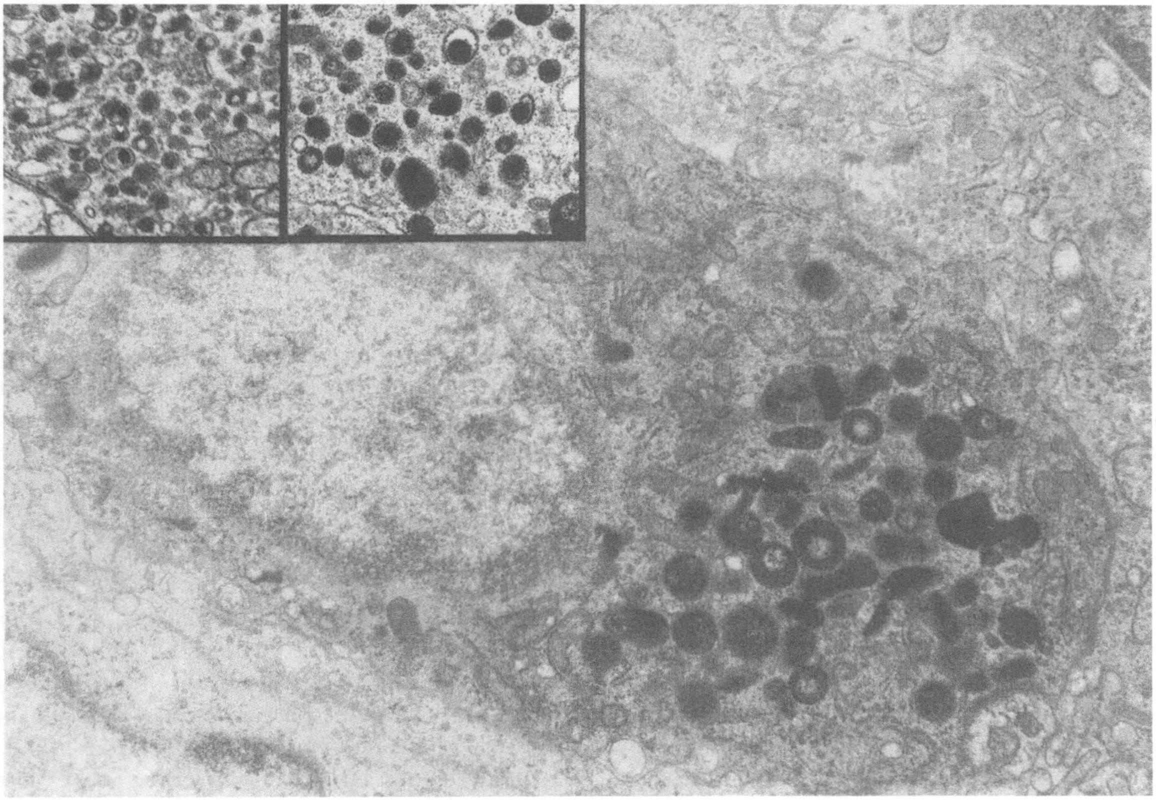

Fig. 12. Electron micrograph of female endocrine-paracrine cell containing large 300 nm sized secretory granules. Other types of secretory granules found in female endocrine-paracrine cells are small round secretory granules 80–120 nm (inset upper left) and intermediate round 80–200 nm (inset upper right) (×25,000).

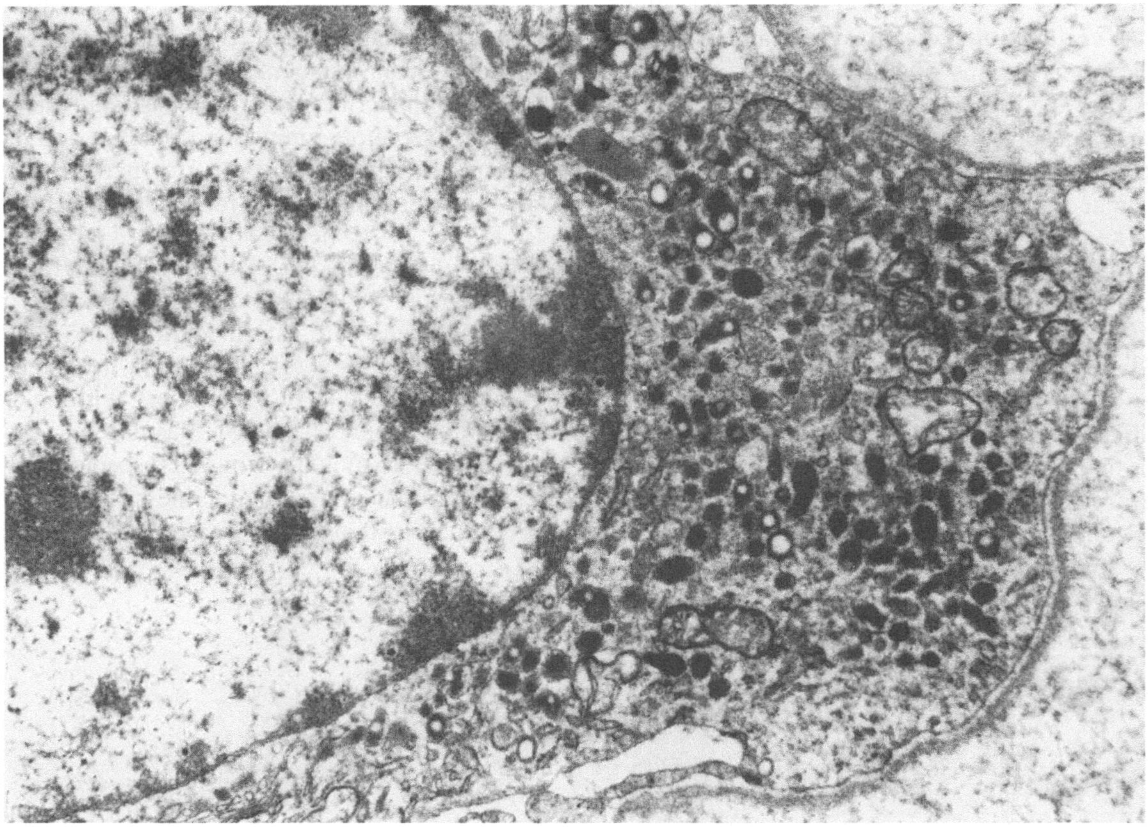

Fig 13 Endocrine-paracrine cell with intermediate pleomorphic secretory granules, PR type 5, matched with a calcitonin immunoreactive endocrine-paracrine cell from a serial Spurr epoxy section (2 5 μm) (×25,000)

Mesy Jensen [20]. Prostate tissue was embedded in Spurr Epoxy resin as well as Lowicryl K4M resin (with an adaptation of large block pop-off technique using low temperature embedding resin) [19]. Immunoelectron microscopy and the "thick/thin section" correlation technique was used to compare calcitonin content with granule morphology. Two secretory granule types (although a continuum between the two could not be excluded) were described: One type contained intermediate pleomorphic secretory granules, which ranged in size from 120 to 360 nm (Fig. 13), and the other type contained smaller round secretory granules, which ranged in size from 80 to 280 nm. Both secretory granule types also immunostained for serotonin with colocalization of calcitonin and serotonin in the same secretory granules (Figs. 14a,b). These calcitonin-positive endocrine-paracrine cell's granules were compared to previous ultrastructural studies on the morphology of secretory granules in human C-cells. There appear to be two C-cell variants with differing secretory granule morphologies [18]; however, neither one closely resembled the calcitionin containing cells in the prostate.

The last article listed in Table 1 was published in 1989 by di Sant'Agnese and de Mesy Jensen [28] and described distinct myelinoid bodies present in a large subpopulation of prostatic and urethral endocrine-paracrine cells (Fig. 6). These bodies had not previously been described in endocrine-paracrine cells of other tissues in the human diffuse neuroendocrine system. However, a single report has identified myelinoid bodies in intestinal EP cells of the mosquito [9].

While some EP cells contained only a few

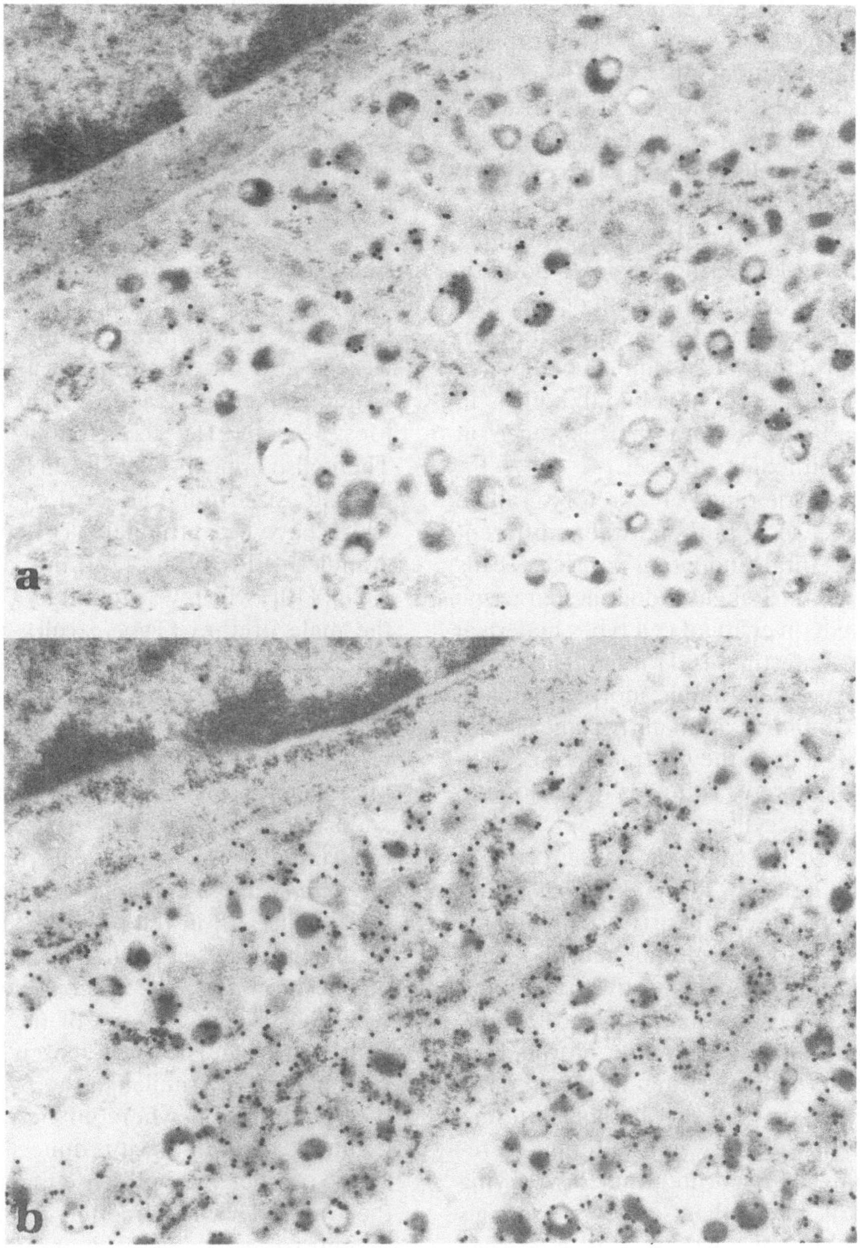

Fig 14 Immunoelectron micrographs of serial thin sections immunostained for (a) calcitonin and (b) serotonin Calcitonin and serotonin are present in the same secretory granules (protein A gold on popped off Lowicryl embedded tissue section ×25 000)

developing myelinoid bodies, others were filled These bodies were composed of either stacked (Zebra bodies) or whorled membranes with both types sometimes present in the same cell It appeared that these myelinoid bodies could fuse together to form larger bodies These bodies appeared to be developing from or in association with lysosomes some of which were in the form of lipofuscin An interesting finding was the apparent fusion of secretory granules with the myelinoid bodies and their presence within the myelinoid bodies. It is believed that this may represent a process termed *crinophagy*, first described by DeDuve in 1969 [17]. This process involves the degradation of excess secretory granules by lysosomes. Crinophagy is known to occur in other endocrine-paracrine cells, such as the pancreatic alpha cells [48] and beta cells [54], and in antral gastrin-producing cells [46]. However, none of these cells were described containing myelinoid bodies. The crinophagic hypothesis was further supported by the frequent decrease or absence of secretory granules in the cytoplasm of cells with prominent myelinoid bodies by the exclusive presence of myelinoid bodies in endocrine-paracrine cells and their absence in other prostatic epithelial cell types.

In summary, a wide range of secretory granule morphologies are seen both between different prostatic and urethral endocrine-paracrine cells and frequently within a single endocrine-paracrine cell. The potential diversity of cell types may rival that in the gastrointestinal (GI) tract. The correlation of ultrastructural granule morphology and amine/peptide content is at an early stage similar to that of the EP cells in the GI tract in the 1960s and 1970s. Much more work needs to be done to further classify these cells.

The PR1–PR9 classification system of di Sant'Agnese and de Mesy Jensen [22] was somewhat arbitrary but a useful heuristic construct to illustrate the wide range of granule morphologies and to serve as a basis for comparative studies and a uniform terminology. Tissue autolysis, fixation, and staining may all affect granule morphology and are a further complicating factor [45,47]. Furthermore, it is not clear whether different "types" of granules, that is, with different secretory storage products, can be intermixed in varying proportions. It is likely that secretory granules may progress through maturational life cycle stages (including involutional stages) with varying amounts of prohormone and cleavage products or different rates of secretional storage, which could influence morphology [46]. Even the bioavailability of biogenic amines and precursor can affect granule morphology. Finally, very pleomorphic granules seen in two-dimensional cross sections may be difficult to distinguish from separate granule types [12]. Much more work needs to be done by immunoelectron microscopy relating specific secretory storage products to specific granules and specific endocrine-paracrine cells in order to more accurately classify these cells.

With all these caveats in mind, certain preliminary conclusions can be drawn concerning the relatively few studies of the normal ultrastructure of prostatic and urethral endocrine-paracrine cells. There appears to be a distinct cell type with small, uniform round granules (PR type 1 of di Sant'Agnese and de Mesy Jensen [22]) in the human prostate, which Casanova et al. [11] (type II cell) also described in the male urethra, and Lendon et al. [44] and di Sant'Agnese and de Mesy Jensen [21] described in the female urethra. There also appears to be a cell "type" with intermediate size round to oval granules, some of which have eccentric halos (PR type 3 and most granules of PR type 4 [22]) in the prostate, Type II cell [10], which was found by Casanova [11] in the male urethra (Type I cell), and also in the female urethra [21]. This is also similar to one of the two cell types with calcitonin immunoreactivity [20]. The other calcitonin immunoreactive cell was consistent with the PR type 6 cell type with intermediate pleomorphic granules. Another endocrine-paracrine cell type was described by Aumüller [6] in the male urethra and *veru montanum* and a similar type of cell is described by Capella [10] in the prostate (Type I cell) and by di Sant'Agnese and de Mesy Jensen [21] in the female urethra. This endocrine-paracrine cell type does not match any of the PR types of di Sant'Agnese and de Mesy Jensen [22]; in fact, it is morphologically similar to the PR type 5 and PR type 9, but somewhere in between in size of granules. In addition, it is quite similar to the PR type 6 cell but without dense inner cores. Finally, the two endocrine-paracrine cell types described by Fetissof et al. [34] in the urethra and prostate do not match well any of the PR1–PR9 cell types of di Sant'Agnese and de Mesy Jensen [22] and may reflect "new cell types." Since the PR1–PR9 classification was introduced, we have observed cells in the human prostate similar to these two cell types.

It should also be noted that a large subpopulation of most if not all cell "types" contain variable numbers of myelinoid and/or "zebra" bodies, which are of unknown nature but may represent a crinophagic process.

It can also be concluded that at least some urethral endocrine-paracrine cells are innervated by efferent autonomic nerves and possible afferent nerves. It is our experience that the male and female urethral endocrine-paracrine cells are more heavily innervated than the prostatic endocrine-paracrine cells, and to some extent the literature supports this, but further studies are necessary.

Lastly, it can be concluded that endocrine-paracrine cells may communicate and regulate each other. Prostatic and urethral endocrine-paracrine cells at times lie side by side, closely apposed with dendritic processes from different endocrine-paracrine cells, frequently making contact with each other.

3. Ultrastructural Studies of Human Neuroendocrine Prostatic Malignancies

Table 2 is a review of the ultrastructural studies of human prostatic malignances with neuroendocrine differentiation. Malignant neoplasms with differentiation of the endocrine-paracrine cell phenotype are defined as having neuroendocrine differentiation. If the entire neoplasm shows this differentiation, it is termed a *neuroendocrine carcinoma*, such as small cell carcinoma (Fig. 15) or a carcinoid tumor. If only some neoplastic cells show this line of differentiation, the tumors are called *adenocarcinoma with focal neuroendocrine differentiation* (Fig. 16).

Wenk et al. in 1977 [66] were the first to publish electron micrographs of neuroendocrine prostatic carcinoma. They reported a case, associated with Cushing's syndrome of locally re-

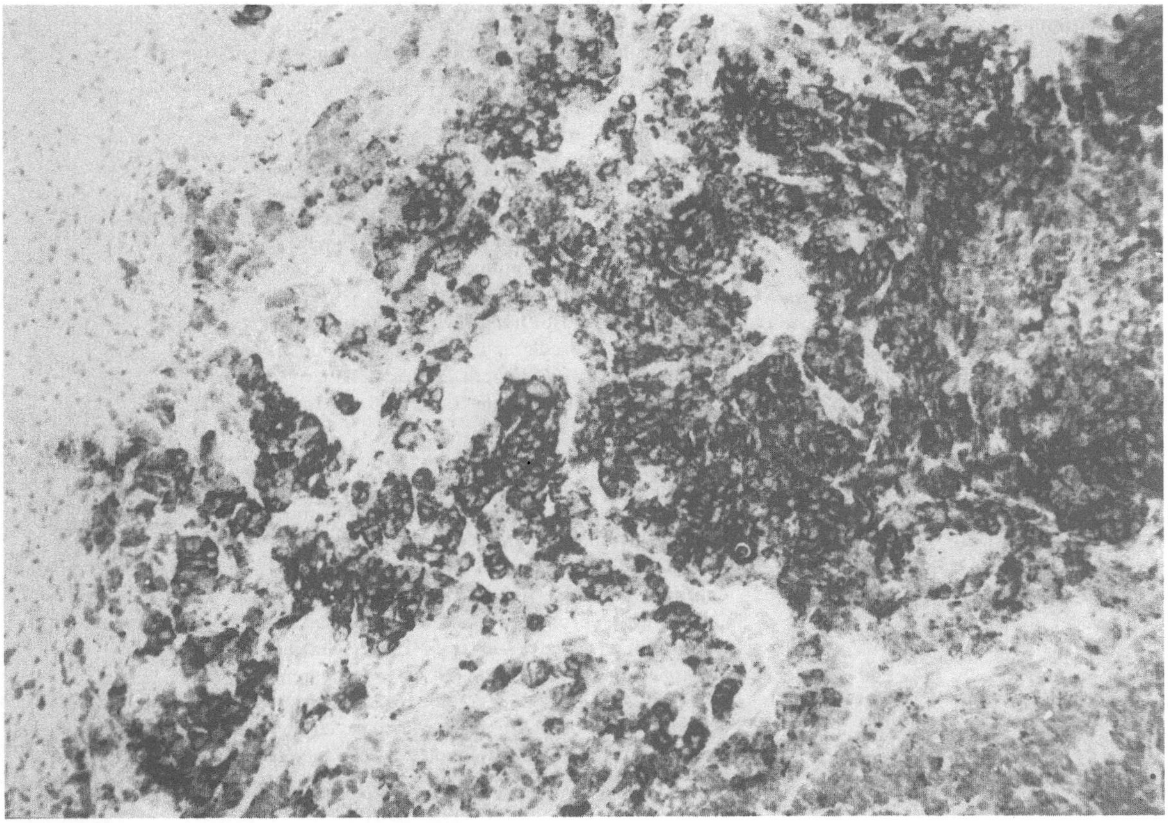

Fig 15 Chromogranin A immunoreactive small cell carcinoma of the prostate (chromogranin A immunoperoxidase, ×55)

Table 2 Ultrastructural studies of human neuroendocrine (NE) prostatic malignancies

Year	Authors	Neoplasm, method, hormone content, & granule morphology
1977	Wenk RE, Bhagavan BS, Levy R, Miller D, Weisburger W [66]	Small cell carcinoma/ACTH-plasma & ICC EM paraffin retrieved tissue (one NE cell illustrated) Intermediate round granules, 140–260 nm (NOS)
1981	Capella C, Usellini L, Buffa R, Frigerio B, Solcia E [10]	Mixed adenocarcinoma-carcinoid, focal NE differentiation/ACTH-plasma & ICC beta-endorphin-ICC EM routine & paraffin retrieved tissue (three NE cells illustrated) Type I — (adenocarcinoma & focal NE diff) intermediate pleomorphic granules, 280–300 nm (NOS) Type II — (NE diff) small, round granules, 147 nm (NOS) Type III — (adenocarcinoma & focal NE diff) large round granules, 350–450 nm (NOS)
1986	Fetissof F, Bruandet P, Arbeille B, Penot J, Marboeuf Y, Le Roux J, Guilloteau D, Beaulieu JL [33]	Focal NE differentiation/calcitonin, NSE, serotonin, hCG-ICC (prior to DES) EM routine (four NE cells illustrated) Large pleomorphic granules, 350 nm (NOS) Large round granules, 500 nm (NOS) Intermediate round granules, 180–300 nm (NOS) Small round granules, 100 nm (NOS)
1987	di Sant'Agnese PA, de Mesy Jensen KL [25]	Focal NE differentiation/bombesin, calcitonin, serotonin-ICC EM large block, pop-off" technique (four NE cells illustrated) Small round, intermediate round, intermediate pleomorphic granules
1987	Ro JY, Tetu B, Ayala AG, Ordonez NG [52]	Small cell with NE differentiation, combined adenocarcinoma-small cell/NSE-ICC EM paraffin retrieved tissue (one NE cell illustrated) Small round granules, 200 nm (NOS)
1988	Turbat-Herrera EA, Herrera Gore I, Lott RL, Grizzle WE, Bonnin JM [61]	Mixed small cell with NE differentiation-adenocarcinoma/NSE, chromogranin, calcitonin, synaptophysin, small cell/ACTH-ICC, PTH-serum EM routine from autopsy (one NE cell illustrated) Small round & intermediate round granules, 100–400 nm (NOS)
1988	Srigley JR, Hartwick WJ, Edwards V, de Harven E [56]	Small cell carcinoma with NE differentiation EM routine (one NE cell illustrated) Intermediate round granules
1990	di Sant'Agnese PA (review) [31]	NE differentiation/serotonin ICC Small cell/chromogranin A, calcitonin-ICC EM large block, "pop-off" technique (three NE cell types illustrated) NE diff—Intermediate pleomorphic granules Small cell—small round granules
1991	Christopher ME, Sefte AD, Sorenson K, Resnick MI [13]	Small cell/NSE chromogranin, synaptophysin-ICC EM routine (no illustration of NE cells in article) Small dense cored granules present in groups of cells
1992	Frydman CP, Bleiweiss IJ, Unger PD, Gordon RE, Brazenas NV [37]	Adenocarcinoma with Paneth cell-like" change EM routine (one NE cell illustrated)—large, round granules
1992	Weaver MG, Abdul-Karim FW, Srigley J, Bostwick DG, Ro JY, Ayala AG [64]	Adenocarcinoma with focal NE differentiation & large eosin granules chromogranin, serotonin-ICC EM paraffin retrieved tissue (one NE cell illustrated) Large pleomorphic granules, 240–480 nm (NOS)
1992	Weaver MG, Abdul-Karim FW, Srigley JR [65]	Adenocarcinoma with focal NE differentiation & large eosin granules/serotonin, chromogranin, NSE-ICC, Small cell with NE differentiation & large eosin granules/chromogranin-ICC EM paraffin retrieved tissue (two NE cells illustrated) Large round, 240–480 nm (NOS) (adenocarcinoma) (similar to PR type 9 granule, di Sant'Agnese & de Mesy Jensen [19] Small round, 80–120 nm (NOS) (small cell) (similar to PR type 1 granule, di Sant'Agnese & de Mesy Jensen [19]

NOS = not otherwise specified, ICC = immunocytochemistry, PIN = prostatic intraepithelial neoplasia, NSE = neuron specific enolase, ACTH = adrenocorticotrophic hormone, hCG = human chorionic gonadotrophin, PTH = parathyroid hormone, DES = diethylstilbestrol, diff = differentiation, eosin = eosinophilic

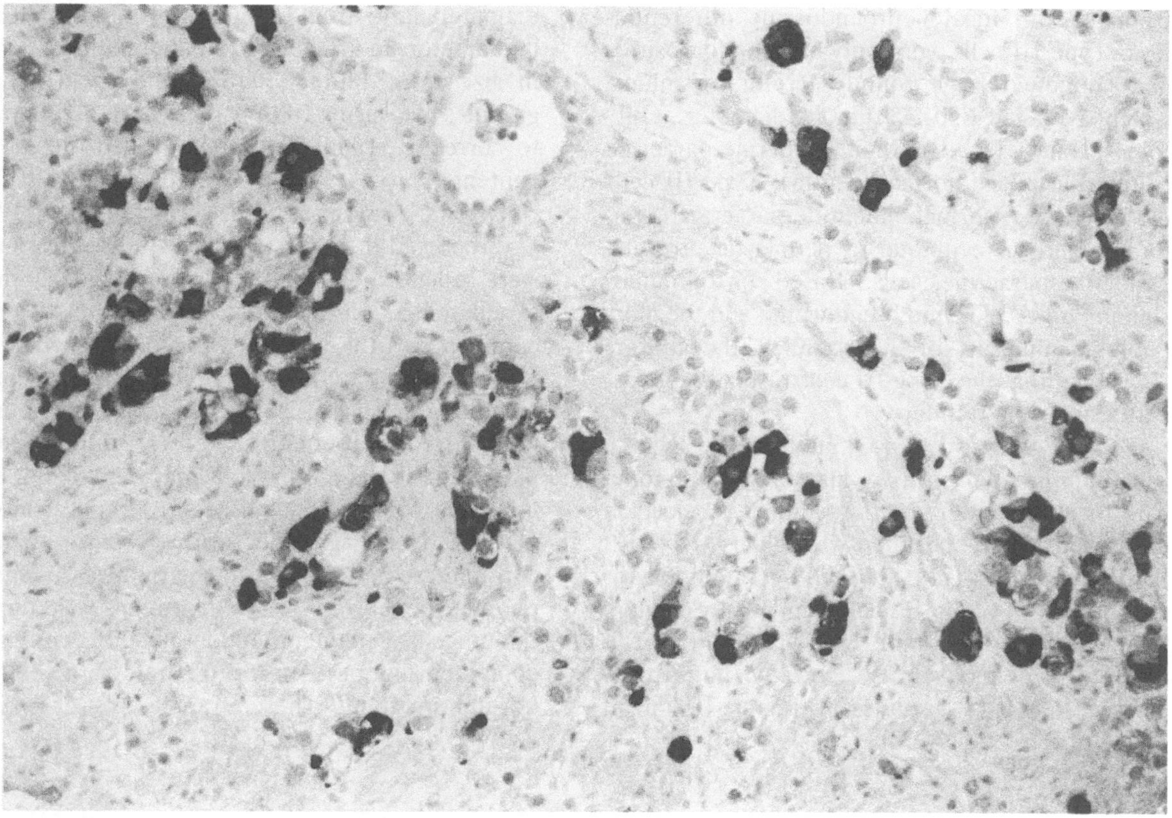

Fig 16 An adenocarcinoma of the prostate with focal neuroendocrine differentiation (serotonin immunoperoxidase, ×125)

current poorly differentiated prostatic carcinoma with a small cell pattern, producing ACTH. Extracts of the autopsy tumor tissue analyzed for ACTH were almost 40 times normal plasma levels. The tumor cells immunostained positively for ACTH. Suboptimally preserved tumor cells were examined by electron microscopy, and one type of cell was identified. These cells contained intermediate, round secretory granules, ranging in size from 140 to 260 nm, with 210 nm the average diameter. It was pointed out by the authors that the granule morphology was "not comparable" to pituitary ACTH cells, not only because of the poor preservation of the tissue, but also because at that point in time ultrastructural studies defining the ultrastructural morphology of ACTH secretory granules were contradictory and incomplete [68].

In 1981, Cappella et al. [10] published an article characterizing endocrine-paracrine cells found in normal and hyperplastic prostates, and neuroendocrine differentiation in the form of mixed prostatic adenocarcinoma-carcinoid tumors, and focal neuroendocrine differentiation in prostatic carcinoma. Using tissue retrieved from paraffin blocks, three morphologic variants of malignant cells with neuroendocrine differentiation were described based on silver stains and secretory granule morphology: Type I cells were found in mixed adenocarcinoma-carcinoid and prostatic carcinoma with focal neuroendocrine differentiation. This type was argyrophil and argentaffin positive and contained intermediate pleomorphic secretory granules, which averaged 248 nm in diameter. Type II cells were present only in prostatic carcinoma with focal neuroendocrine differentiation. These cells were also argyrophil and argentaffin positive and contained small round to oval secretory granules averaging 123 nm in diameter. Type III cells were found exclusively in adenocarcinomas with focal neuroendocrine differentiation. Type III cells were only argyrophil positive and contained large round secretory granules, which averaged 350–450 nm in diameter. Only Types I and II had normal endocrine-paracrine counterparts (see normal section). Type III cells did not have a normal endocrine-paracrine counterpart and were unique to neoplastic prostatic endocrine-paracrine cells. Based on immunostaining for ACTH and b-endorphin and the morphologic similarity of the granules, the authors concluded that the Type III cells resembled corticotrophs of the pituitary.

Fetissof et al. in 1986 [33] published a case of a calcitonin-immunoreactive prostatic carcinoma with focal NE differentiation studied by electron microscopy. This specimen was taken after DES therapy and was not studied by immunocytochemistry. Prior biopsies had been focally positive for calcitonin, serotonin, and HCG. Four cell types were defined ultrastructurally: large pleomorphic secretory granules averaging 350 nm in diameter, large round granules averaging 500 nm in diameter, intermediate round granules ranging in size from 180 to 300 nm, and small round granules measuring 100 nm. There was no attempt to correlate granule morphology with hormone content.

Di Sant'Agnese and de Mesy Jensen in 1987 [25] reported the ultrastructural study of five prostatic adenocarcinomas (four from radical prostatectomies and one from a metastatic prostate carcinoma to the testicle) with focal neuroendocrine differentiation. The large-block "pop-off" technique [27] was used to locate cells with neuroendocrine differentiation. Cells resembling normal endocrine-paracrine cell types were identified, including cells with small round granules, intermediate round granules with eccentric halos, and intermediate pleomorphic granules. No morphometric analysis of the granules was done. Other cells with neuroendocrine differentiation contained unique secretory granules not seen in normal prostate. These granules were round,

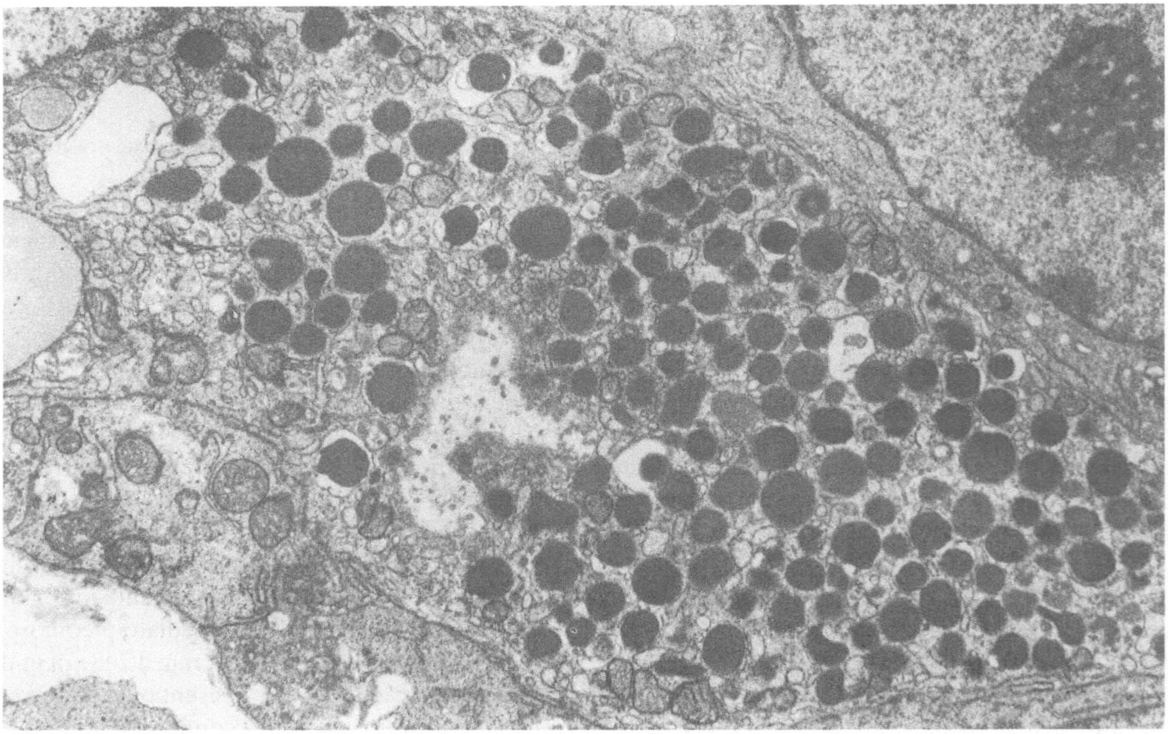

Fig 17 Electron micrograph of an adenocarcinoma with focal neuroendocrine differentiation demonstrating a malignant cell with neuroendocrine differentiation and large, generally round secretory granules These granules are visible as bright red granules on hematoxylin and eosin sections, and have therefore been referred to as "Paneth cell-like" (×11,500)

intermediate sized, and moderately electron dense.

Several reports (ranging from one to seven cases each) studying the ultrastructure of small cell carcinoma of the prostate appeared in the late 1980s and early 1990s [13,30,52,56,60]. Some cases showed NE differentiation by immunocytochemistry and electron microscopy and others did not. In general tumors with neurosecretory granules were positive for neuron specific enolase (NSE), and negative for prostatic specific antigen (PSA) and prostatic acid phosphatase (PAP), whereas those without neurosecretory granules and/or NSE negative were often positive for PSA and PAP. Neurosecretory granules tended to be sparse and generally small and round.

A review published in 1990 by di Sant'Agnese in *Progress in Reproductive and Urinary Tract Pathology* [31] illustrated the further ultrastructural findings from prostatic carcinomas with focal neuroendocrine differentiation and prostatic small cell carcinoma. The prostatic carcinomas with focal neuroendocrine differentiation contained intermediate pleomorphic secretory granules, which were morphologically similar to PR type 4 [22]. These cells were immunocytochemically positive for serotonin. In the small cell carcinoma, neuroendocrine cells contained small round secretory granules. The majority of the tumor cells were positive for serotonin and strongly positive for chromogranin A.

Unfortunately, the term *Paneth cell-like* change or metaplasia has been applied to normal and hyperplastic prostatic cells as well as cells with neuroendocrine differentiation in prostatic carcinoma [37,64,65]. We recommend that this change be described as "NE cells containing large eosinophilic granules." In normal or hyperplastic prostate, the granules are apically oriented, resemble serous granules, and are negative for neuroendocrine antigens and lysozyme but positive for PSA and PAP [37, 64]. In carcinomas, cells with large eosinophilic granules are seen and appear to represent focal neuroendocrine differentiation with the cells containing large neurosecretory granules (Fig. 17) [64,65]. These granules were interpreted as serous secretory granules by others [37] since the cells were PSA and PAP positive, although they were negative for a-1-antitrypsin and lysozyme by immunocytochemistry. Immunocytochemical neuroendocrine markers were not performed. We feel that most likely this interpretation is incorrect and these cells represent focal neuroendocrine differentiation.

4. Concluding Remarks

In summary, certain conclusions can be drawn from these studies. Small cell carcinomas of the prostate, which account for approximately 1–2% of prostatic malignancies, may or may not show neuroendocrine differentiation. Those that do generally have sparse small round granules are similar to the normal PR1 endocrine-paracrine cell counterpart [22]. These findings are consistent with the size and distribution of neurosecretory granules in small cell neuroendocrine carcinomas arising in other organ systems.

Prostatic adenocarcinomas with focal neuroendocrine differentiation have a wide range of neurosecretory granules morphology. In part these granules and cell types resemble those seen in normal prostate, and this recapitulates the wide range of granule morphology and multiple cell types seen in the normal prostate. To further complicate the picture, granule morphologies and cell types that do not resemble any known normal types are also seen. This may reflect the rarity of the normal counterparts and, therefore, the absence of any published description. This may also reflect abnormal granule formation or packaging of ectopic secretory products associated with neoplastic transformation [39].

References

1 Abrahamsson PA, Lilja H Partial characterization of a thyroid-stimulating hormone-like peptide in neuroendocrine cells of the human prostate gland Prostate 14 71–81, 1989
2 Abrahamsson PA, Wadstrom LB, Alumets J, Falkmer S, Grimelius L Peptide-, hormone- and serotonin-immunoreactive cells in normal and hyperplastic prostate glands Pathol Res Pract 181 675–683, 1986
3 Abrahamsson PA, Wadstrom LB, Alumets J, Falkmer S, Grimelius L Peptide-, hormone- and serotonin-immunoreactive tumour cells in carcinoma of the prostate Pathol Res Pract 182 298–307, 1987
4 Abrahamsson PA, Falkmer S, Falt K, Grimelius L The course of neuroendocrine differentiation in prostatic car-

cinomas An immunohistochemical study testing chromogranin A as an "endocrine marker" Pathol Res Pract 185 373–380, 1989
5 Almagro UA, Thieu TM, Remeniuk E, Kneck B, Strumpf K Argyrophilic, "carcinoid-like" prostatic carcinoma Arch Pathol Lab Med 110 916–919, 1986
6 Aumuller G, Metz W, Grube D Elektronen- und fluoreszenzmikroskopische untersuchungen an der memschlichen prostata Verh Anat Ges 70 895–903, 1976
7 Azzopardi JG, Evans DJ Argentaffin cells in prostatic carcinoma Differentiation from lipofuchsin and melanin in prostatic epithelium J Pathol 104 247–251, 1971
8 Bishop A, Polak J Gut endocrine and neural peptides Endocrinol Pathol 1 4–24, 1990
9 Brown MR, Raikhel AS, Arden OL Ultrastructure of midgut endocrine cells in the adult mosquito, *Aedes aegypti* Tissue Cell 17 709–721, 1985
10 Capella C, Usellini L, Buffa R, Frigerio B, Solicia E The endocrine component of prostatic carcinomas, mixed adenocarcinoma-carcinoid tumours and non-tumour prostate Histochemical and ultrastructural identification of the endocrine cells Histopathology 5 175–192, 1981
11 Casanova S, Corrado F, Vignoli G Endocrine-like cells in the epithelium of the human male urethra J Submicr Cytol 6 435–438, 1974
12 Childs G, Ellison DG, Garner LL An immunocytochemist's view of gonadotropin storage in the adult male rat Cytochemical and morphological heterogeneity in serially sectioned gonadotropes Am J Anat 158 397–409, 1980
13 Christopher M, Seftel A, Sorenson K, Resnick M Small cell carcinoma of the genitourinary tract An immunohistochemical, electron microscopic, and clinicopathological study J Urol 146 382–388, 1991
14 Cohen RJ, Glezerson G, Haffejee Z, Afrika D Prostatic carcinoma Histological and immunohistological factors affecting prognosis Br J Urol 66 405–410, 1990
15 Cutz E Neuroendocrine cells of the lung An overview of morphologic characteristics and development Exp Lung Res 3 185–208, 1982
16 Dauge MC, Grossin M, Doumecq-Lacoste JM, Vinceneux P, Delmas V, Bocquet L Tumeur "carcinoide" de la prostate Une nouvelle observation anatomoclinique avec revue de la litterature Arch Anat Cytol Path 33 73–79, 1985
17 DeDuve C The lysosome in retrospect In Lysosomes in Biology and Pathology, Vol 2 JT Dingle, FB Fell (eds) Amsterdam North-Holland, 1969, pp 3–37
18 De Lellis RA, Nunnemacher G, Wolfe HJ C-cell hyperplasia An ultrastructural analysis Lab Invest 36 237–248, 1977
19 de Mesy Jensen, di Sant'Agnese PA Large block embedding and "pop-off" technique for immunoelectron microscopy Applications to prostatic endocrine-paracrine cells Ultrastruct Pathol 16 51–59, 1992
20 di Sant Agnese PA, de Mesy Jensen KL Calcitonin, katacalcin and calcitonin gene-related peptide in the human prostate An immunocytochemical and immunoelectron microscopic study Arch Pathol Lab Med 113 790, 1989
21 di Sant'Agnese PA, de Mesy Jensen KL Endocrine-paracrine (APUD) cells of the human female urethra and paraurethral ducts J Urol 137 1250–1254, 1987
22 di Sant'Agnese PA, de Mesy Jensen KL Endocrine-paracrine cells of the prostate and prostatic urethra An ultrastructural study Hum Pathol 15 1034–1041, 1984
23 di Sant'Agnese PA, de Mesy Jensen KL Human prostatic endocrine-paracrine (APUD) cells Distributional analysis with a comparison of serotonin and neuron-specific enolase immunoreactivity and silver stains Arch Pathol Lab Med 109 607–612, 1985
24 di Sant'Agnese PA, de Mesy Jensen KL Somatostatin and/or somatostatinlike immunoreactive endocrine-paracrine cells in the human prostate gland Arch Pathol Lab Med 108 693–696, 1984
25 di Sant'Agnese PA, de Mesy Jensen KL Neuroendocrine differentiation in prostatic carcinoma Hum Pathol 18 849–856, 1987
26 di Sant'Agnese PA Calcitoninlike immunoreactive and bombesinlike immunoreactive endocrine-paracrine cells of the human prostate Arch Pathol Lab Med 110 412–415, 1986
27 di Sant'Agnese PA, de Mesy Jensen KL Diagnostic electron microscopy on reembedded ("popped off") areas of large Spurr epoxy sections Ultrastruct Pathol 6 247–253, 1984
28 di Sant'Agnese PA, de Mesy Jensen KL Myelinoid bodies in endocrine-paracrine (neuroendocrine, APUD) cells of the prostatourethral region J Submicrosc Cytol Pathol 21 557–564, 1989
29 di Sant'Agnese PA Endocrine aspects of the prostate In Bloodworth's Endocrine Pathology, 3rd ed J Lechago, V Gould (eds) In press
30 di Sant'Agnese PA Neuroendocrine differentiation in carcinoma of the prostate Cancer 70 (Suppl) 254–268, 1992
31 di Sant'Agnese PA Prostatic endocrine-paracrine cells and neuroendocrine differentiation in prostatic carcinoma In Progress in Reproductive and Urinary Tract Pathology, Vol II I Damjanov, AH Cohen, SE Mills, RH Young (eds) New York W W Norton, 1990, pp 87–108
32 Fetissof F, Bertrand G, Guilloteau D, Dubois MP, Lanson Y, Arbeille B Calcitonin immunoreactive cells in prostate gland and cloacal derived tissues Virchows Arch A Pathol Anat Histopathol 409 523–533, 1986
33 Fetissof F, Bruandet P, Arbeille B, Lanson, Y, Boivin F, Jobard P Calcitonin-secreting carcinomas of the prostate An immunohistochemical and ultrastructural analysis Am J Surg Pathol 10 702–710, 1986
34 Fetissof F, Dubois MP, Arbeille-Brassart B, Lanson Y, Boivin F, Yoband P Endocrine cells in the prostate gland, urothelium and Brenner tumors Immunohistological and ultrastructural studies Virchows Arch A Pathol Anat Histopathol 42 53–64, 1983
35 Feyrter F Uber das urogenitale helle-zellen system des menschen Mikr Anat Forsch 57 324–344, 1951
36 Feyrter F Uber diffuse endocrine epithelial organe Lepzig J A Barth, 1938
37 Frydman CP, Bleiweiss IJ, Unger PD, Gordon RE, Brazenas NV Paneth cell-like metaplasia of the prostate

gland Arch Pathol Lab Med 116 274–276, 1992
38 Gnessi L, Ulisse S, Fabbri A, et al Isolation of a human seminal plasma peptide with bombesin-like activity Fertil Steril 51 1034–1039, 1989
39 Gould VE Neuroendocrineomas and neuroendocrine carcinomas, APUD-cell system neoplasms and their aberrant secretory activities Pathol Annu, 1977, p 33
40 Grube D The endocrine cells of the digestive system Amines, peptides and modes of action Anat Embryol 175 151–162, 1986
41 Kadmon D, Thompson T, Lynch G, Scardino P Elevated plasma chromogranin-A concentrations in prostatic carcinoma J Urol 146 358–361, 1991
42 Kazzaz BA Argentaffin and argyrophil cells in the prostate J Pathol 112 189–193, 1974
43 Larsson LI On the possible existence of multiple endocrine, paracrine and neurocrine messengers in secretory cell systems Invest Cell Pathol 3 73–85, 1980
44 Lendon RG, Dixon JS, Gosling JA The distribution of endocrine-like cells in the human male and female urethral epithelium Experientia 32 377–378, 1976
45 Mortensen NJ, McC, Morris JF The effect of fixation conditions on the ultrastructural appearance of gastrin cell granules in the rat gastric pyloric antrum Cell Tissue Res 176-251-263, 1977
46 Nielsen HO, Hage E The antral gastrin-producing cells in duodenal ulcer patients An ultrastructural study before and during treatment with cimetidine Virchows Arch A Pathol Anat Histopathol 406 271–277 1985
47 Nordmann JJ Ultrastructural appearance of neurosecretory granules in the sinus gland of the crab after different fixation procedures Cell Tissue Res 185 557–563, 1977
48 Orci L, Junod R, Pictet A, Renold E, Rouiller C Granulolysis in A cells of endocrine pancreas in spontaneous and experimental diabetes in animals J Cell Biol 38 462–466, 1968
49 Pearse AGE The cytochemistry and ultrastructure of polypeptide hormone-producing cells of the APUD series and the embryologic, physiologic, and pathologic implications of the concept J Histochem Cytochem 17 303–313, 1969
50 Pearse AGE The APUD cell concept and its implications in pathology Pathol Annu 9 27, 1974
51 Pretl K Zur frage der endokrinie der menschlichen vorsteherdruse Virchows Arch A Pathol Anat Histopathol 312 392–404, 1944
52 Ro JY, Tetu B, Ayala AG, Ordonez NG Small cell carcinoma of the prostate Immunohistochemical and electron microscopic studies of 18 cases Cancer 59 977–982, 1987
53 Sasaki A, Yoshinaga K Immunoreactive somatostatin in male reproductive system in humans J Clin Endocrinol Metab 68 996–999, 1989
54 Schnell AH, Swenne I, Borg LAH Lysosomes and pancreatic islet function A quantitative estimation of crinophagy in the mouse pancreatic B-cell Cell Tissue Res 252 9–15, 1988
55 Sjoberg HE, Arver S, Bucht E High concentration of immunoreactive calcitonin of prostatic origin in human semen Acta Physiol Scand 110 101–102, 1980
56 Srigley JR, Hartwick WJ, Edwards V, deHarven E Selected ultrastructural aspects of urothelial and prostatic tumors Ultrastruct Pathol 12 49–65, 1988
57 Stratton M, Evans DJ, Lambert IA Prostatic adenocarcinoma evolving into carcinoid Selective effect of hormonal treatment J Clin Pathol 39 750–756, 1986
58 Sunday M, Kaplan L Motoyama E, Chin W, Spindel E Biology of disease Gastrin releasing peptide (mammalian bombesin) gene expression in health and disease Lab Invest 59 5–24, 1988
59 Tarle M, Rados N Investigation on serum neurone-specific enolase in prostate cancer diagnosis and monitoring Comparative study of a multiple tumor marker assay Prostate 18 ••–••, 1991
60 Tetu B, Ro JY, Ayala AG, et al Small cell carcinoma of the prostate part I A clinicopathologic study of 20 cases Cancer 59 1803–1809 1987
61 Turbat-Herrera EA Herrera GA, Gore I, Lott RL, Griwzle WE, Bonnin YM Neuroendocrine differentiation in prostatic carcinomas A retrospective autopsy study Arch Pathol Lab Med 112 1100–1106, 1988
62 Ulisse S, Gnessi L, Fabbri A et al Bombesin-like immunoreactivity in human seminal fluid Regul Pept 19 143, 1987
63 Wasserstein PW, Goldman RL Diffuse carcinoid of prostate Urology 18 407–409, 1981
64 Weaver MG, Abdul-Karim FW Srigley J, Bostwick DG, Ro JY, Ayala AG Paneth cell like change of the prostate gland A histological, immunohistochemical, and electron microscopic study Am J Surg Pathol 16 62–68, 1992
65 Weaver MG, Abdul-Karim FW, Srigley JR Paneth cell-like change and small cell carcinoma of the prostate Two divergent forms of prostatic neuroendocrine differentiation Am J Surg Pathol 16 1013–1016, 1992
66 Wenk RE, Bhagavan BS Levy R, et al Ectopic ACTH, prostatic oat cell carcinoma and marked hypernatremia Cancer 40 773–778, 1977
67 Yamada T Local regulatory actions of gastrointestinal peptides In Physiology of the Gastrointestinal Tract, 2nd ed LR Johnson (ed) New York Raven Press, 1987, pp 131–142
68 Yoshimura F A new concept of anterior pituitary cell classification in the rat based on both cell differentiation and secretory cycle In Pars Distalis of the Pituitary Gland — Structure, Function, and Regulation F Yoshimura, A Gorbman (eds) Elsevier Science, 1986, pp ••–••

CHAPTER 9

Human Bulbourethral and Urethral Glands

FRANCESCA TESTA-RIVA, ALESSANDRO RIVA, TERENZIO CONGIU,
ANTONELLO DE LISA, & PIETRO M. MOTTA

1. Introduction

Studies on the fine structure of the bulbourethral glands have been restricted largely to animals [12,14,15,20,29,30,59,60]. A few works were carried out on human bulbourethral (BU) glands by transmission electron microscopy (TEM) [17, 38,43,45] and, more recently, two studies [42,44] were published by our group to correlate TEM with scanning electron microscopic (SEM) findings in order to describe the general configuration of this gland in man. Comparison of our results with those reported by the above authors has clearly shown that the human BU glands possess, like other human accessory sex organs [2,6,18,31,33, 41,43,45], some distinctive characteristics [44], even with regard to the more closely related species [29].

Very little information is available on the cytoarchitecture and functional role of the urethral glands in man, apart from a few histochemical data [19,50] obtained with the light microscope and some brief reports of our group [35,43,45,46] with TEM and SEM.

By the use of techniques [11,28,54] that allow the removal of connective tissue and basal lamina, coupled with refinements of methods for exposure of lateral cell surfaces [13,23–25,35,37,47], and by a newly introduced procedure for visualization of cellular organelles [34], we provide in the present chapter more detailed information on the three-dimensional (3D) morphology and the cytoarchitecture of the parenchymal components of human bulbourethral and urethral glands.

2. Bulbourethral Glands

The bulbourethral (BU, Cowper's) glands are small paired, androgen dependent organs [57], placed within the two layers of the urogenital diaphragm. The BU glands, which are homologous to Bartholin glands of the female [48,52], are enclosed, in fact, in the striated muscle fibers of the *sphincter uretrae* and *transversus perinei profundus*. Each gland is divided into several lobules and opens with a single duct onto the floor of the cavernous part of the urethra. The lobules consist [3,8,52,53] of tubuloalveolar secretory portions that drain directly or through short ducts (ductuli) into wide cavities called *ampullae*, which probably act as reservoirs of secretion [3]. Excretory ducts originate from ampullae of the various lobules and join to form the long (4–5 cm) main excretory duct (MED). Ductuli, ampullae, excretory ducts, and MED together constitute the excretory portion.

The secretions of the BU glands are released in the early ejaculatory phase, contributing to the first fraction of the seminal plasma [52]. Since, however, they mix with the much larger prostatic secretion, it is still uncertain which compounds [26] the BU glands secrete or their specific function, apart from the rather trivial function of lubricating the cavernous urethra [52].

2.1. Secretory Portion

Following the removal of interlobular connective tissue by the HCl-collagenase method [11], the

Riva, A., Testa Riva, F., and Motta, P.M., (eds.), Ultrastructure of the Male Urogenital Glands: Prostate, Seminal Vesicles, Urethral, and Bulbourethral Glands. *ISBN 0-7923-2800-0.*

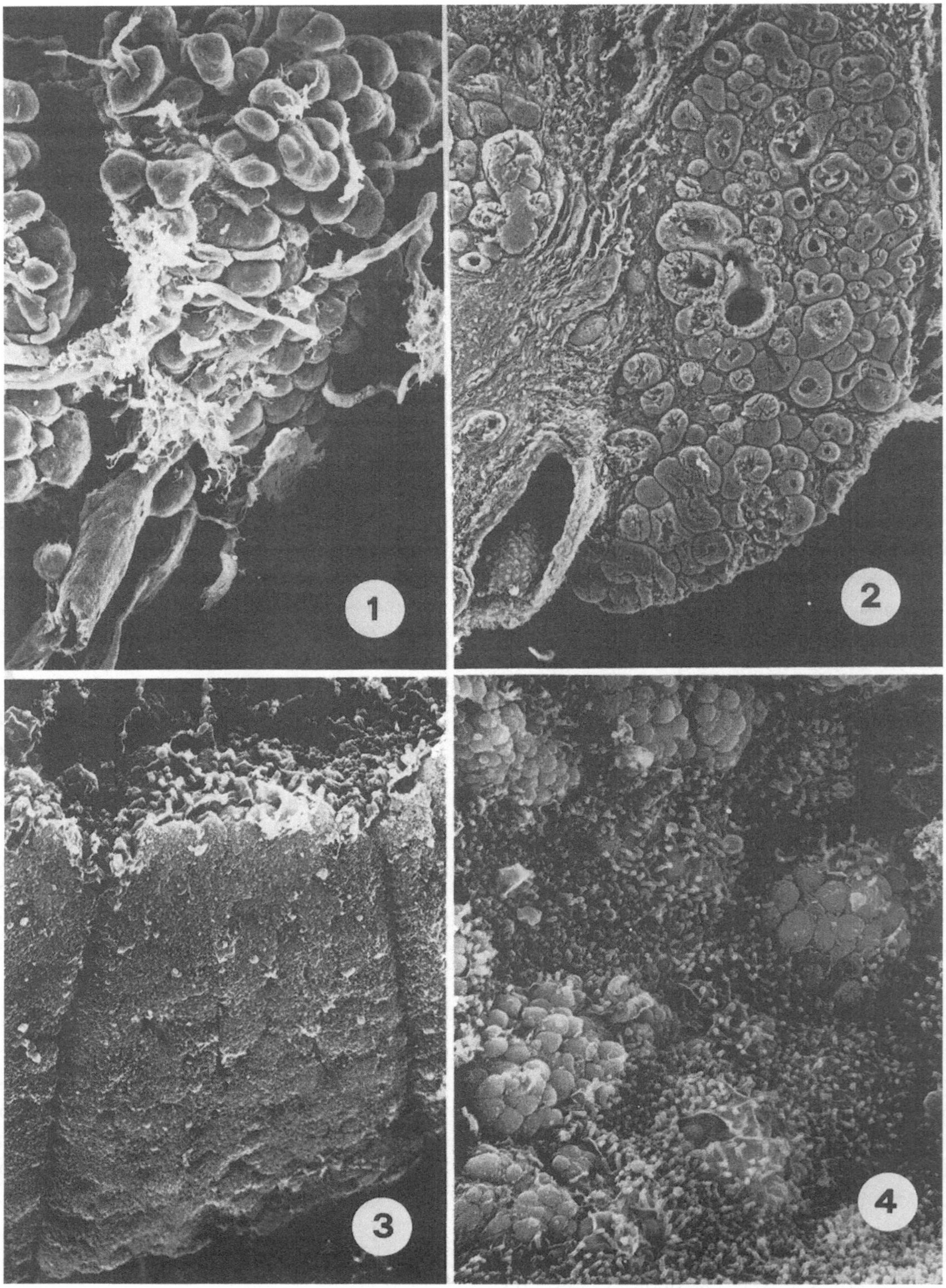
1
2
3
4

glands appear to be composed of short tubules (Fig. 1), more or less coiled, that sometimes bifurcate. The tubules join each other, even at right angles, and are often dilated into alveoli at their blind ends (Fig. 1). No constricted segments, resembling the intercalated ducts of salivary glands [36], are observed. Similar findings (Fig. 2) are seen under low magnification of sectioned glands subjected to the osmium maceration method [34].

By SEM, cells filled with secretion appear pyramidal or cylindrical in shape with rather straight outlines (Fig. 3). Their lateral surfaces, possibly with relationship to the secretory content, may be either smooth or covered by frondlike expansions oriented at random. Apices of mucous cells appear to be covered with microvillosities (Fig. 3) and, in sites where the maceration process has removed the apical plasmalemma, the spherical shape of secretory droplets is evident (Fig. 4).

At TEM, tubuli and alveoli consist of mucous cells at various stages of their secretory cycle. Cells filled with secretion (Fig. 5) are by far the most numerous but, interspersed with them, cells in an early phase of the cycle (with scarce mucus) and cells in intermediate stages are also observed [44]. The nuclei, with sparse clumps of heterochromatin, are compressed at the cell base and generally exhibit an irregular profile. The nucleolus is often recognizable. The scarce ground cytoplasm is located mainly around the nucleus and along the cellular borders, also forming thin trabeculae among the mucous granules (Fig. 5). A small Golgi apparatus, scarce elements of the rough endoplasmic reticulum (RER), and a few small mitochondria are noticeable in these cytoplasmic strands (Fig. 5). The mucous droplets are the most distinctive elements in this maturation stage and often seem to coalesce into large masses of mucus by fusing their limiting membranes at multiple points (Fig. 5). A dark spherical body may be noticed at the periphery of some droplets, more frequently in the smallest ones (Fig. 5).

As revealed by previous histochemical investigations [38,51], the mucous droplets consist of an acidic mucin, particularly rich in carboxyl (sialic) groups and containing [42,45] the blood group antigens (BGS), suggesting that the human BU glands secrete these substances into the semen. The mucous droplets may be discharged individually into the lumen by means of typical exocytosis. This process can involve the consecutive release of vertically aligned granules forming intracellular canaliculi [44]. On the other hand, fusion of large masses of mucus with the apical plasmalemma can occur at different sites, and mucus, as well as fragments of cells, are discharged into the lumen. This mechanism of secretion may be regarded as an apocrine process similar to that described in the Bartholin glands [48]. Narrow intercellular canaliculi with short microvilli and indentations, possibly related to exocytosis, are also observed.

An additional secretory component is represented by filamentous bodies [56] described in 1917 by Schaffer [49] in the human Cowper's and Bartholin's glands under the name of *attraktosomen* because of its ability to attract secretory material. With the advent of electron microscopy, the filamentous bodies were detected in most human mucous glands [40], with the exception of goblet cells. They are absent from serous cells and from the mucous cells of most animals. At TEM these bodies have an irregular outline and vary greatly in size and shape (Fig. 5). They are membrane bound and exhibit a filamentous content with some intermingled densities. Lipid droplets of different sizes are often found in close proximity to the filamentous bodies [44]. The latter may fuse together and

←

Fig 1 SEM of lobule of a bulbourethral gland (BU) observed after removal of connective tissue by the HCl-collagenase method The secretory tubules are often dilated into alveoli Note an excretory duct in the lower left corner (×220)

Fig 2 SEM of sectioned lobule of BU gland treated with the osmium maceration method Tubuli and alveoli show a narrow lumen, while that of ampullae (arrows) is much wider A sectioned excretory duct is seen in the lower left corner (×88)

Fig 3 SEM, osmium maceration method, of bulbourethral gland A sectioned secretory cell filled with mucus exhibits lateral straight outlines and an apex covered with microvillosities (×8800)

Fig 4 SEM, osmium maceration method of bulbourethral gland Apexes of secretory cells, seen from the lumen, appear covered with microvilli In the sites where the apical plasmalemma has been removed, the spherical secretory droplets are evident (×3850)

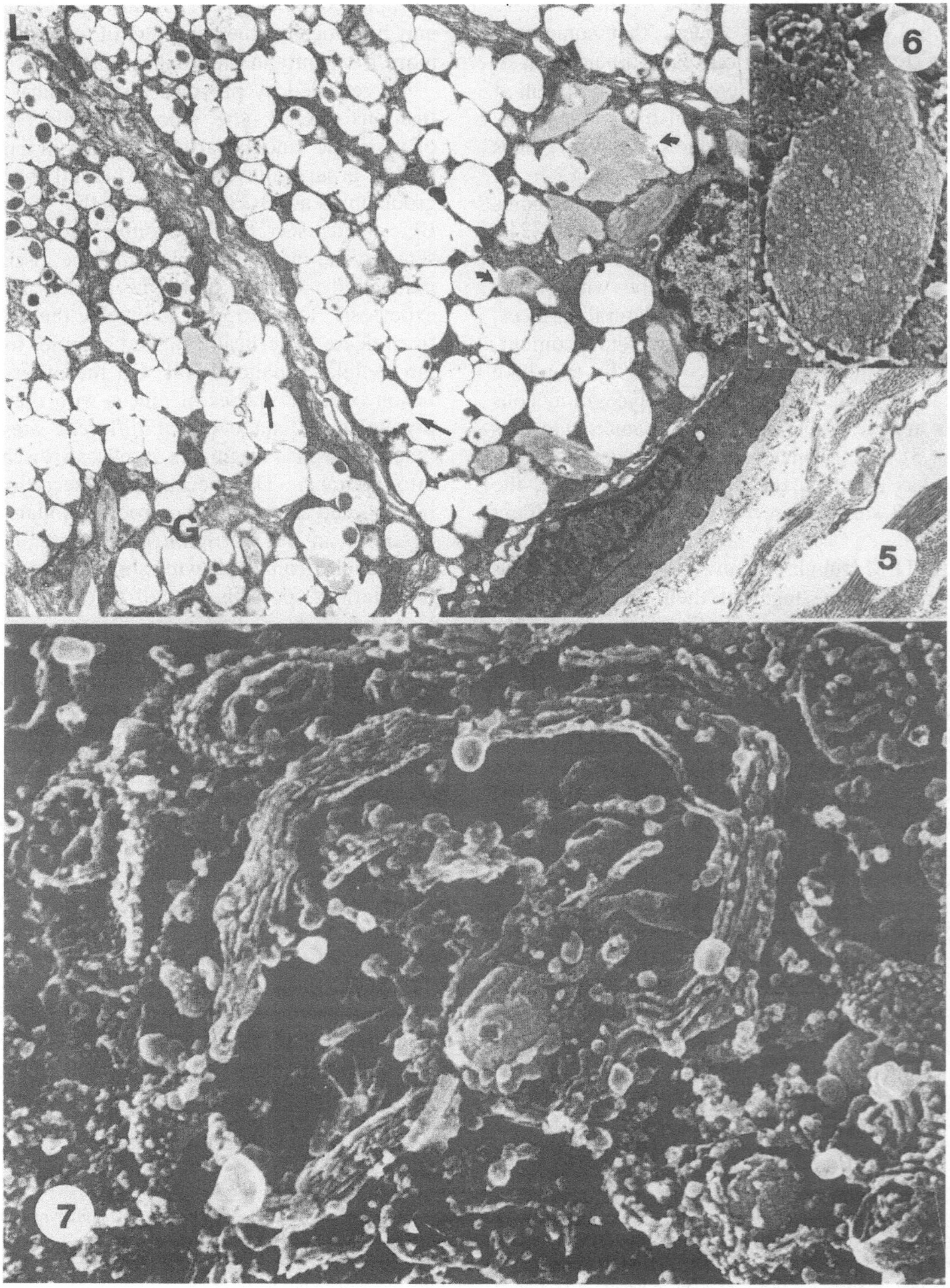
L
6
G
5
7

with mucous droplets at multiple points of their contour, giving rise to large masses of secretory material in which the filamentous texture gradually disappears The filamentous bodies are mostly located in the basal region of the cell, especially in mature stages, but some may also be encountered in more apical positions Images of direct exocytosis of these bodies into the lumen, however, have not been observed By SEM the filamentous bodies were appreciable only in osmium macerated specimens (Fig 6), where, although devoid of filamentous structure, they looked less granular than the adjoining mucous droplets From an histochemical point of view, it is not established whether the filamentous body content is the same in all different localizations or if it varies, like the mucous droplets, according to the gland being considered A neutral mucin was demonstrated [16] in filamentous bodies of human salivary glands, which are morphologically indistinguishable from those observed here At the light microscope level, however, previous studies on human BU glands [38] were not able to show histochemical differences between filamentous bodies and mucous droplets in which an acidic mucin was demonstrated On the other hand, a lack of reactivity for BGS is observed in these bodies of BU glands [42,45], as well as in those of human salivary glands [7] It appears that their filamentous content is discharged into the lumen after fusion with the mucus of the secretory droplets The same process is also reported in the submucosal glands of the human nasal sinuses [56] and in human salivary glands [36,39]

Cells in an early phase of their secretory cycle show ovoidal nuclei and mucous droplets that are generally smaller and localized in the apical cytoplasm [44] The Golgi apparatus is well developed and with the osmium maceration method [34,55] its internal 3D ultrastructure can be easily seen (Fig 7) With this method many mitochondria exhibit cristae that are tubular in shape (Fig 7) It must be noted that some authors [21,58] maintain that in rat tissues mitochondria studied with the same method exhibit mostly tubular cristae Filamentous bodies are also present and generally have a supranuclear position

Rare cells filled with mitochondria and of unknown function are observed both by TEM and SEM among secretory mucous cells This is a finding also common with human epididymis [32]

Myoepithelial cells (mec) are placed between the basal lamina and the secretory cells in tubules and alveoli (Fig 5) They do not form a continuous layer around parenchymal cells, since cytoplasmic processes of the latter reach the basal lamina at many points By TEM mec appear very thin and often with flattened nuclei (Fig 5) Their cytoplasm is filled with microfilaments, and numerous dense bodies are distributed among them (Fig 5) On the stromal side they show a lot of focal densities, probably corresponding to hemidesmosomes, whereas on the parenchymal side they are joined to secretory cells by means of desmosomes Their basal contour may be only slight wavy or show irregular thin processes, which project toward the connective tissue In any case, the basal lamina follows the plasmalemma point by point

Mec of Cowper s glands have been described by SEM in the Japanese monkey [29], where they exhibit an elongated, belt- or spindle-shaped body with short processes interdigitating with those of adjacent cells On the other hand, mec of human Cowper s glands are hardly recognizable at SEM After digestion of the basal lamina, in fact, the surface of secretory endpieces appears covered with numerous thin parallel processes (Fig 8), which intermingle so intricately that it is not possible to define the exact outline of each cell nor to distinguish the mec from the secretory cells As observed by TEM, processes of secretory

←

Fig 5 TEM of bulbourethral gland Mature mucous cells crowded with secretory droplets often coalescing (arrows) Many droplets exhibit a small dense spherule Note the irregularly shaped filamentous bodies which in some places are seen fusing with mucous droplets (small arrows) A portion of myoepithelial cell (mec) with a dense filamentous cytoplasm is seen in between the basal lamina and the secretory cells G = Golgi apparatus L = lumen (×7700)

Fig 6 SEM of bulbourethral gland A filamentous body seen after the osmium maceration procedure (×19 800)

Fig 7 SEM osmium maceration method of bulbourethral gland 3D image of a well developed Golgi apparatus Some mitochondria (arrows) with tubular cristae are also present (×19 800)

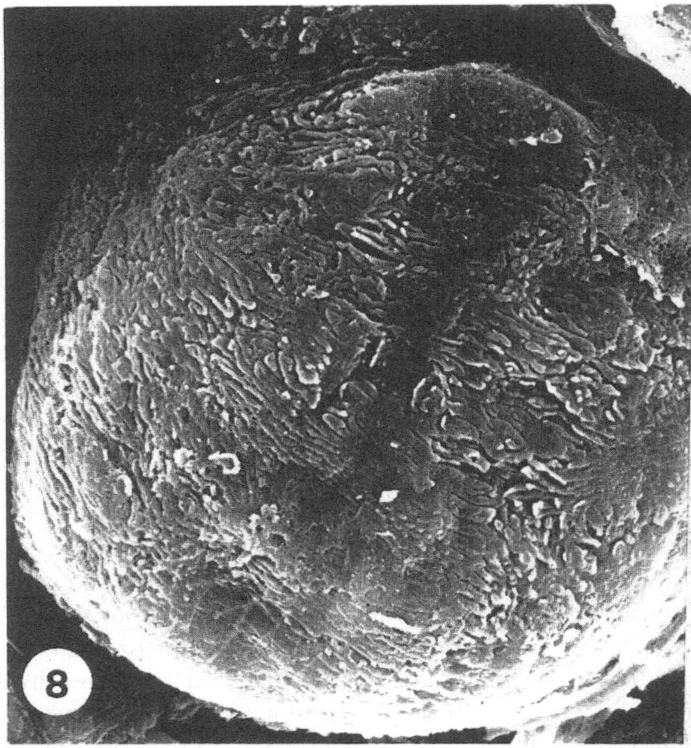
8

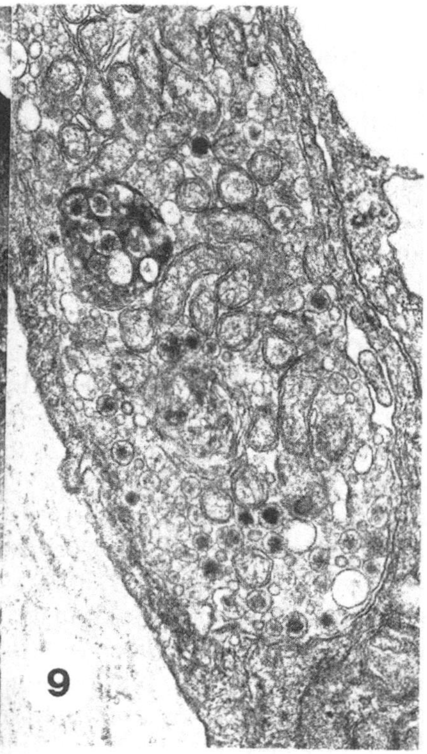
9

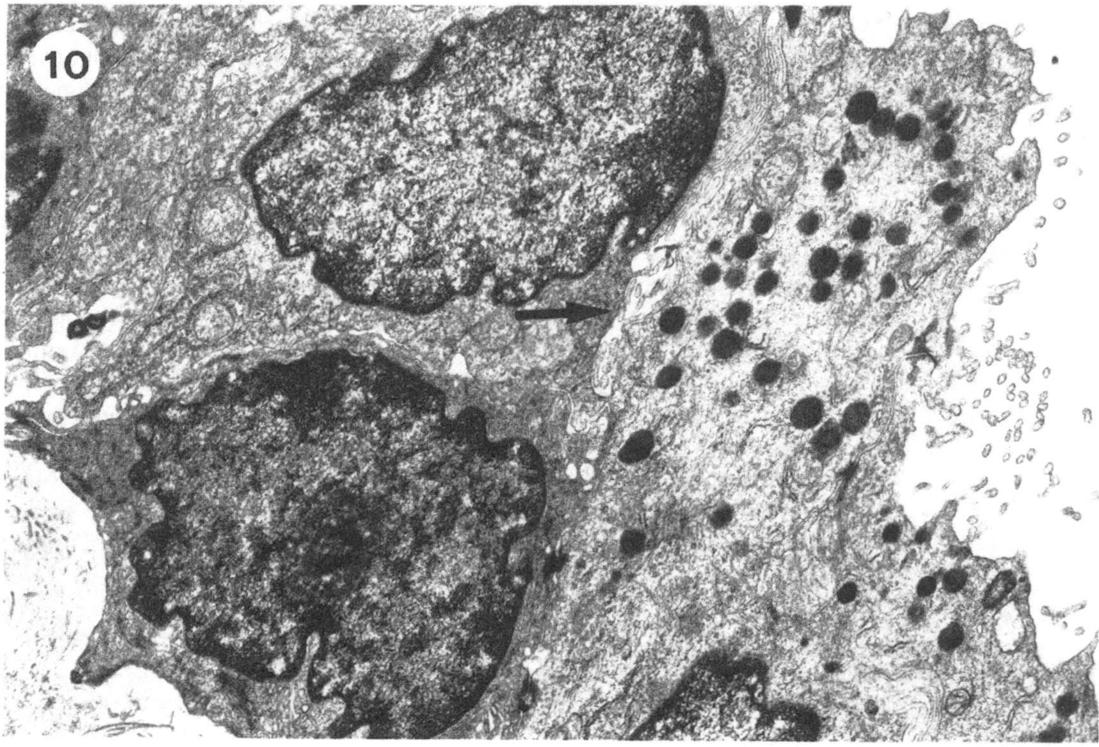
10

cells reach the basal lamina and frequently show an irregular stromal contour, similar to that of adjacent myoepithelial cells.

Free mononuclear cells are often observed within the epithelium. They are identified as immunocompetent cells [27], but their role in defense against local infections is still unclear. Some plasmacells are also found in the lamina propria of the connective tissue.

In a few instances, in all the portions of human BU glands (MED included), we have observed with TEM rare basally placed cells with vesicles of various sizes and densities (Fig. 9). Although far less numerous, these cells strongly resemble the endocrinelike cells present in the secretory epithelium of human urethral glands.

2.2. *Excretory Portion*

The transition between the secretory and excretory portion is gradual, and mucous cells, isolated or in small groups, are encountered among ductal cells as well. The small ducts (ductuli), ampullae, and excretory ducts are lined by a simple epithelium with flattened, cuboidal, or columnar cells that, particularly in excretory ducts, are disposed in a pseudostratified manner. The cellular apex is rich in microvilli and sometimes bulges into the lumen [44]. The nucleus often has an irregular profile and may exhibit some deep indentations. A well-developed nucleolus is frequently observed. Irregular short cisternae of the RER are sparse or are disposed around mitochondria that are quite numerous and scattered in the cytoplasm. Many free ribosomes are also present. A small Golgi apparatus is generally placed in the proximity of the nucleus. Thin mec processes are sometimes recognizable around ductal cells.

The intercellular spaces are narrow in tracts where desmosomes are seen connecting adjacent ductal cells, but at certain sites (Fig. 10) they enlarge to form intercellular channels into which many thin cytoplasmic folds project. Furthermore, the basolateral contours of these cells appear, by TEM, to be quite irregular with extensive interdigitations of frondlike cellular processes [44]. The intercellular dilated channels and folded cell membranes are considered to be devices for intercellular and transepithelial transport in the type I cells of the periurethral glandular complex of the male water buffalo [1]. It is interesting to note that in water buffalo bulbourethral glands, the type I cells are found preferentially near the ductular collecting cavities. Therefore, it is possible to speculate that a similar function may also be ascribed to the analogous ductal cells of human Cowper's glands.

A number of ductal cells contain dense rounded granules (Fig. 10), which are membrane bounded, do not coalesce, and seem to be secreted by an exocytotic mechanism. They are few in number and may be scattered throughout the cell or placed in the apical cytoplasm (Fig. 10). The cytoplasmic organelles are similar to those of other ductal cells. Since we have never found filamentous bodies in these cells, it seems improbable that they represent an immature stage of mucous cells. On the other hand, cells with dense granules cannot be considered to be serous cells because they possess a synthetic apparatus (i.e., RER, Golgi) that is scarcely developed, unlike those of typical serous cells [39].

By SEM the MED (Fig. 11) appears lined by a cylindrical stratified epithelium. Cells resting on the basal lamina are cuboidal and have, at TEM, a dark cytoplasm with mitochondria and a few other organelles [42]. In the middle and superficial layers of the epithelium, the cells, which are tall and elongated, possess more abundant organelles and have numerous lateral folds (Fig. 11), which project into dilated intercellular spaces. Seen from the lumen by SEM, apices of MED

←

Fig 8 SEM of bulbourethral gland A secretory tubule seen after digestion of the basal lamina Its surface exhibits many interdigitating processes belonging to mec and secretory cells (×4400)

Fig 9 TEM of bulbourethral gland Portion of an endocrinelike cell with rounded vesicles of different size, sometimes containing a dense core (×30,800)

Fig 10 TEM of bulbourethral gland ductal cells with dense rounded granules in their apical cytoplasm The arrow indicates the section of an intercellular channel into which many thin cytoplasmic folds project (×15,400)

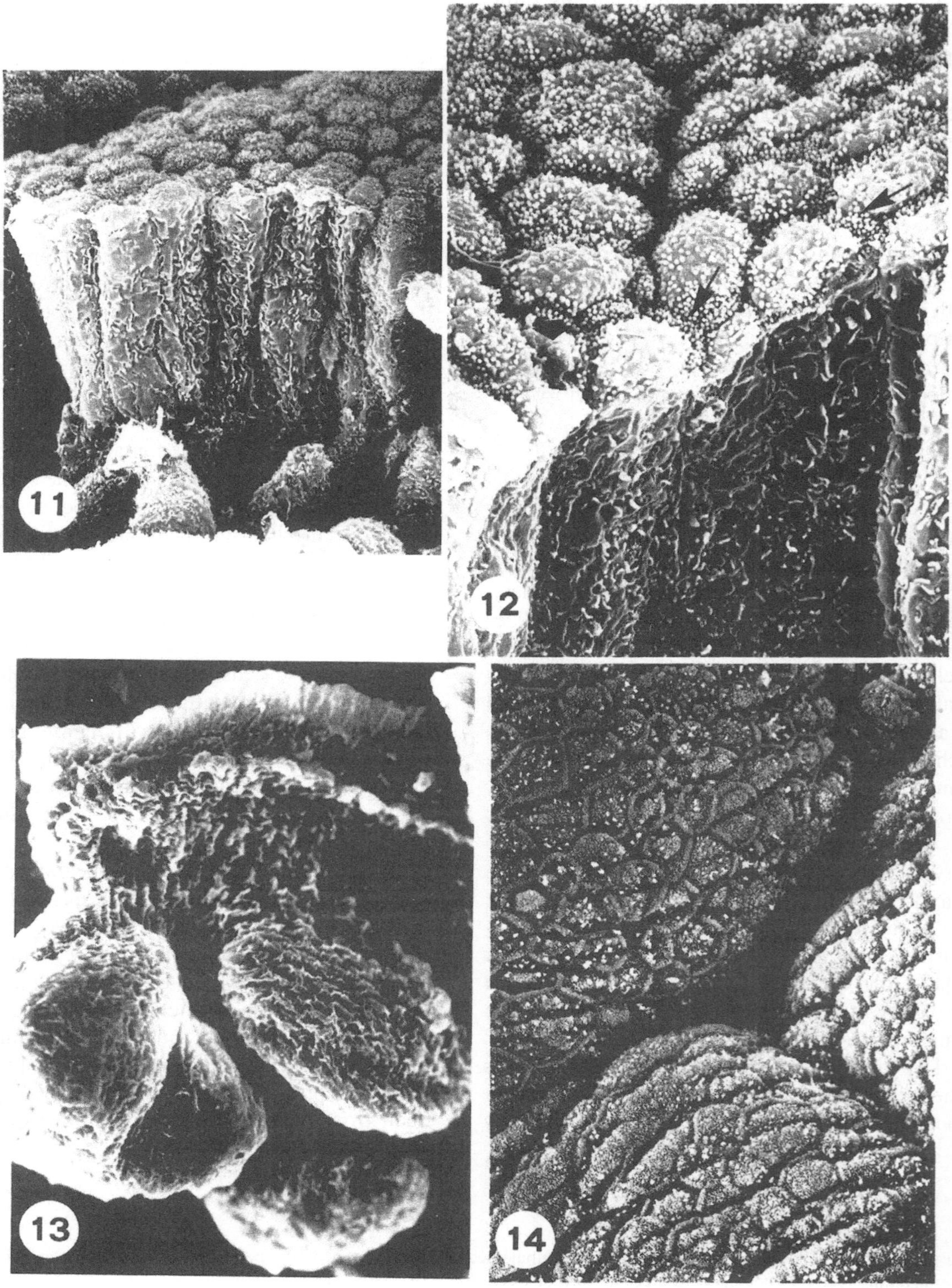
11
12
13
14

superficial cells show sparse microvillosities, among which cytoplasmic protrusions are seen (Fig. 12). The cell boundaries appear prominent and are accentuated by closely disposed microvilli (Fig. 12). By TEM these cells [42] show numerous mitochondria, a well-developed Golgi apparatus, and short profiles of rough endoplasmic reticulum. Characteristically, their cytoplasm contains small secretory granules, whose appearance and density vary greatly [42]. Some granules are homogenous with clear or moderately dense matrix, and others show a small dark eccentric body or have a larger electron-dense portion. Though some cells exhibit only one kind of secretory granules, most cells house granules with different substructures [42]. Our standard histochemical tests, carried out at the light microscopic (LM) level, show that the apical zone of superficial cells contain an acidic mucin rich in carboxylic groups, similar to that present in mucous cells of the human BU [51] and urethral [46,50] glands. On the other hand, the ultrastructural appearances of granules of MED superficial cells seem to be typical. These granules, in fact, differ morphologically not only from mucous droplets and ductal secretory granules of BU glands (previously described in this paper), but also from those of mucus-secreting cells of human Bartholin gland ducts [48]. Although distinctly smaller, they bear a certain resemblance to the secretory granules of human urethral glands (see forward). Cells of the latter glands, however, contain many filamentous bodies, which we are unable to find in cells of bulbourethral MED. Other histochemical studies are needed, but these results may also suggest that the MED adds some peculiar secretory component to the secretion of BU glands besides those originating from mucous droplets, filamentous bodies, and granules of the ductal cells.

3. Urethral Glands

The human urethral glands, first described by Littré in 1719 [22], are simple or ramified tubulo-alveolar glands present all along the penile urethra but particular numerous in its superior wall. There are also occasional secretory cells, isolated or in groups, interspersed within the epithelial lining of the urethra. They originate from the endoderm of the urogenital sinus [9] and seem to be androgen dependent organs [5]. Like the bulbourethral, the urethral glands contribute with their secretion to the first fraction of the human ejaculate, where they mix with the prostatic fluid [26].

By SEM, after removal of extracellular material, the glands look like tubulo-alveolar outpocketings of the cavernous urethral epithelium (Fig. 13). Their stromal surface is slightly wavy and exhibits small folds. No myoepithelial cells are found. The glandular endpieces open into the urethral lumen through a narrow canal whose outlet appears as a deep invagination of the urethral lining (Fig. 14).

By TEM the epithelium of the urethral glands is generally pseudostratified with principal exocrine cells (Figs. 15 and 16) and small basal cells (Fig. 17). Endocrinelike cells, resting on the basal lamina, are also observed (Figs. 18 and 19). In fractured specimens, by SEM, the principal cells appear tall and columnar in shape, their lateral surfaces exhibit thin irregular folds, and the apices are covered by a variable number of short microvilli. At TEM these cells are filled, in their supranuclear cytoplasm, with secretory granules that exhibit different morphological features (Fig. 15). Usually they contain an irregular, globular dense mass surrounded by a clear portion with granulo-fibrillar material. Sometimes the dark portion occupies almost the

←

Fig 11 SEM of epithelium of the bulbourethral gland main excretory duct (MED) seen after exposure of lateral surfaces of adjacent cells Cells of the superficial layer show numerous lateral folds disposed at random (×1430)

Fig 12 SEM of the bulbourethral gland Superficial cells of MED seen from the lumen An apical protrusion is indicated (arrowhead) Note the prominent cell boundaries marked by tightly packed microvilli (arrows) (×4400)

Fig 13 SEM of urethral glands seen from the stromal side following removal of the connective tissue and basal lamina The upper portion of the figure shows the epithelium of the urethra (×700)

Fig 14 SEM of deep invagination of the urethral epithelium corresponding to the outlet of a urethral gland The apexes of superficial cells are marked by protruding polygonal lines covered with microvilli (×880)

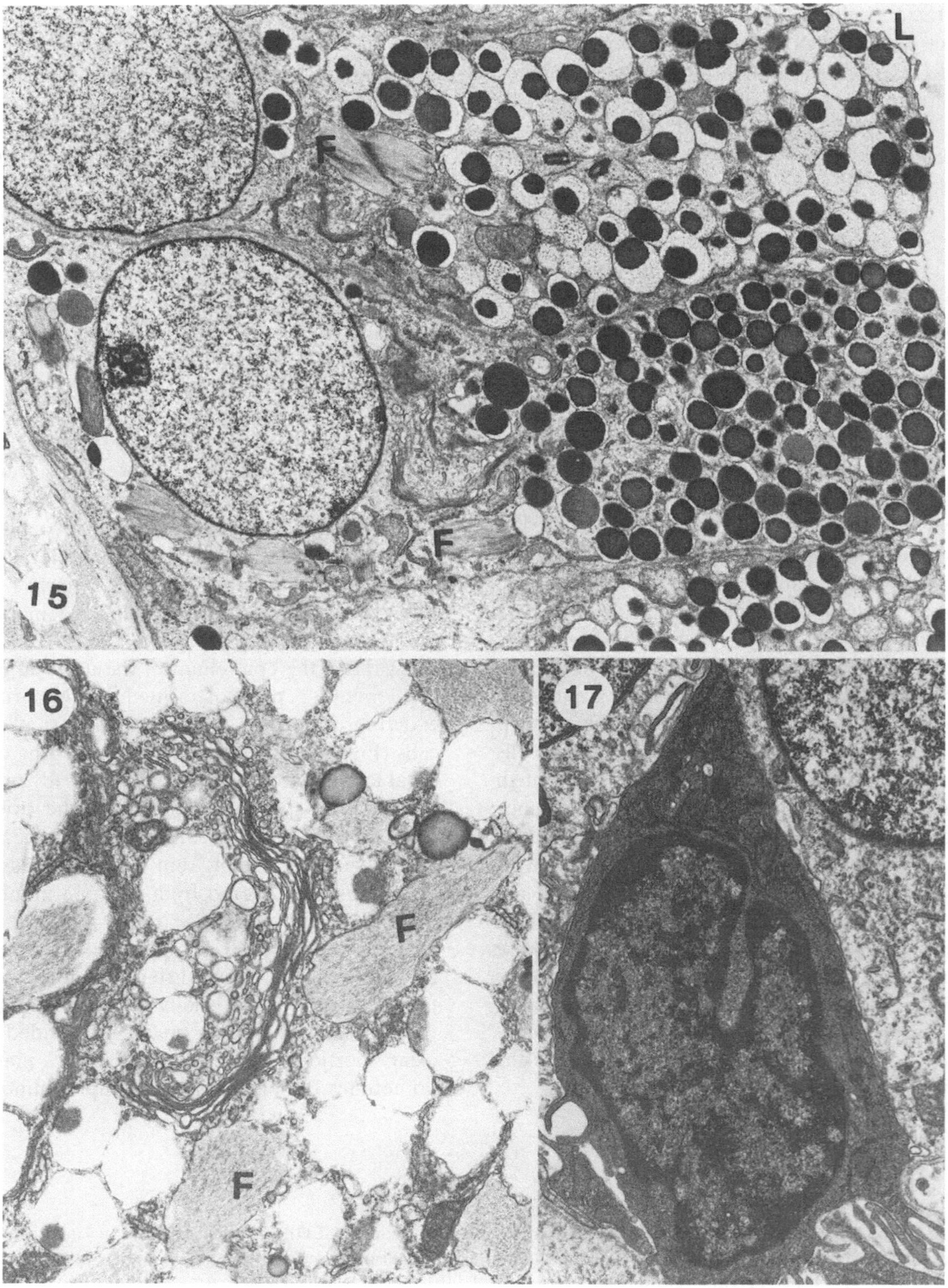

Fig. 15. TEM of principal cells of urethral glands. F = filamentous bodies; L = lumen (×7700).
Fig. 16. TEM of urethral gland. Golgi apparatus and filamentous bodies in a principal cell. F = filamentous bodies (×15,400).
Fig. 17. TEM of urethral gland. Basal cell, which in this case exhibits a dark cytoplasm (×15,400).

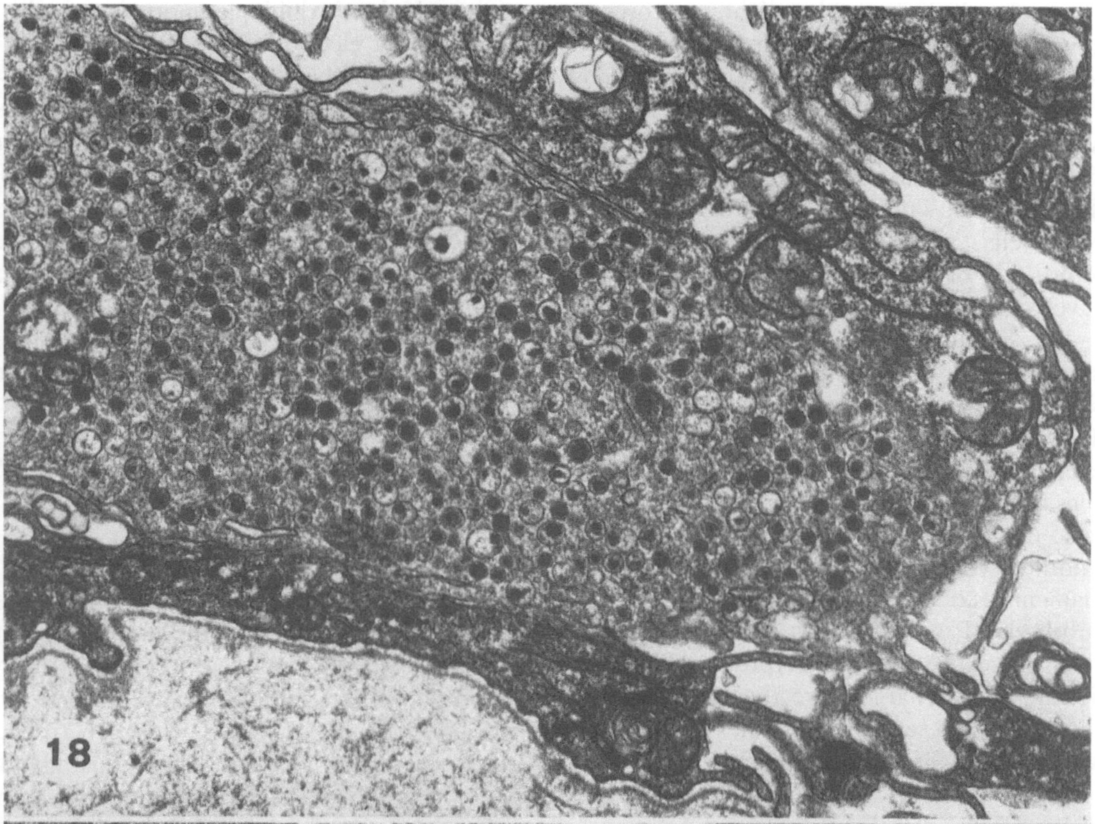

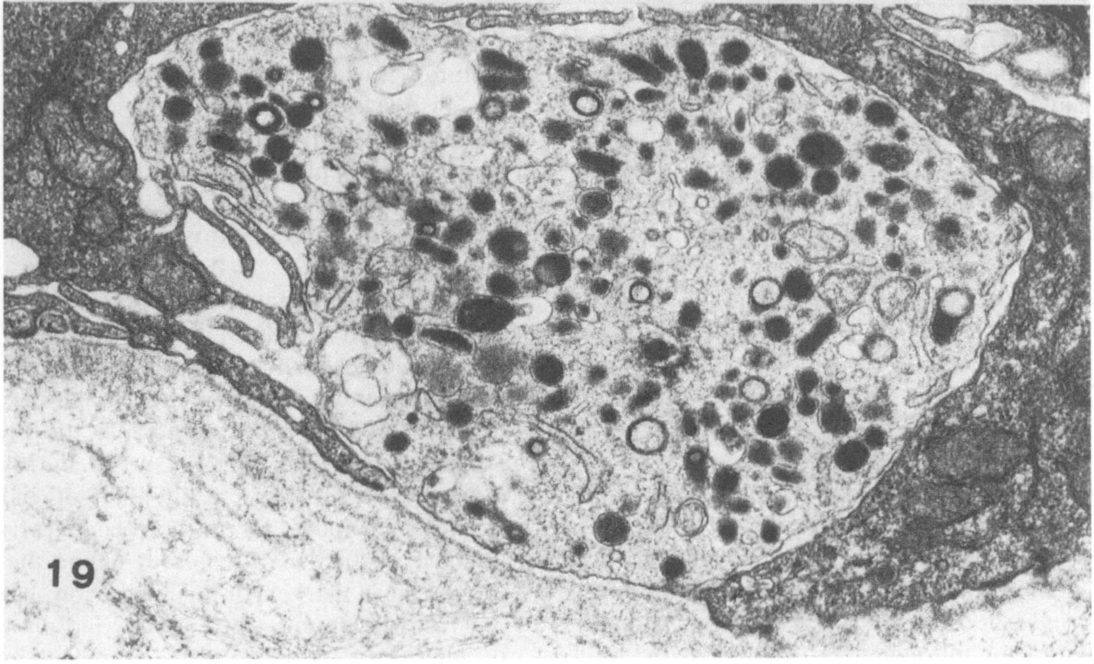

Fig 18 TEM of urethral gland Portion of an endocrinelike cell with mostly rounded granules containing a dense core (×24 000)

Fig 19 TEM of urethral gland Portion of an endocrinelike cell showing pleomorphic granules with various densities (×31 000)

entire granule, and sometimes it is very small. An histochemical study by light microscopy demonstrated [50] that these granules contain an acidic glycoprotein. Even if the urethral glands are considered of the mucous type [19], their secretory granules do not accumulate to the extent characteristic of mucous glands and show less tendency to fuse with each other than in typical mucous cells, such as, for example, mature secretory cells of bulbourethral glands. As a rule, however, the darker granules do not coalesce, while the lighter ones often fuse their limiting membranes at several points.

Nuclei are generally ovoid and euchromatic with an evident nucleolus (Fig. 15). A well-developed Golgi apparatus (Fig. 16) and scattered profiles of RER, often surrounding mitochondria, are also observed.

Another secretory component is represented by filamentous bodies (Figs. 15 and 16) similar to those observed in BU glands and other human mucous glands. As described previously, these bodies are not discharged directly into the lumen but coalesce with secretory granules before exocytosis. Large aggregates of filamentous bodies and lipid droplets are sometimes noticed in the basal cytoplasm.

In a few instances we have found cells endowed only with dark granules and apparently devoid of filamentous bodies. The hypothesis that these cells might represent another cellular type is tempting but no proof is currently available to verify this. The basal cells (Fig. 17) are flattened with a filamentous cytoplasm and their nucleus has clumps of heterochromatin. Their plasmalemma exhibits short, irregular folds but lacks the tapering processes typical of myoepithelial cells.

The endocrinelike (EL) cells (Figs. 18 and 19) are more numerous here than in bulbourethral glands. At least in our sections, they are basally oriented and never reach the glandular lumen, that is, appear to be of the closed type. Previous reports on human male urethra [4,10] and prostate [10] demonstrated several types of endocrine-paracrine cells on the basis of the secretory granule morphology and staining characteristics. In urethral glands the EL cells show a variety of small granules of different size and density. Some cells contain a population of mostly rounded granules with a dense core of variable size (Fig. 18), and others exhibit pleomorphic granules (Fig. 19) with an electron-dense core in various positions, eventually surrounded by a lucent halo. Cells with very few small, dense granules are rarely observed. In the absence of histochemical or immunohistochemical data we cannot, at present, give any suggestion as to the function of these cells. However, by analogy with the importance of this kind of cell in the gastrointestinal apparatus in both physiological and pathological conditions, we believe that EL cells of urethral glands may play a significant role as well (see also Chapter 8).

4. Concluding Remarks

Findings reported here demonstrate the cytoarchitecture of the human BU and male urethral glands, organs that, like the prostate gland, are functionally connected with both the urinary and reproductive systems. In general, secretory cells of both glands seem to be closely related to the cells of other human mucous glands, as demonstrated, *inter alia*, by the presence of the filamentous bodies and their ability to secrete BGS. A more detailed analysis of their cytological features, however, shows that secretory cells of the two glands bear distinctive characteristics. Moreover, the BU glands, besides the mucous and the myoepithelial cells, house, especially in their excretory portion, a population of cells endowed with dark secretory granules of unknown nature.

A finding not previously reported is the presence in both glands of endocrine cells. These cells, which seem to be more numerous in the urethral glands, appear quite similar to those demonstrated by other authors in the prostate glands and urethral lining. Due to the obvious difficulty in obtaining a number of bioptical specimens suitable for ultracytochemical study, we have so far been unable to define the main cytochemical markers of their secretion. Even so, our results demonstrate the many morphological peculiarities of these glands, even with respect to the homologous organs of closely related mammals. Their morphological features are at variance with those of the human prostate, a gland with which they also share an endodermal origin and sensitivity to sex hormons. Thus, a better understanding of their cytophysiology may be useful not only to clarify the functional meaning of their contribution to human semen, but also to increase our understanding of why their pathology is so different from that of the prostate gland.

Acknowledgments

This work was supported by grants from Consiglio Nazionale delle Ricerche and Ministero dell'Università e della Ricerca Scientifica e Tecnologica. We thank Mrs. Silvana Bernardini Foddis and Mr. Alessandro Cadau for their valuable technical assistance.

References

1 Abou-Elmagd A, Wrobel KH The periurethral glandular complex in the water buffalo An ultrastructural, histological and lectin-histochemical study Arch Histol Cytol 52 501–512, 1989
2 Aumuller G Prostate Gland and Seminal Vesicles Berlin Springer, 1979
3 Braus H Uber den feineren Bau der Glandula bulbourethralis (Cowperschen Druse) des Menschen Anat Anz 17 381–397, 1900
4 Casanova S, Corrado F, Vignoli G Endocrine-like cells in the epithelium of the human male urethra J Submicrosc Cytol 6 435–438, 1974
5 Coffey DS Androgen action and the sex accessory tissues In The Physiology of Reproduction E Knobil, JD Neil (eds) New York Raven Press, 1988, pp 1081–1119
6 Cossu M, Marcello MF, Usai E, Testa Riva F, Riva A Fine structure of the epithelium of the human ejaculatory duct Acta Anat 116 225–233, 1983
7 Cossu M, Riva A, Lantini MS Subcellular localization of blood group substances ABH in human salivary glands J Histochem Cytochem 38 1165–1172, 1990
8 Cowdry EV Special Cytology, Vol III New York Hoeber, 1932
9 De Kretser DM, Temple-Smith PD, Kerr JB Disturbance in Male Fertility Bandhauer K, Frich J (eds) Berlin Springer, 1982
10 Di Sant'Agnese PA, De Mesy Jensen KL Endocrine-paracrine cells of the prostate and prostatic urethra An ultrastructural study Hum Pathol 15 1034–1041, 1984
11 Evan AP, Dail WG, Damrose D, Palmer G Scanning electron microscopy of cell surfaces following removal of extracellular material Anat Rec 185 435–446, 1976
12 Feagans WM, Belt WD, Sheridan MN Fine structure of the acinar cell in the hamster bulbourethral gland Acta Anat 52 273–281, 1963
13 Gattone V II, Conforti J A method for obtaining lateral surfaces of renal tubular cells for scanning electron microscopy J Electr Microsc Techn 2 283–284, 1985
14 Geuze JJ, Slot JW Synthesis and secretion of glycoprotein in rat bulbourethral (Cowper's) glands II Modes of mucus secretion after stimulation by copulation Am J Anat 152 391–418, 1978
15 Grzycki S, Latalski M Observations on the fine structure of rat bulbourethral gland cell Z Mikrosk Anat Forsch 80 191–202, 1969
16 Harrison JD, Auger DW, Paterson KL, Rowley PS A Mucin histochemistry of submandibular and parotid salivary glands of man Light and electron microscopy Histochem J 19 555–564, 1987
17 Hellgren L, Mylius E, Vincent J The ultrastructure of the human bulbourethral gland J Submicrosc Cytol 14 683–689, 1982
18 Hoffer AP The ultrastructure of the ductus deferens in man Bio Reprod 14 425–433, 1976
19 Holbhuber KJ Histochemische Untersuchungen am Sekret der Urethraldrusen bei Mensch und einigen Saugern Acta Histochem 33 331–346, 1969
20 Holm-Nielsen E The bulbourethral gland of the rat Fine structure and histochemistry Anat Anz 139 254–263, 1976
21 Lea PJ, Hollenberg MJ Mitochondrial structure revealed by high-resolution scanning electron microscopy Am J Anat 184 245–257, 1989
22 Littre A Description de l'uretre de l'homme Hist Acad Sci Ann 1700 (Paris) 1700 311–316, 1719
23 Low FN Microdissection by ultrasonication for scanning electron microscopy In Cells and Tissues A Three Dimensional Approach by Modern Techniques in Microscopy PM Motta (ed) New York Alan R Liss, 1989, pp 571–580
24 Low FN, McClugage SG Jr Microdissection by ultrasonication Scanning electron microscopy of the epithelial basal lamina of the alimentary canal in the rat Am J Anat 169 137–147, 1984
25 Maggioni A, Caggiati A, Macchiarelli G Scanning electron microscopy of microvessels and perivascular cells in different organs after KOH digestion In Cells and Tissues A Three Dimensional Approach by Modern Techniques in Microscopy PM Motta (ed) New York Alan R Liss, 1989, pp 469–474
26 Mann T, Lutwak-Mann C Male Reproductive Function and Semen Berlin Springer-Verlag, 1981
27 Migliari R, Riva A, Lantini MS, Melis M, Usai E Diffuse Lymphoid tissue associated with the human bulbourethral gland An immunohistologic characterization J Androl 13 337–341, 1992
28 Miller BS, Woods RI, Bohlen HG, Evan AP A new morphological procedure of viewing microvessels A scanning electron microscopic study of the vasculature of the small intestine Anat Rec 203 493–503, 1982
29 Murakami M, Sugita A, Abe J, Hamasaki M, Shimada T SEM observation of some exocrine glands, with special reference to configuration of the associated myoepithelial cells Biomed Res 2(Suppl) 99–102, 1981
30 Nogueira JC Estudo histologico e ultramicroscopico da

glandula bulbouretral de gato (*Felis domestica*) adulto Arg Esc Vet 22 175–177, 1970
31 Orlandini GE, Holstein AF La differenziazione e la progressione degli spermatozoi nell'uomo Arch Ital Anat Embriol S91 11–39, 1986
32 Palacios J, Regadera J, Nistal M, Paniagua R Apical mitochondria-rich cells in the human epididymis An ultrastructural, enzymohistochemical, and immunohistochemical study Anat Rec 231 82–88, 1991
33 Riva A Fine structure of human seminal vesicle epithelium J Anat 102 71–86, 1967
34 Riva A, Congiu T, Faa G The application of the OsO_4 maceration method to the study of human bioptic material A procedure avoiding freeze-fracture Microsc Res Techn 26 526–527, 1993
35 Riva A, Lantini MS, Migliari R, Scarpa R, Cossu M A correlative TEM-SEM study of the human urethral glands Bull Assoc Anat 75 73–76, 1991
36 Riva A, Lantini MS, Testa Riva F Normal human salivary glands In Ultrastructure of the Extraparietal Glands of the Digestive Tract PM Motta (ed) Boston Kluwer Academic, 1989, pp 53–74
37 Riva A, Mallardi V, Lantini MS, Valentino L, Testa Riva F 3D microanatomy of human parotid gland Bull Assoc Anat 75 171–175, 1991
38 Riva A, Sirigu P, Testa Riva F, Usai E Fine structure and histochemistry of epithelial cells of the human bulbourethral glands Acta Anat 111 125–126, 1981
39 Riva A, Tandler B Salivari ghiandole In Enciclopedia Medica Italiana, Vol 13, 2nd ed Firenze Utet-Sansoni Edizioni Scientifiche, 1986, pp 1729–1744
40 Riva A, Tandler B, Testa Riva F Ultrastructural observations on human sublingual gland Am J Anat 181 385–392, 1988
41 Riva A, Testa Riva F, Usai E, Cossu M The ampulla ductus deferentis in man, as viewed by SEM and TEM Arch Androl 8 157–164, 1982
42 Riva A, Usai E, Cossu M, Lantini MS, Scarpa R, Testa-Riva F Ultrastructure of human bulbourethral glands and of their main excretory ducts Arch Androl 24 177–184, 1990
43 Riva A, Usai E, Cossu M, Scarpa R, Testa Riva F Anatomia ultrastrutturale delle ghiandole annesse all'apparato genitale dell'uomo In Attualita in Andrologia R Giorgino, G Abbaticchio (eds) Bologna Monduzzi Editore, 1984, pp 1–12
44 Riva A, Usai E, Cossu M, Scarpa R, Testa Riva F The human bulbourethral glands A transmission electron microscopy and scanning electron microscopy study J Androl 9 133–141, 1988
45 Riva A, Usai E, Scarpa R, Cossu M, Lantini MS Fine structure of the accessory glands of the human male genital tract In Developments in Ultrastructure of Reproduction Progress in Clinical and Biological Research, Vol 296 PM Motta (ed) New York Alan R Liss, 1989, pp 233–240
46 Riva A, Usai E, Scarpa R, Lantini MS, Valentino L, Testa Riva F Fine structure of human urethral glands In IV International Congress of Andrology, Miniposters Serono Symposium Review M Serio (ed) Rome Ares-Serono Symposia, 1989, p 331
47 Riva A, Zaccheo D, Testa Riva F A SEM study of the human parotid and submandibular glands Proceedings of the XIth International Congress on Electron Microscopy, Kyoto, 1986, pp 2863–2864
48 Rorat E, Ferenczy A, Richart RM Human Bartholin gland, duct and duct cyst Arch Pathol 99 367–374, 1975
49 Schaffer J Beitrage zur Histologie menschlicher Organe VIII Glandula bulbo-urethralis (Cowper) und vestibularis major (Bartholini) Sitzgsberg Akad Wiss Wien, Math-Naturwiss 1915–1917, K1 III 126 27–45
50 Sirigu P, Turno F, Perra MT, Usai E, Hafez ESE Histochemistry of human urethral glands Arch Androl 26 43–51, 1991
51 Sirigu P, Turno F, Usai E, Perra MT Histochemical study of the human bulbourethral (Cowper's) glands Andrologia 25 293–299, 1993
52 Spring-Mills E, Hafez ESE The bulbourethral glands In Male Accessory Sex Glands E Spring-Mills, ESE Hafez (eds) Amsterdam North Holland, Elsevier, 1980, pp 93–99
53 Stieve H Die Bulbourethraldruse In Handbuch der mikroskopischen Anatomie des Menschen, Vol VII W Mollendorf (ed) Berlin Springer-Verlag, 1930, pp 272–278
54 Takahashi-Iwanaga H, Fujita T Application of an NaOH macerating method to a scanning electron microscopic observation of Ito cells in the rat liver Arch Histol Jpn 49 349–357, 1986
55 Tanaka K, Mitshuishima A A preparation method for observing intracellular structures by scanning electron microscopy J Microsc 133 213–222, 1984
56 Vidic B, Tandler B Ultrastructure of the secretory cells of the submucosal glands in the human maxillary sinuses J Morphol 150 167–182, 1976
57 Williams-Ashman HG Perspectives in the male sexual physiology of eutherian mammals In Physiology of Reproduction E Knobil, J Neill (eds) New York Raven Press 1988, pp 727–775
58 Winslow JL, Hollenberg MJ, Lea PJ Resolution limit of serial sections for 3D reconstruction of tubular cristae in rat liver mitochondria J Electron Microsc Techn 18 241–248, 1991
59 Wrobel KH Morphologische Untersuchungen an der Glandula bulbourethralis der Katze Z Zellforsch 101 607–620, 1969
60 Wrobel KH Studies on the ultrastructure and histochemistry of the bulbourethral gland in the goat Z Zellforsch 108 582–596, 1970

CHAPTER 10

ABH and Lewis Antigens in Human Male Accessory Sex Glands

MARGHERITA COSSU, MARIA SERENELLA LANTINI, & ROBERTO MIGLIARI

1. Introduction

Antigenic properties of human semen are due to sperm surface antigens produced by germinal cells during spermatogenesis (intrinsic antigens) and to those of seminal plasma. The latter are in part serum proteins, in part substances common to semen and other body fluids, and in part seminal plasma-specific antigens [15]. They are supplied by the male accessory sex organs and can be absorbed on the sperm surface (sperm-coating antigens). An example of sperm-coating antigens is ABH antigens, first found on spermatozoa by Landsteiner and Levine [14] and in seminal plasma by Edwards et al. [6]. ABH antigens are expressed in erythrocytes and in the cell membranes of endothelia and of a variety of tissues, and enter in the composition of several secretions such as saliva, milk, tears, and digestive juices [22]. Their antigenic determinants consist of a few sugars linked to a precursor molecule by distinct glycosyltransferases coded by the ABO, H, and Se genes [19]. Two α-2-L fucosyltransferases (coded by the Se and H genes) lead to H antigen formation; the α-3-N acetylgalactosaminyltransferase (coded by the A gene) converts H into A antigen; the α-3-D galactosyltransferase (coded by the B gene) converts H into B antigen. In addition, the ABO system is strictly related to the Lewis system, which controls the expression of Le-a and Le-b antigens in tissues and secretions. The Le gene codes for a α-4-L fucosyltransferase, which adds a fucose to H substance or to its precursor, giving rise to Le-b or Le-a substances, respectively. Figure 1 illustrates the substrates and enzymes involved in the synthesis of ABH and Lewis antigens; Figure 2 summarizes the interactions between ABO, Se, and Lewis systems. Individuals are grouped into secretors and nonsecretors based upon the presence or not of ABH substances in their saliva. The secretor status is routinely determined testing the Le-b antigen in blood and saliva, in that it can be exclusively found in secretors, although a minority of them lacking Le-b exists (Fig. 2).

Genetic control of the expression of ABH and related antigens has been proposed to vary, with some exceptions, according to the embryological origin of each tissue: The ectodermal tissues express them independently on the Se and Le genes, while endodermal derivatives produce ABH and/or Lewis antigens in subjects who inherited the Se and/or Le alleles [18]. Blood group antigen expression also varies in the different developmental stages of embryonic tissues [30], in the different maturative phases of adult tissues [19], and in a number of epithelial tumors, such as carcinomas of the breast, uterus, mouth, prostate, and bladder [5,7,9,10,12,33].

Human semen contains relatively high concentrations of blood group substances, whose secretion is generally ascribed to the prostate and seminal vesicles [1,2,15], although this assumption has not been supported by evidence. A postembedding immunogold staining (IGS) method, standardized in a recent study on salivary glands [4], seemed to be the most reliable to reveal the secretory blood group antigens in human male

Riva, A., Testa Riva, F., and Motta, P.M., (eds.), Ultrastructure of Male Urogenital Glands: Prostate, Seminal Vesicles, Urethral, and Bulbourethral Glands ISBN 0-7923-2800-0

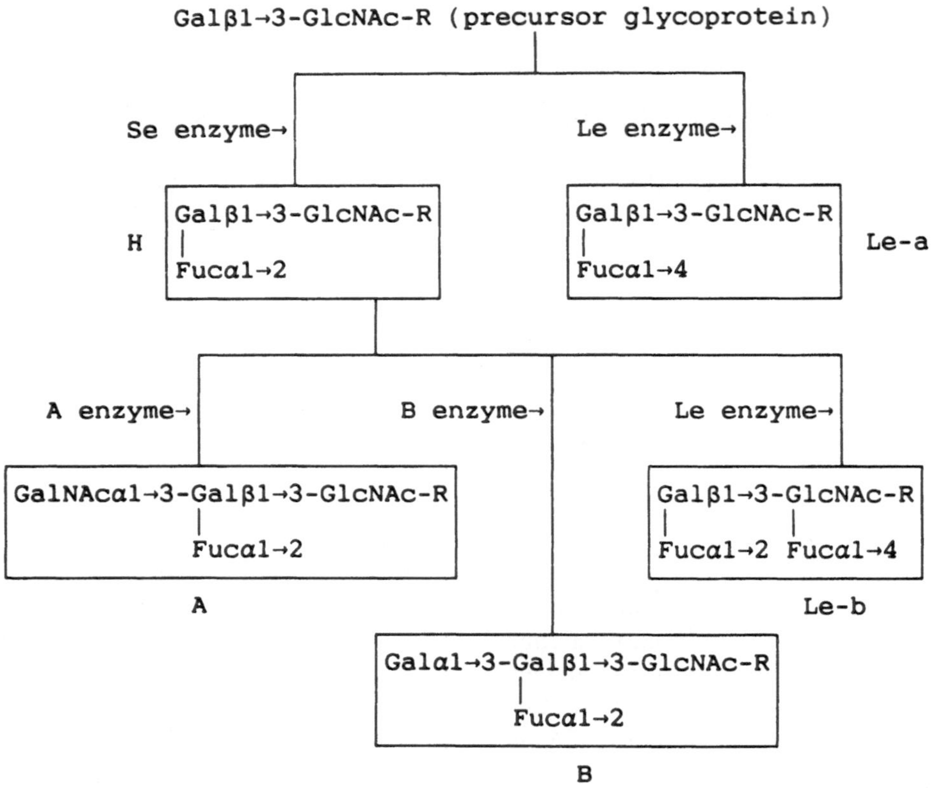

Fig 1 Synthetic pathway for the A, B, H, Le-a, and Le-b antigen formation

genes	Le	le
A, Se	A, H, Le-a, Le-b	A, H
A, se	Le-a	/
B, Se	B, H, Le-a, Le-b	B, H
B, se	Le-a	/
0, Se	H, Le-a, Le-b	H
0, se	Le-a	/

Fig 2 Substances present in secretions depending upon the alleles of the AB0, Se, and Lewis systems inherited

→

Fig 3 Cowper's gland from a type A subject, treated with anti-A antibody Mucous droplets are intensely labeled, while the filamentous bodies (arrowheads) and a myoepithelial cell (me) appear unreactive Gold particle ∅ 30 nm (×7500)
Fig 4 Littre's gland from a type O subject, treated with anti-H antibody Antigen labeling is restricted to the secretory granules, which fill the cytoplasm of principal cells Gold particle ∅ 30 nm (×7500)
Fig 5 Littre's gland from a type B subject, treated with anti-B antibody The endocrine cell (ec) is unreactive Gold particle ∅ 30 nm (×7500)
Fig 6 Mucous cell of Cowper's gland from a type A subject Double labeling of A antigen (gold particle ∅ 30 nm) and Le-b antigen (gold particle ∅ 10 nm) in secretory droplets and Golgi saccules (×18,500)

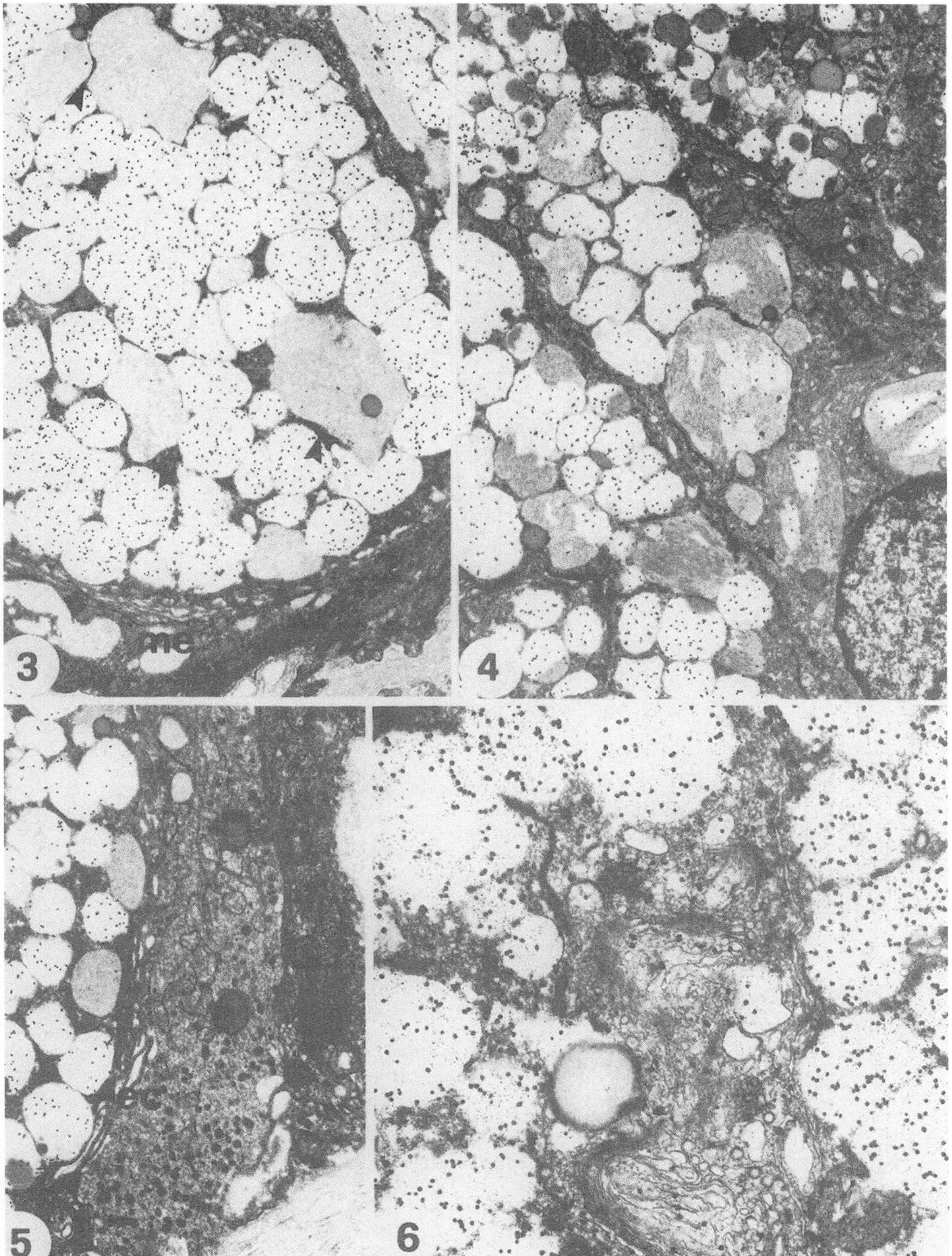
3
me
4
5
ec
6

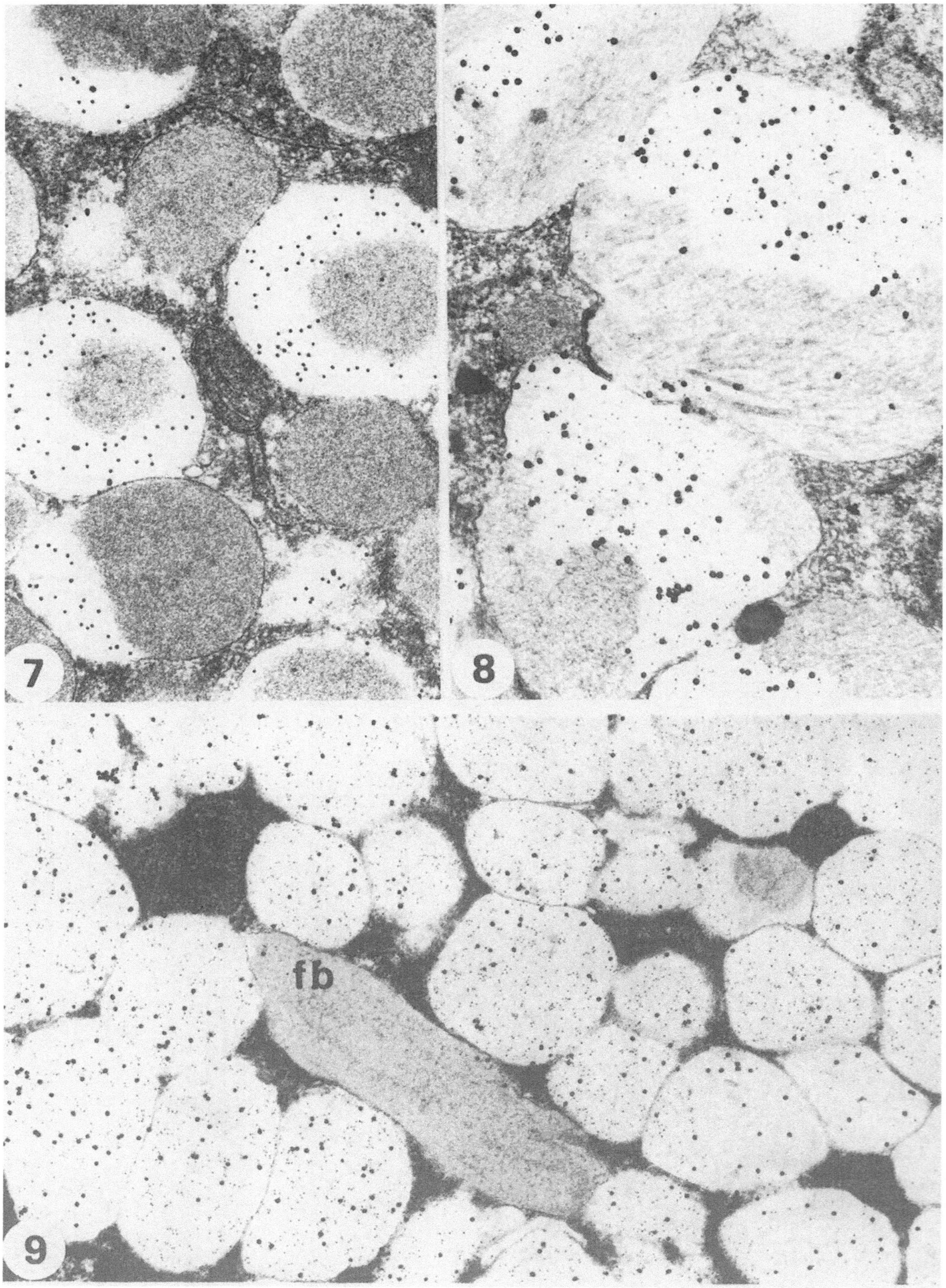
7
8
9
fb

accessory sex glands. This method can be applied on routinely prepared (fixed in half-strength Karnovsky, osmicated, and Epon embedded) samples, with the great advantage of obtaining both optimal ultrastructural tissue preservation and precise intracellular localization of labeling. The results shown here have been obtained by means of this method, using mouse monoclonal antibodies specific for A, B, H, Le-a, and Le-b blood group antigens, and gold conjugated anti-mouse antibodies.

2. Prostate, Seminal Vesicle, and Deferential Ampulla

The belief that seminal blood group antigens are supplied by seminal vesicle and prostate arose when Szulman [29] first found ABH antigens in some prostatic acini and in a few seminal vesicle cells. More recently, demonstration of ABH and Lewis antigens was provided in normal and pathological prostatic parenchyma at the light microscope level [7,31,32,34], but these studies were focused on the blood group antigens as cell surface antigens and their altered expression in cancerous lesions. With the IGS method we found no cell showing ABH or Lewis labeling in prostate, seminal vesicle, and deferential ampulla, although we examined a great number of sections obtained from different zones of each gland. However, the contrast between such results and the above cited data is only apparent if we consider that the IGS method applied on osmicated and Epon embedded tissues selectively stains the secretory blood group antigens, while it does not reveal those associated with the cell surface [3]. Therefore, the absence of labeling with this method does not allow exclusion of the presence of blood group antigens as membrane associated molecules, for their binding sites are probably lost or blocked during sample preparation. On the other hand, failure to reveal labeling in secretory granules suggests that blood group antigens are not secreted by these glands and that the notion that prostate and seminal vesicle are the chief sources of seminal blood group substances must be reevaluated.

3. Bulbourethral (Cowper's) and Urethral (Littré's) Glands

Cowper's and Littré's glands have never been considered as possible sources of seminal antigens until our preliminary data indicated the presence of ABH substances in their secreting cells [23,25, 26]. On the basis of further experiments, we can offer a detailed view of the distribution pattern of the secretory ABH and Lewis antigens in Cowper's and Littré's glands. Blood group substances have been found only in the mucous cells of Cowper's glands and in the principal cells of Littré's glands, while ductal, myoepithelial, endocrine, and other secreting cells are always negative (Figs. 3–5). In positive cells, immunoreactivity is confined to secretory granules and Golgi saccules, while all other cell structures, including filamentous bodies, are completely unstained (Figs. 3–12). Within the granules, immunolabeling is restricted to the pale matrix, and this is especially evident in Littré's gland cells, whose granules have a more evident dark component [23,26] (Figs. 4, 7, and 12). This fine localization of antigen reactivity is still appreciable in those secretory granules fused with filamentous bodies but not completely mixed with them (Figs. 4, 8, and 10). A similar intragranular localization of blood group antigens has been described in the mucous cells of human salivary glands [3,4], where a correspondence between blood group antigens and acidic mucins distribution is likely

←

Fig 7 Principal cell of Littré's gland from a type A subject, treated with anti-A antibody Secretory granules show an unlabeled dark component and a positive pale matrix Gold particle ∅ 15 nm (×32,000)

Fig 8 Principal cell of Littré's gland from a type 0 subject Double labeling of H antigen (gold particle ∅ 30 nm) and Le-b antigen (gold particle ∅ 10 nm) in secretory granules fused with filamentous bodies The filamentous material devoid of labeling and the pale matrix endowed with both antigens are clearly recognizable (×32,000)

Fig 9 Mucous cell of Cowper's gland from a type A subject Double labeling of A antigen (gold particle ∅ 10 nm) and H antigen (gold particle ∅ 30 nm) A antigen appears much more intensely labeled than H fb = filamentous body (×18,000)

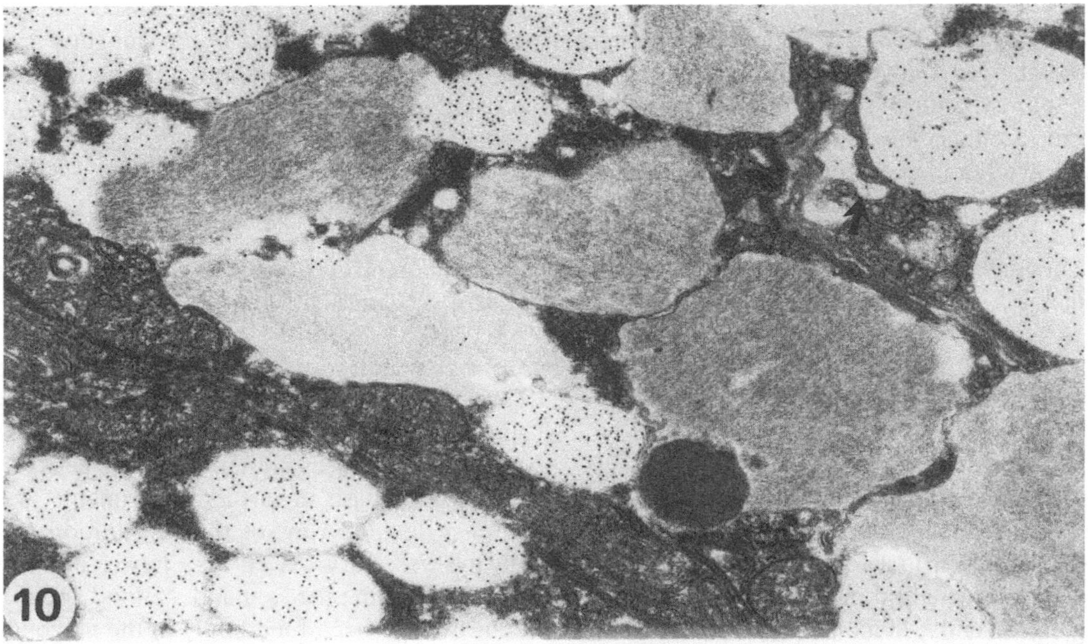
10

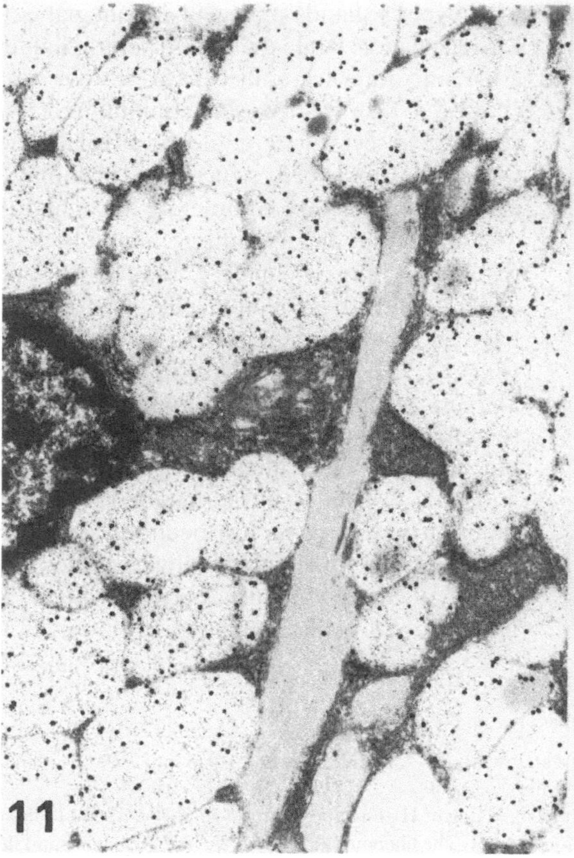
11

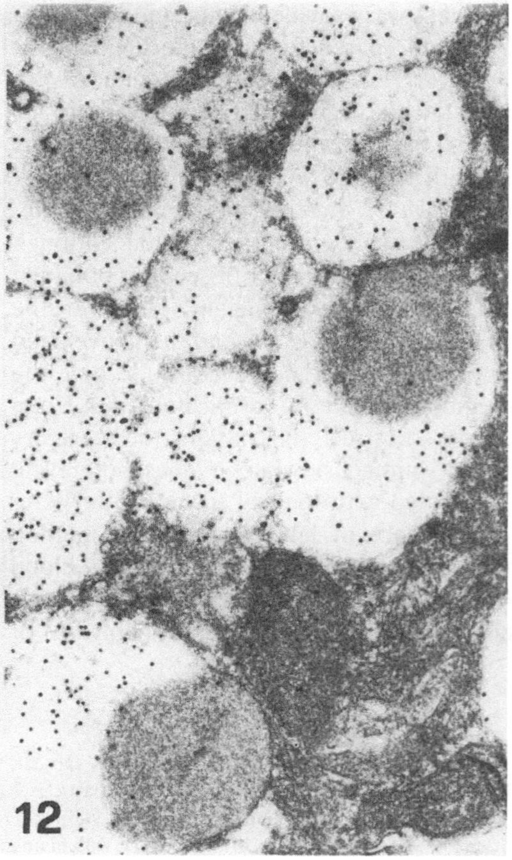
12

[8]. Histochemical data reveal acidic mucins in Cowper's and Littré's glands cells [24,27,28], but not their ultrastructural localization, so that we actually ignore if the lack of immunolabeling in filamentous bodies corresponds, as in salivary glands, to a lack in acidic mucins.

The anti-blood group antigen A, B, and H antibodies label the granules dependent on the blood group phenotype of the donors. A antigen intensely reacts in glands of type A donors, B antigen in those of B donors, and H antigen in those of the 0 type donors (Figs. 3–9). In addition, moderate labeling of H is revealed in glands of A and B subjects as well. In these subjects, double labeling experiments show that A or B coexist with H, although H appeared much more weakly stained (Fig. 9). We found neither the mosaicism at the cellular level reported in human pancreas [11], Brunner's glands [13], and other epithelia [19], where A-rich cells do not contain H and vice versa, nor the mosaicism at the granular level described in the same cell in human salivary [16] and cervical glands [17]. The mosaiclike distribution of ABH antigens has been ascribed to differences in the cellular or granular maturative processes, that is, A- or B-rich elements would correspond to the later phases, and H-rich elements to the earlier ones. Since in Cowper's and Littré's glands we found, at most, a heterogeneous distribution pattern for ABH substances, we think that their mucous cells convert H into A or B beginning in early phases, although a certain amount of H remains and is secreted as such.

Lewis antigens, as ABH, are present in human epithelia and in secretions such as milk and saliva [22]. Studies concerning these antigens chiefly deal with their altered distribution as surface antigens in neoplastic tissues [9,10,20,34], while their expression in normal epithelia and secretions has received scarce attention. Thus far no literature data document their presence in human semen. The present results demonstrate that Cowper's and Littré's glands secrete both Le-a and Le-b antigens, which therefore must be considered to be normal components of the human seminal plasma.

The distribution of these antigens in Cowper's and Littré's glands reflects well the general rules governing the expression, which is strictly dependent on their secretor status (Fig. 2). Since we had no information on the patients' secretor status, we considered those individuals whose glands exhibited labeled ABH to be secretors, and those whose glands were negative to probably be nonsecretors. In secretors, both Le-a and Le-b are found in the same sites where ABH are revealed: Le-a very faintly, and Le-b rather strongly labeled (Figs. 6, 8, 10, and 11). To explain this difference in reactivity, it must be borne in mind that in secretors the substrate of Lewis enzyme that forms Le-a, namely, the precursor glycoprotein, is also used by the Se enzyme to form H substance (Fig. 1), and possibly because of a lower affinity of Lewis enzyme for this substrate, the resulting Le-a is rather scarce. By contrast, the Lewis enzyme might have a high affinity for H substance as a substrate to form Le-b antigen, which in fact appears intensely labeled. In nonsecretors only Le-a is consistently labeled in secretory granules (Fig. 12). The abundance of Le-a in nonsecretors, who lack Se enzyme, may be explained by considering that the Lewis enzyme has all the precursor glycoprotein needed to form Le-a antigen at its disposal.

The physiological significance of the blood group substances secreted by Cowper's and Littré's glands is completely unknown. As mucin components, they could merely play a role in lubricating the urethral walls, but a more specific function could be assigned to them as sperm-coating antigens, since they modify the antigenicity of the sperm surface after ejaculation.

←

Fig 10 Mucous cells of Cowper's gland from a type 0 subject, treated with anti-Le-b antibody Mucous droplets and Golgi saccules (arrow) are the only sites of immunoreaction Gold particle ∅ 15 nm (×31,000)

Fig 11 Mucous cell of Cowper's gland from a type 0 subject Double labeling of Le-a antigen (gold particle ∅ 30 nm) and Le-b antigen (gold particle ∅ 10 nm) Le-b antigen appears much more intensely labeled than Le-a (×16,500)

Fig 12 Principal cell of Littré's gland from a presumed nonsecretor, type 0 subject, treated with anti Le-a-antibody Le-a antigen, the only found in this subject, appears abundant in the pale matrix of the secretory granules Gold particle ∅ 15 nm (×30,500)

Such modifications might be of some importance in determining male infertility due to sperm autoimmunity [1,15]. Moreover, seminal and sperm-coating antigens are thought to interact with specific antibodies of cervical secretions [21], but the suggested importance of these interactions as a possible cause of infertility has been not demonstrated.

4. Concluding Remarks

The IGS method has enabled us to demonstrate that seminal ABH antigens are not secreted by the prostate or seminal vesicle, but are supplied by Cowper's and Littré's glands, depending on the blood group type and secretor status. Another important finding is that Lewis antigens are also secreted by Cowper's and Littré's glands, being the first demonstration that Lewis antigens are normal components of human seminal plasma.

On the basis of these results, the functional role of these glands in reproductive physiology appears more relevant than that hitherto ascribed to them, since their secretion not only protects and lubricates the urethral walls, but also supplies some antigenic properties to seminal plasma.

Acknowledgments

This work was supported by the Consiglio Nazionale delle Ricerche (C.N.R.) and the Ministero dell'Università e della Ricerca Scientifica e Tecnologica (M.U.R.S.T.). We gratefully acknowledge Dr. Marina Quartu for her constant help in editing and Mrs. Silvana Bernardini for her expert technical assistance.

References

1 Ablin RJ Immunologic properties of sex accessory tissue components In Male Accessory Sex Organs Structure and Function in Mammals D Brandes (ed) New York Academic Press, 1974, pp 434–460

2 Boettcher G Blood group antigens in seminal plasma, and the nature of human sperm-coating antigen In Immunology and Reproduction RG Edwards (ed) London International Planned Parenthood Federation, 1969, pp 148–167

3 Cossu M, Floris A, Lantini MS An immunohistochemical study of ABH antigens in human submandibular glands at the light and electron microscopic levels Eur J Histochem 36 489–499, 1992

4 Cossu M, Riva A, Lantini MS Subcellular localization of blood group substances ABH in human salivary glands J Histochem Cytochem 38 1165–1172, 1990

5 Dabelsteen E, Pindborg JJ Loss of epithelial blood group substance A in oral carcinomas Acta Pathol Microbiol Scand Sect A 81 435–444, 1973

6 Edwards RG, Ferguson LC, Combs RRA Blood group antigens on human spermatozoa J Reprod Fertil 7 153–161, 1964

7 Gupta RK Schuster R, Christian WD Loss of isoantigens A and H in prostate Am J Pathol 70 439–448, 1973

8 Harrison JD, Auger W, Paterson KL, Rawley PSA Mucin histochemistry of submandibular and parotid salivary glands of man Light and electron microscopy Histochem J 19 555–564 1987

9 Idikio HA, Manickavel V Lewis blood antigens (a and b) in human breast tissues Cancer 68 1303–1308, 1991

10 Inoue M Sasagawa T, Saito J, Shimizu H, Ueda G, Tanizawa O, Nakajama M Expression of blood group antigens A, B, H, Lewis-a and Lewis-b in fetal, normal, and malignant tissues of the uterine endometrium Cancer 60 2985–2993, 1987

11 Ito N, Nishi K, Nakajima M, Matsuda Y, Ishitani A, Mizumoto J, Hirota T Localization of blood group antigens in human pancreas with lectin-horseradish peroxidase conjugates Acta Histochem Cytochem 19 205–218, 1986

12 Juhl BR, Hartzen SH, Hainau B A, B, H antigen expression in transitional cell carcinomas of the urinary bladder Cancer 57 1768–1775, 1986

13 Kent SP The demonstration and distribution of water soluble blood group 0(H)antigen in tissue sections using a fluorescein labelled extract of *Ulex europaeus* seed J Histochem Cytochem 12 591–599, 1964

14 Landsteiner K, Levine P On group specific substances in human spermatozoa J Immunol 12 415–418, 1926

15 Mann T, Lutwak-Mann C Male Reproductive Function and Semen Berlin Springer Verlag, 1981, p 324

16 Nakajima M, Ito N, Nishi K, Okamura Y, Hirota T Immunogold labeling of blood-group antigens in human salivary glands using monoclonal antibodies and the streptavidin-biotin technique Histochemistry 87 539–543, 1987

17 Okamura Y Heterogeneity of the blood group ABH antigens and variation in the expression of these antigens of secretory granules in human cervical glands An electron microscopic observation using lectins and monoclonal antibodies Histochemistry 94 489–496, 1990

18 Oriol R Tissular expression of ABH and Lewis antigens in humans and animals Expected value of different animal models in the study of AB0-incompatible organ transplants Transplant Proc 20 4416–4420, 1987

19 Oriol R, Mollicone R, Coullin P, Dalix AM, Candelier JJ Genetic regulation of the expression of ABH and Lewis antigens in tissues APMIS 100 28–38, 1992

20 Orntoft TF, Nielsen MJS, Wolf H, Olsen TS, Clausen H,

Hakomori S Dabelsteen E Blood group AB0 and Lewis antigen expression during neoplastic progression of human urothelium Cancer 60 2641–2648 1987

21 Parish WE Carron Brown JA Richards CB The detection of antibodies to spermatozoa and to blood group antigens in cervical mucus J Reprod Fertil 13 469–477 1967

22 Pittiglio DH Genetics and Biochemistry of A B H and Lewis Antigens In Blood Group Systems ABH and Lewis ME Wallace FL Gibbs (eds) Arlington VA American Association of Blood Banks 1986 pp 1–50

23 Riva A Lantini MS Migliari R Scarpa R Cossu M A correlative TEM SEM study of the human urethral glands Bull Assoc Anat 75 73–76 1991

24 Riva A Sirigu P Testa Riva F Usai E Fine structure and histochemistry of epithelial cells of the human bulbourethral glands Acta Anat 111 125–126 1981

25 Riva A Usai E Cossu M Lantini MS Scarpa R Testa Riva F Ultrastructure of human bulbourethral glands and of their main excretory ducts Arch Androl 24 177–184 1990

26 Riva A Usai E Scarpa R Cossu M Lantini MS Fine structure of the accessory glands of the human male genital tract In Developments in Ultrastructure of Reproduction Progress in Clinical and Biological Research Vol 296 PM Motta (ed) New York Alan R Liss 1989 pp 233–240

27 Sirigu P Perra MT Human bulbourethral glands Histochemical parameters Mol Androl 1 226–231 1989

28 Sirigu P Turno F Perra MT Usai E Hafez ESE The human urethral glands An histochemical study Arch Androl 26 37–47 1990

29 Szulman AE The histological distribution of blood group substances A and B in man J Exp Med 111 785–800 1960

30 Szulman AE Evolution of ABH blood group antigens during embryogenesis Ann Inst Pasteur/Immunol 138 845–847 1987

31 Vowden P Lowe AD Lennox ES Bleehen NM Are blood group isoantigens lost from malignant prostatic epithelium? Immunohistochemical support for the preservation of the H isoantigen Br J Cancer 53 307–312 1986

32 Walker PD Karnik S De Kernion JB Pramberg JC Cell surface blood group antigens in prostatic carcinoma Am J Clin Pathol 81 503 506 1984

33 Weistein RS Coon J Alroy J Davidsohn I Tissue associated blood group antigens in human tumors In Diagnostic Immunohistochemistry RD DeLellis (ed) New York Masson 1981 pp 239–261

34 Young WW Mills SE Lippert MC Ahmed P Lau SK Deletion of antigens of the Lewis a/b blood group family in human prostatic carcinoma Am J Pathol 131 578 586 1988

CHAPTER 11

Autonomic Innervation of the Human Male Accessory Sex Glands

ANNIKKI VAALASTI

1. Introduction

The human male accessory sex glands receive autonomic innervation from both the sympathetic and parasympathetic nervous system. The sympathetic fibers are derived from the last thoracic and upper lumbar segments via the hypogastric and presacral nerves and the parasympathetic fibers via the pelvic nerves from the sacral segments [39]. The cell bodies of the postganglionic sympathetic as well as parasympathetic nerves are located in the hypogastric or main pelvic ganglia, situated on the lateral aspects of the bladder neck, seminal vesicles, and prostate [14, 23,27,29,30,39]. In humans, instead of a solid ganglion, numerous small clusters of nerve cells are distributed in the pelvic plexus [22,24,39]. This type of sympathetic innervation with a peripherally located ganglion is not seen in any other organ and is referred to as *short adrenergic neurons* [24,39]. In addition to the classical adrenergic and cholinergic nerves, nerves containing various polypeptides have also been demonstrated in the genitals. The peptidergic nerves obviously represent subpopulations of sympathetic and parasympathetic nerves, since peptide transmitters have been shown to be colocalized in both the adrenergic and cholinergic nerves [46].

Much of our present knowledge of genital innervation is based on studies using different laboratory animals, since only a few investigations have been carried out in man. However, the general arrangement of innervation is similar in different species, including man [3,7,39] and results concerning animals can mostly be generalized to humans.

2. Classification and Ultrastructure of Autonomic Nerve Terminals

The ultrastructural characteristics of adrenergic and cholinergic nerve terminals are generally established. Axons containing a predominance of small granular vesicles (SGV), 40–60 nm in diameter, and a few large granular vesicles (LGV), 80–120 nm in diameter, are considered adrenergic [37]. Numerous small agranular vesicles (SAV), 40–60 nm in diameter, and a few LGVs are characteristic of cholinergic axons (Figs. 1 and 5) [13]. These morphological features of the synaptic vesicles are best preserved after potassium permanganate fixation [37]. The transmitter substances adrenaline and acetylcholine are stored in the SGVs and SAVs, respectively. A third type of nerve terminal characterized by numerous LGVs (Figs. 2 and 7) was named the *p-type* terminal by Baumgarten and coworkers [8]. Later these p-type terminals were considered to represent purinergic [12] or peptidergic [8] nerves. With modern electron microscopic immunocytochemical techniques, the localization of neuropeptides in the LGV has been established [46]. Now that neuropeptides have been shown to be colocalized in both adrenergic and cholinergic terminals, the existence of a morphologically separate peptidergic terminal may be questioned.

Riva, A., Testa Riva, F., and Motta, P.M., (eds.), Ultrastructure of Male Urogenital Glands Prostate, Seminal Vesicles, Urethral, and Bulbourethral Glands © *1994 Kluwer Academic Publishers ISBN 0-7923-2800-0 All rights reserved*

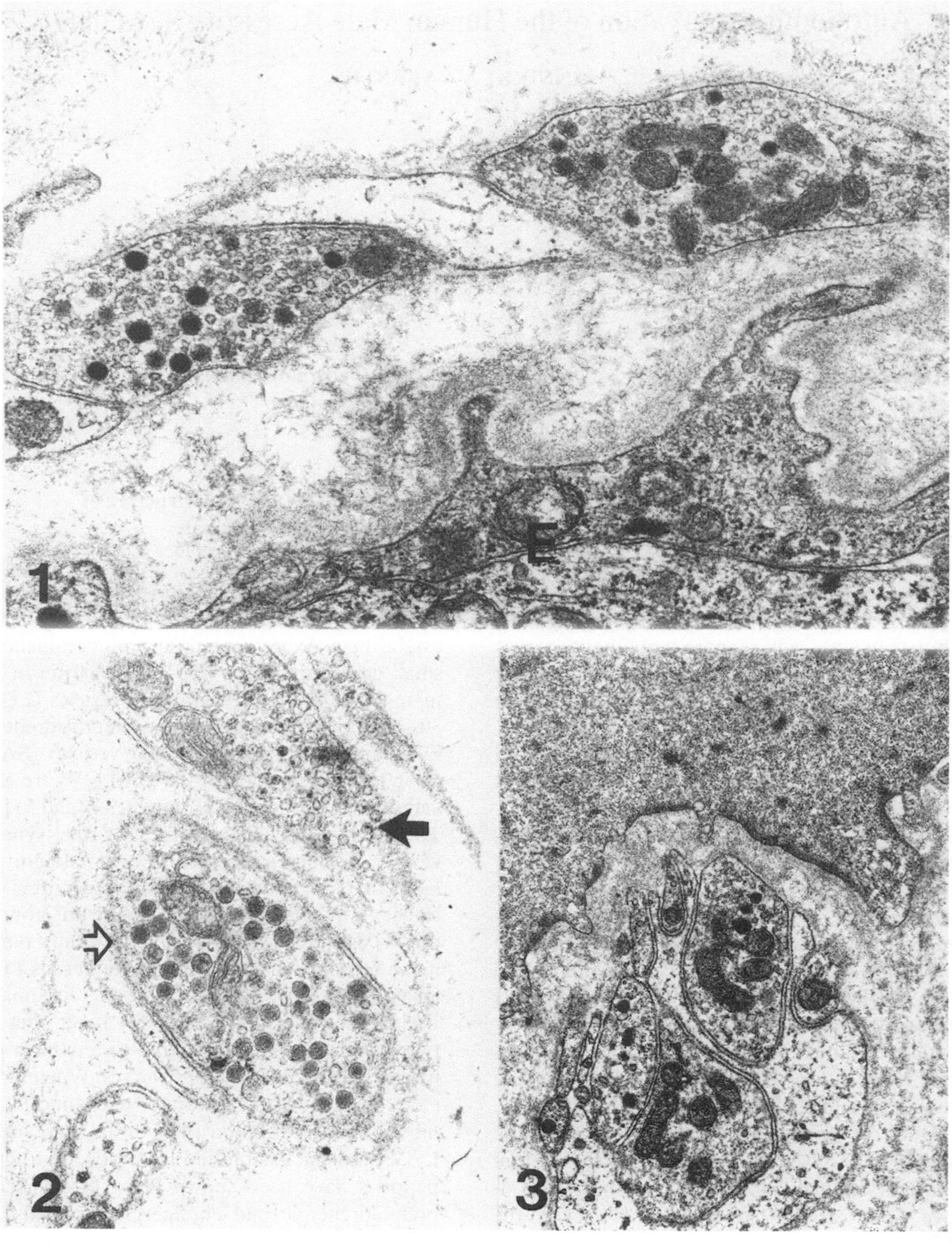
1
E
2
3

3. Adrenergic Innervation of the Male Accessory Sex Glands

The male genital organs are especially richly supplied by sympathetic adrenergic nerves, which provide mainly motor innervation to the prostate, seminal vesicle, and vas deferens. Accordingly, most neurons in the hypogastric or main pelvic ganglion show catecholamine histofluorescence [3,23,24,36,47] or tyrosine hydroxylase immunoreactivity [26].

Adrenergic innervation of the vas deferens has been extensively studied in different laboratory animals using histochemical techniques [17,33, 34,39,47], since it serves as a good model of short adrenergic neurons and their neuromuscular relations. A dense plexus of varicose adrenergic nerves has been demonstrated throughout the smooth muscle layers, as well as around blood vessels. The arrangement of adrenergic nerves in the human vas deferens is similar but the innervation is less dense [1,9,38]. The amount of adrenergic terminals increases from the epididymal end of the vas deferens towards the prostatic end [9,33]. Electron microscopic studies using rat [17,37], guinea pig [3,15], or human [9] vas deferens have confirmed the light microscopic results. Large bundles of nonmyelinated nerve fibers enclosed in a Schwann cell are seen in the adventitia [9]. Adrenergic nerve endings or terminal axons, which represent varicosities seen in the light microscope, are filled with SGVs, occasional LGVs, mitochondria, and glycogen particles, as described in detail by Baumgarten and coworkers [9]. The terminal axons are partly or totally devoid of Schwann cells. In the human vas deferens most smooth muscle cells are assumed to be in contact with one or more adrenergic nerve terminals. Some of the adrenergic axons are in close contact with smooth muscle cells or may be partly wrapped by processes of smooth muscle cells. However, more frequently several hundred nanometers separate nerve terminals from the muscle cells (Fig. 3). No postsynaptic specializations of smooth muscle membranes are seen. Most perivascular axons are also adrenergic [9].

Also in the seminal vesicle adrenergic innervation is mainly confined to the smooth muscle layer, as demonstrated in various animal species [3,32–34,39,47,48]. The innervation of the human seminal vesicle is less well documented than that of laboratory animals [4]. Also in the human seminal vesicle adrenergic innervation is most abundant in the muscular wall (Fig. 4). The very few electron microscopic studies made of the innervation of seminal vesicles confirm the light microscopic findings. In the guinea pig [3,15] and rabbit [16] seminal vesicles, adrenergic axon terminals, filled with dense-core vesicles, are distributed throughout the muscle layer. The only electron microscopic data available on the innervation of human seminal vesicle are from Aumüller [4]. However, it seems that the innervation of the human seminal vesicle does not differ essentially from that of other species.

Adrenergic innervation of the prostate has received much more attention than innervation of the other accessory sex glands. Numerous light microscopic studies have shown a rich adrenergic innervation of smooth muscle of the prostate in different laboratory mammals [4,33,34,39,41]. Results concerning the adrenergic innervation of the human prostate are somewhat contradictory. Sparse adrenergic innervation of the human prostatic stroma has been described by Baumgarten and coworkers [7] and Shirai and coworkers [38]. The material of both studies, however, consisted of tissue from prostatic hyperplasia, not normal tissue. Age-dependent reduction of prostatic innervation has previously been described by Casas [14]. Higgins and Gosling [24] found no regional variation in the distribution of autonomic nerves between different prostatic lobes in humans. Vaalasti and Hervonen have described human pros-

←

Fig. 1. Electron micrograph showing two cholinergic-type axons filled with numerous SAVs, some LGVs, and mitochondria, lying beneath prostatic epithelium (E) (×30,000).

Fig. 2. Electron micrograph of a p-type terminal (open arrow) containing mainly LGVs and a typical adrenergic terminal containing SGVs (arrow) (×31,600).

Fig. 3. Several axons within the same Schwann cell in the human vas deferens. The dense-cores of the synaptic vesicles are poorly preserved. The gap between the axons and the smooth muscle cells is several hundred nanometers (×16,000).

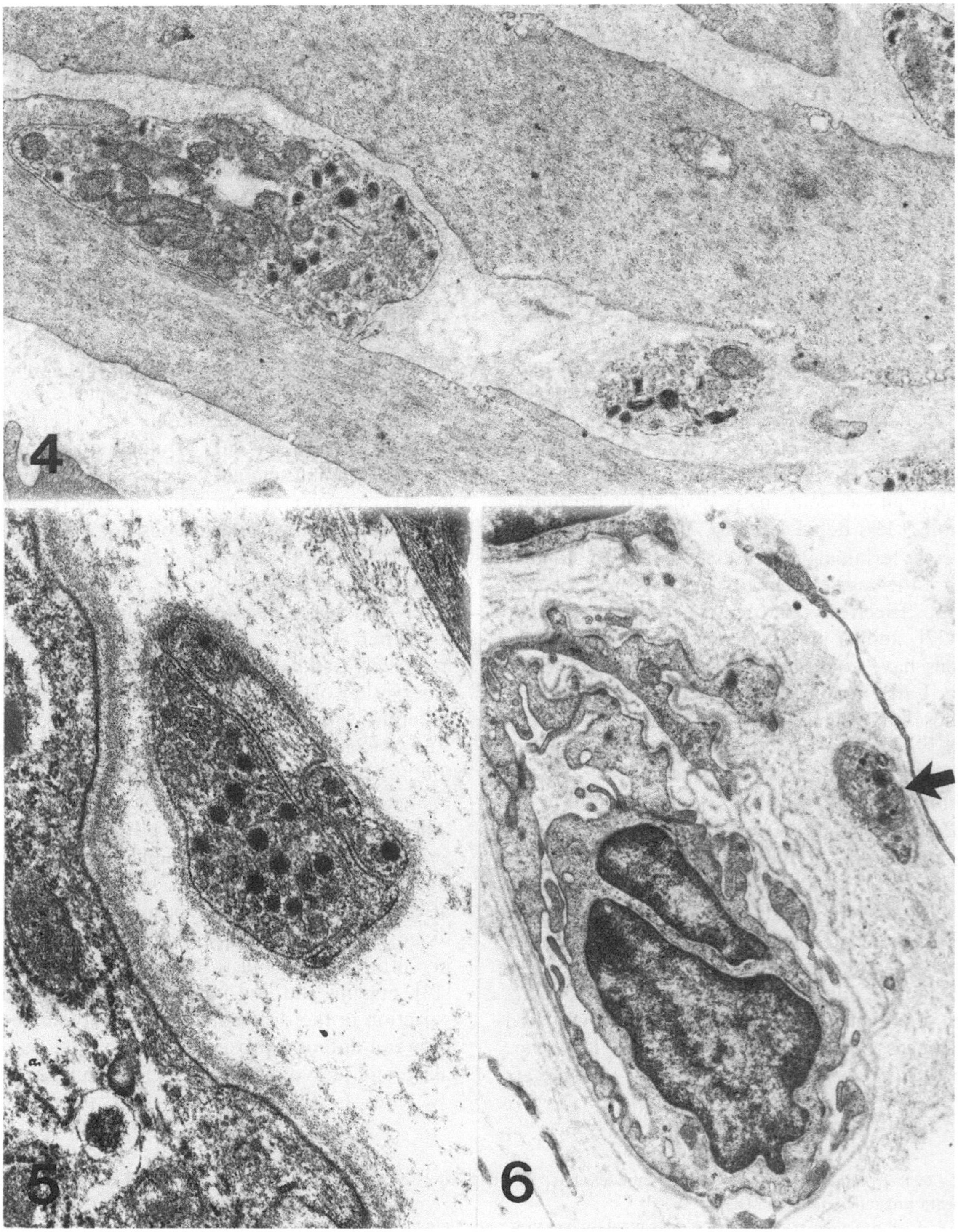
4
5
6

tatic innervation on both light [42] and electron microscopic level [43] Typical adrenergic nerve terminals were abundant among smooth muscle cells in normal prostatic tissue but were only rarely seen in hyperplastic prostates The exact classification of terminals into adrenergic and cholinergic was made using specimens fixed with potassium permanganate Although this fixative preserves well the dense-core vesicles of adrenergic axons, it preserves the fine structure of other cells less satisfactorily In specimens immersion fixed with glutaraldehyde, it is often difficult to differentiate adrenergic from cholinergic axons Occasionally very intimate neuromuscular contacts can be seen in the human prostate, although most frequently a gap of 100 nm or more is seen (Fig 7) Adrenergic axons often run together with cholinergic axons within the same Schwann cell Accumulations of lipofuscin pigment are rarely seen in the Schwann cells and are probably degenerative features (Fig 8) Nerve endings aroung blood vessels of the human prostate (Fig 6) are mainly of the cholinergic type

4. Cholinergic Innervation of the Male Accessory Sex Glands

The distribution of parasympathetic cholinergic nerves in the male genital organs has long been poorly known, probably in the absence of unanimously accepted methods for identification of cholinergic nerves Acetylcholinesterase (AChE) activity, which can also be demonstrated on electron microscopic level, has been used as a marker for cholinergic nerves However, a weak AChE activity may sometimes be found also in adrenergic nerves and especially in ganglion cells Classification based on the morphology of synaptic vesicles has also its limitations, since factors such as fixation, functional state of a nerve fiber, etc can modify the appearance of the terminal [7] The following data must be interpreted bearing in mind these limitations

The presence of cholinergic nerves in the rat vas deferens has recently been questioned [26] despite electron microscopic demonstration of cholinergic-type terminals [17,37] and AChE-containing nerve fibers in the vas deferens In the human vas deferens, AChE activity and catecholamine fluorescence have been shown to exist in separate populations of nerves [1,38] The AChE-positive, presumably cholinergic nerves, are found preferentially subepithelially in the mucosa of the vas deferens [1] Electron microscopy of the human vas deferens confirms the presence of cholinergic-type terminals, but their exact neuroeffector contacts remain to be studied in detail [7] No direct innervation of the vas deferens epithelium has been demonstrated [7,20]

In the seminal vesicles of the guinea pig and rat [3,32] AChE-containing nerve fibers have been found mainly in the submucosa, with only occasional fibers in the inner muscular layers [32, 48] Electron microscopic examination reveals cholinergic-type axons subepithelially also in humans (Fig 5) In addition, Aumuller [4] has demonstrated neuroglandular synapses in human seminal vesicle Similar results have been obtained from studies on guinea pigs and rabbits [3,16]

A dense plexus of AChE-positive nerves has been demonstrated in the prostate of various animals [41] as well as man [18,24,38,42] The preferential localization of cholinergic-type nerve terminals in association with the glandular epithelium has been shown in ultrastructural studies [21,41,43] No direct contacts between glandular cells and nerve terminals have been demonstrated in the rat [21,41] or human [43] prostate Nerve terminals are seen underlying the basal lamina of the epithelium but are never seen to penetrate it (Fig 1) In the human prostate cholinergic-type axons are also seen in close contact with smooth muscle cells and around blood vessels (Fig 6)

←

Fig 4 Electron micrograph showing several axons adjacent to smooth muscle cells in the human seminal vesicle Processes of the smooth muscle cell partly encircle the axons (×21 000)

Fig 5 Cholinergic type axon lying beneath the epithelium in the human seminal vesicle (×32 000)

Fig 6 Electron micrograph of the human prostate showing a small capillary and a cholinergic nerve ending (arrow) (×10 500)

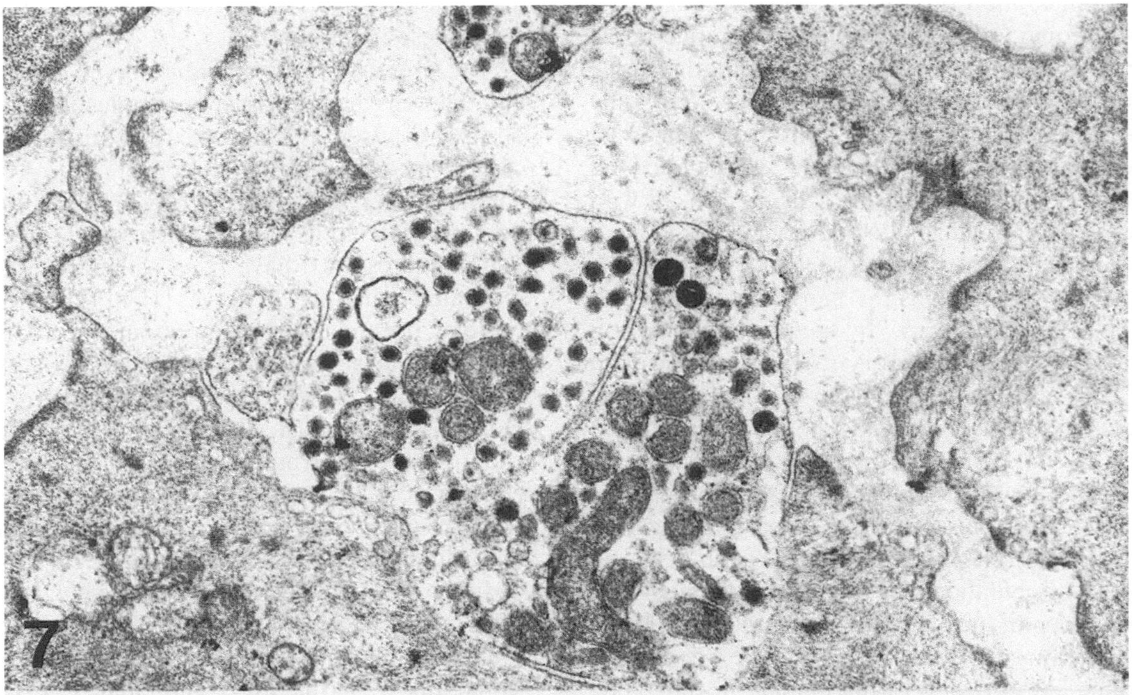
7

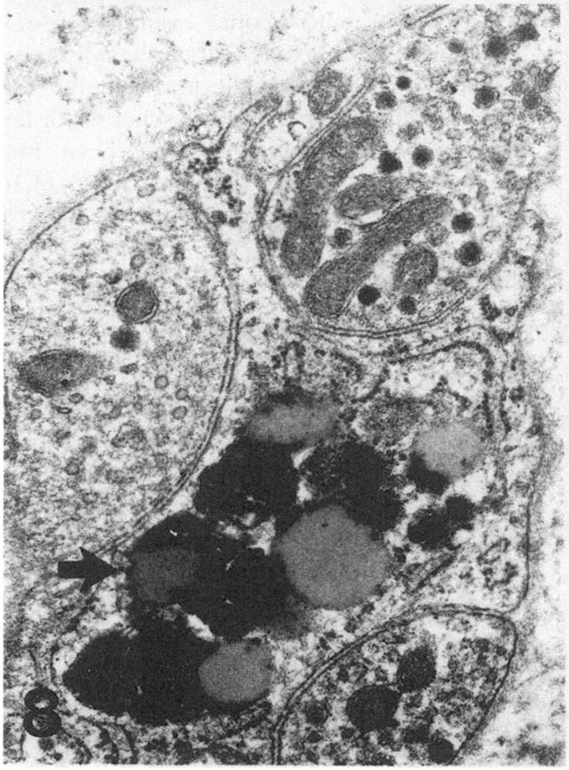
8

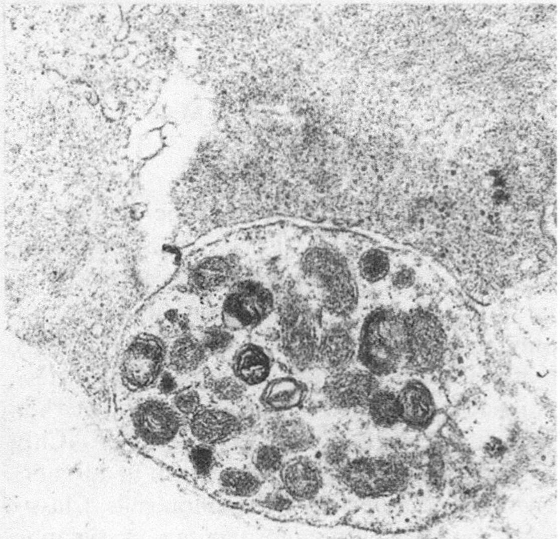
9

5. Peptidergic Innervation of the Male Accessory Sex Glands

The existence of a nonadrenergic and noncholinergic innervation in the male genital tract has been suggested on the basis of numerous functional and morphological studies P-type axons [8] containing mainly LGVs have been described also in the human prostate (Figs 2 and 7) [43] It has been suggested that these p-type axons represent peptidergic nerves [46] However, it has since been shown using double-labeling immunocytochemical methods that neuropeptides are stored in the LGVs of adrenergic and cholinergic nerves [46] Thus the p-type terminals do not necessarily represent a separate entity but only a morphological variation of adrenergic or cholinergic terminals

The number of neuropeptides demonstrated in the male genital tract has increased rapidly Vasoactive intestinal polypeptide (VIP) [1,2,26, 28,31,32,35,40,44,45,48], enkephalin [5,25,35, 44,45], substance P [35,40,48], neuropeptide Y (NPY) [26,32,35], galanin [6,26,35], calcitonin gene-related peptide (CGRP), and somatostatin (H Tainio, personal communication) have been found in nerves of the human genital tract Furthermore, it has been shown that VIP is mainly colocalized in cholinergic nerves in the submucosa, especially in the vas deferens and seminal vesicle [1,24,32,48] NPY seems to coexist in the adrenergic nerves innervating smooth muscle cells [24,32,48] Data on the occurrence and distribution of the other peptides, especially substance P, somatostatin, and CGRP, are contradictory The distribution of peptidergic nerves is probably species specific and the use of different antisera may also give conflicting results

Only a few electron microscopic studies have been published on the peptidergic innervation of the male genital organs Vaalasti and coworkers [45] described the distribution of VIP- and enkephalin-immunoreactive nerves in the human genital tract (Figs 10–12) VIP-immunoreactive nerves were located subepithelially in the vas deferens and seminal vasicle (Fig 11), but in the prostate they were also adjacent to smooth muscle cells No direct neuroepithelial contacts were seen Throughout the genital tract VIP-immunoreactive nerves are seen around blood vessels Similar results have been presented on the rat seminal vesicle by Yuri [48] and on the guinea pig vas deferens by Feher and Burnstock [20] NPY-immunoreactive as well as enkephalin-immunoreactive nerves have been found in close contract with smooth muscle cells [20,45,48] Immunoreactivity to all these peptides has been located in the LGVs (Fig 12) Diffuse staining frequently seen in the axoplasm may be artifactual (Fig 10) No ultrastructural data on the colocalization of various peptides in the same axons in the human genitals are available

The presence of afferent (sensory) nerves in the genital tract has been suggested by numerous authors Nerve endings containing numerous mitochondria are seen in the human prostate [43] and morphologically they resemble sensory endings seen in other tissues (Fig 9)

6. Functional Aspects and Conclusions

Functional as well as morphological data have confirmed the presence of multiple neuronal control mechanisms in the human genital tract As a general rule adrenergic innervation is responsible for control of contractile activity in the vas deferens, seminal vesicles, and prostate [10,11] The cholinergic nerves are of minor importance in motor control Secretory activity of the accessory genital glands is mainly under parasympathetic control [11,19] An intact autonomic innervation is necessary for the maturation and transport of spermatozoa

←

Fig 7 P type axon filled with numerous LGVs in close contact with a smooth muscle cells in the human prostate (×30 000)

Fig 8 Accumulations of lipofuscin pigment (arrow) are frequently seen in the cytoplasm of Schwann cells These most probably represent degenerative features (×30 000)

Fig 9 Electron micrograph showing a nerve terminal full of mitochondria and only a few synaptic vesicles This type of terminal may represent sensory nerve endings (×32 000)

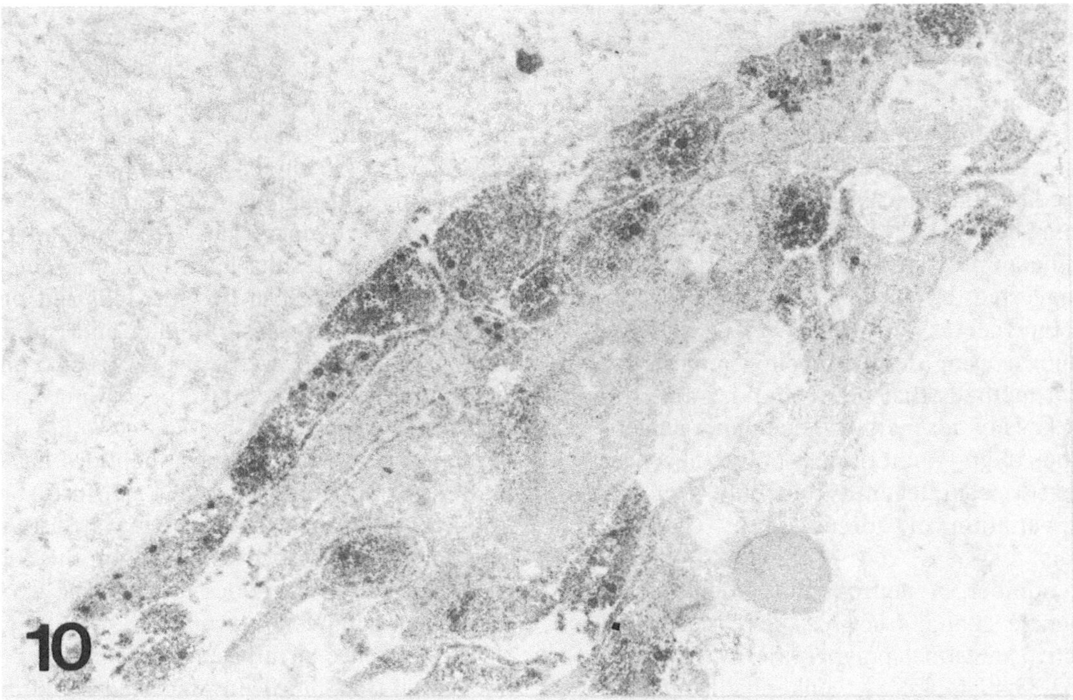
10

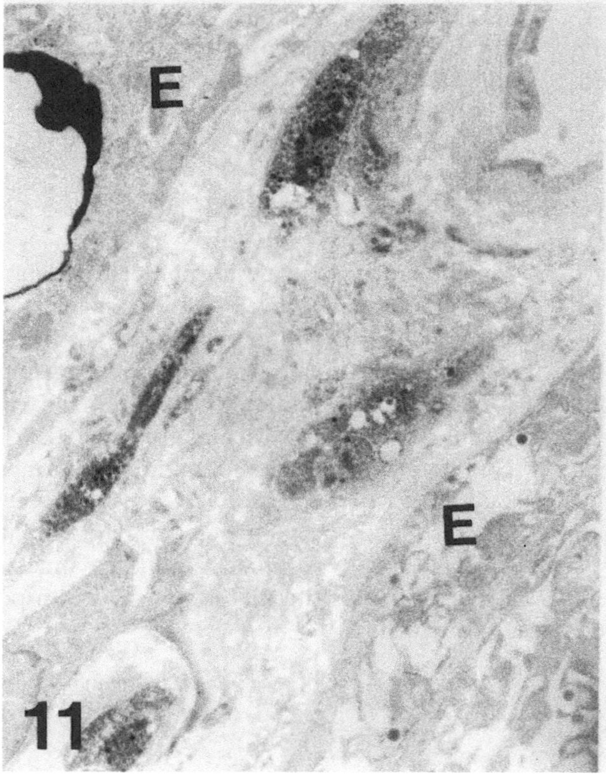
E
E
11

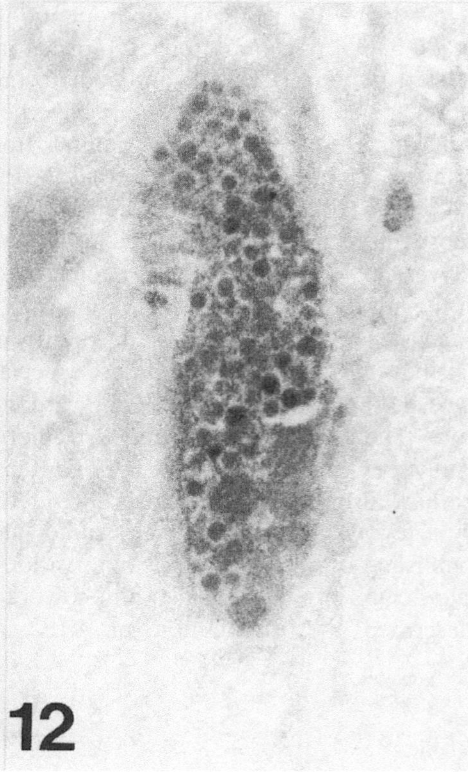
12

The role of peptidergic innervation is still poorly understood. Certain neuropeptides may act as true transmitters, whereas others may just modulate the release and degradation of other transmitters [35,40]. It has been suggested that the peptidergic nerves may play a role in the control of secretory activity, smooth muscle contractility, and regulation of blood flow [35,40], but further studies are needed to confirm these functions. Peptides of the tachykinin family (substance P) and CGRP are preferentially found in sensory nerves. Neurogenic inflammation is caused when these peptides are released from the sensory nerve terminals. It remains to be elucidated if nerves containing substance P or CGRP might be of importance in inflammatory diseases of the genital tract, too.

References

1 Alm P On the autonomic innervation of the human vas deferens Brain Res Bull 9 673–677, 1982
2 Alm P, Alumets J, Håkanson R, Owman C, Sjoberg NO, Sundler F, Walles B Origin and distribution of VIP (vasoactive intestinal polypeptide)-nerves in the genito-urinary tract Cell Tissue Res 205 337–347, 1980
3 Al-Zuhair A, Gosling JA, Dixon JS Observations on the structure and autonomic innervation of the guinea-pig seminal vesicle and ductus deferens J Anat 120 81–93, 1975
4 Aumuller G Prostate gland and seminal vesicles In Handbuch der mikroskopischen Anatomie des Menschen 7 Bd, 6 Teil A Oksche, L Vollrath (eds) Berlin Springer, 1979
5 Aumuller G, Jungblut T, Malek B, Konrad S, Weihe E Regional distribution of opioidergic nerves in human and canine prostates Prostate 14 279–288, 1989
6 Bauer FE, Christofides ND, Hacker GW, Blank MA, Polak JM, Bloom SR Distribution of galanin in the genito-urinary tract of man and rat Peptides 7 5–10, 1986
7 Baumgarten HG, Falck B, Holstein AF, Owman C, Owman T Adrenergic innervation of the human testis, epididymis, ductus deferens and prostate A fluorescence microscopic and fluorimetric study Z Zellforsch 90 81–95, 1968
8 Baumgarten HG, Holstein AF, Owman C Auerbach's plexus of mammals and man Electron microscopic identification of three different types of neuronal processes in myenteric ganglia of the large intestine from Rhesus monkeys, guinea-pigs and man Z Zellforsch 106 376–397, 1970
9 Baumgarten HG, Holstein AF, Rosengren E Arrangement, ultrastructure and adrenergic innervation of smooth musculature of the ductuli efferentes, ductus epididymis and ductus deferens of man Z Zellforsch 120 37–79, 1971
10 Bruschini H, Schmidt RA, Tanagho A Studies on the physiology of the vas deferens Invest Urol 15 112–116, 1977
11 Bruschini H, Schmidt RA, Tanagho A Neurologic control of prostatic secretion in the dog Invest Urol 15 288–291, 1978
12 Burnstock G Purinergic nerves Pharmacol Rev 24 509–581, 1972
13 Burnstock G, Iwayama T Fine structural identification of autonomic nerves and their relation to smooth muscle Prog Brain Res 34 389–404, 1971
14 Casas AP Die Innervation der menschlichen Vorsteherdruse Z Mikrosk Anat Forsch 64 608–633, 1958
15 Clementi F, Naimzada KM, Mantegazza P Study of the nerve endings in the vas deferens and seminal vesicle of the guinea pig Int J Neuropharmac 8 399–403, 1969
16 Dent J, Hodson N, Selhi H Ultrastructural differentiation of fibre types in rabbit seminal vesicles J Physiol 217 7p–9p, 1971
17 Dixon JS, Gosling JA The distribution of autonomic nerves in the musculature of the rat vas deferens A light and electron microscope investigation J Comp Neurol 146 175–188, 1972
18 Dunzendorfer U, Jonas D, Weber W The autonomic innervation of the human prostate Histochemistry of acetylcholinesterase in the normal and pathologic states Urol Res 4 29–31, 1976
19 Farrel JI, Lyman Y A study of the secretory nerves of, and the action of certain drugs on the prostate gland Am J Physiol 118 64–70, 1937
20 Feher E, Burnstock G Ultrastructural identification of vasoactive intestinal polypeptide and neuropeptide Y-containing nerve fibres in the vas deferens of the guinea-pig J Auton Nerv Syst 19 235–242, 1987

←

Fig 10 A thick nerve bundle from the human prostate after immunohistochemical demonstration of VIP immunoreactivity using the PAP method The dark reaction product is seen in the LGVs and also diffusely in the axoplasm No staining on grids has been used (×13,500)

Fig 11 Electron micrograph showing VIP-immunoreactive nerve terminals in the human seminal vesicle VIP-immunoreactive terminals are seen subepithelially (E = epithelium) PAP method, no staining on grids (×7900)

Fig 12 A higher magnification of a VIP-immunoreactive nerve terminal in the human prostate The LGVs are mostly dark stained PAP method, no staining on grids (×22,400)

21 Flickinger CJ The fine structure of the interstitial tissue of the rat prostate Am J Anat 134 107–126, 1972
22 Gorg A, Werner S Lichtmikroskopische und elektronenoptische Studien zur normalen und pathologischen Histologie der Prostata unter besonderer Berucksichtigung des Nervensystems Acta Neuroweget (Wien) 29 203–219, 1966
23 Gosling JA, Thompson SA A neurohistochemical and histological study of peripheral autonomic neurons of the human bladder neck and prostate Urol Int 32 269–276, 1977
24 Higgins JRA, Gosling JA Studies on the structure and intrinsic innervation of the normal human prostate Prostate 2(Suppl) 5–16, 1989
25 Jungblut T, Aumuller G, Malek B, Melchior H Age-dependency and regional distribution of enkephalinergic nerves in human prostate Urol Int 44 352–356, 1989
26 Keast JR Location and peptide content of pelvic neurons supplying the muscle and lamina propria of the rat vas deferens J Auton Nerv Syst 40 1–12, 1992
27 Kolossow NG, Polykarpova GA Versuch einer experimentell-morphologischen Analyse des Nerveapparates der Prostata Z Anat Entwickl 106 98–106, 1937
28 Lange W, Unger J Peptidergic innervation within the prostate gland and seminal vesicle Urol Res 18 337–340, 1990
29 Langley JN, Anderson HK The innervation of the pelvic and adjoining viscera Part IV The internal generative organs Part V Position of the nerve cells on the course of the efferent nerve fibers J Physiol (Lond) 18 122–139, 1895
30 Langley JN, Anderson HK The innervation of the pelvic and adjoining viscera Part VI Anatomical observations J Physiol (Lond) 20 372–406, 1896
31 Larsson LI, Fahrenkrug J, Schaffalitzky de Muckadell OB Occurrence of nerves containing vasoactive intestinal polypeptide immunoreactivity in the male genital tract Life Sci 21 503–508, 1977
32 Moss HE, Crowe R, Burnstock G The seminal vesicle in eight week streptozotocin-induced diabetic rats Adrenergic cholinergic and peptidergic innervation J Urol 138 1273–1278, 1987
33 Norberg KA, Risley PL, Ungerstedt U Adrenergic innervation of the male reproductive ducts in some mammals I The distribution of adrenergic nerves Z Zellforsch 76 278–286, 1967
34 Owman C, Sjostrand NO Short adrenergic neurons and catecholamine containing cells in vas deferens and accessory male genital glands of different mammals Z Zellforsch 66 300–320, 1965
35 Owman C, Stjernquist M Origin, distribution, and functional aspects of aminergic and peptidergic nerves in the male and female reproductive tracts In Handbook of Chemical Neuroanatomy, Vol 6 The Peripheral Nervous System A Bjorklund, T Hokfelt, C Owman (eds) Amsterdam Elsevier, 1988, pp 445–544
36 Partanen M Development, ageing and neuroendocrine characteristics of the hypogastric (main pelvic) ganglion of the rat Acta Univ Tamperensis Ser A 112 1–60, 1980
37 Richardson KG Electron microscopic identification of autonomic nerve endings Nature 210 756, 1966
38 Shirai M, Sasaki K, Rikimaru A A histochemical investigation of the distribution of adrenergic and cholinergic nerves in the human male genital organs Tohoku J Ex Med 111 281–291, 1973
39 Sjostrand NO The adrenergic innervation of the vas deferens and the accessory male genital glands Acta Physiol Scand 65(Suppl 257) 1–82, 1965
40 Stjernquist M, Håkanson R, Leander S, Owman C, Sundler F, Uddman R Immunohistochemical localization of substance P, vasoactive intestinal polypeptide and gastrin-releasing peptide in vas deferens and seminal vesicle, and the effect of these and eight other neuropeptides on resting tension and neurally evoked contractile activity Regul Peptides 7 67–86, 1983
41 Vaalasti A, Hervonen A Innervation of the ventral prostate of the rat Am J Anat 154 231–244, 1979
42 Vaalasti A, Hervonen A Autonomic innervation of the human prostate Invest Urol 17 293–297, 1980
43 Vaalasti A, Hervonen A Nerve endings in the human prostate Am J Anat 157 41–47, 1980
44 Vaalasti A, Linnoila I, Hervonen A Immunohistochemical demonstration of VIP, met^5-enkephalin immunoreactive nerve fibres in the prostate and seminal vesicles Histochemistry 66 89–98, 1980
45 Vaalasti A, Tainio H, Pelto-Huikko M, Hervonen A Light and electron microscope demonstration of VIP- and enkephaline-immunoreactive nerves in the human male genito-urinary tract Anat Rec 215 21–27, 1986
46 Varndell IM, Polak JM The ultrastructure of peptide-containing neurons In Handbook of Chemical Neuroanatomy, Vol 6 The Peripheral Nervous System A Bjorklund, T Hokfelt, C Owman (eds) Amsterdam Elsevier, 1988, pp 143–159
47 Wakade AR, Kirpekar SM Chemical and histochemical studies on the sympathetic innervation of the vas deferens and seminal vesicle of the guinea-pig J Pharmacol Exp Ther 178 432–441, 1971
48 Yuri K Immunohistochemical and enzyme histochemical localization of peptidergic, aminergic and cholinergic nerve fibers in the rat seminal vesicle J Urol 143 194–198, 1990

Index